Diagnosis and Treatment of
Cardiac Arrhythmias

To our wives Hazel and Patricia, for their patience and encouragement during the preparation of this edition.

Publishers' Note

The publishers regret that Dr. Stock died during the final stages of preparation of this book.

Diagnosis and Treatment of Cardiac Arrhythmias

Third Edition

J. P. P. STOCK
M.D., F.R.C.P., F.A.C.C.
Consultant Cardiologist
North Staffordshire
Hospital Group

and

D. O. WILLIAMS
M.B., Ch.B., M.R.C.P. (Ed. & Lond.)
Honorary Senior Registrar in Cardiology
Queen Elizabeth Hospital
Birmingham

Butterworths

ENGLAND: BUTTERWORTH & CO. (PUBLISHERS) LTD.
LONDON: 88 Kingsway, WC2B 6AB

AUSTRALIA: BUTTERWORTHS PTY. LTD.
SYDNEY: 586 Pacific Highway, 2067
MELBOURNE: 343 Little Collins Street, 3000
BRISBANE: 240 Queen Street, 4000

CANADA: BUTTERWORTH & CO. (CANADA) LTD.
ONTARIO: 2265 Midland Avenue, Scarborough, M1P 4S1

NEW ZEALAND: BUTTERWORTHS OF NEW ZEALAND LTD.
WELLINGTON: 26–28 Waring Taylor Street, 1

SOUTH AFRICA: BUTTERWORTH & CO. (SOUTH AFRICA) (PTY.) LTD.
DURBAN: 152–154 Gale Street

First Edition 1969
Second Edition 1970
Third Edition 1974

Suggested UDC number: 616·12–008·318

ISBN 0 407 14752 7

Text set in 10/11 pt. Monotype Baskerville, printed by letterpress,
and bound in Great Britain at The Pitman Press, Bath

CONTENTS

INTRODUCTION TO THE THIRD EDITION

The general plan of the previous editions has been retained. A new chapter on His Bundle Electrography has been included. This was intended to provide a general introduction to an aspect of electrocardiography which is rapidly expanding. Many illustrative examples have been included in this chapter and throughout the text, where His Bundle Electrography has contributed to our appreciation and understanding of clinical arrhythmias.

The anatomy of the conduction system and the concepts of the hemi-blocks have been discussed in greater detail. Guidelines for the differentiation of aberrant conduction from ventricular ectopy have been enlarged. The mechanism of re-entry in the initiation of arrhythmias has been considered in depth and sections on Sick Sinus Syndrome, Sinus Parasystole and Atrial Dissociation have been included. The chapter on the Wolff–Parkinson–White Syndrome has been enlarged to discuss the electrophysiological analysis of this syndrome and its variants. The chapter on drug therapy has been updated and the role of cardiac pacing in the treatment of arrhythmias discussed.

Dr H. J. L. Marriott and Dr Chamberlain have kindly given permission for the reproduction of *Figures 6.4* and *14.17*.

As with the previous editions, Mrs O. Adams has again provided invaluable help and secretarial assistance during the preparation of this third edition.

INTRODUCTION TO THE SECOND EDITION

Knowledge of the mechanisms responsible for disorders of cardiac rhythm continues to grow rapidly and at the same time new drugs and improved electrical techniques are increasing our ability to treat them successfully. Inevitably the second edition is enlarged and much has been re-written. A new chapter has been added on the Wolff–Parkinson–White syndrome and its associated arrhythmias. Apart from this, the general plan of the book has remained unchanged.

In Chapter 1, the internodal tracts whose existence has been fully confirmed are described. In the introduction to the first edition, it was remarked that the subject of arrhythmias had unfortunately become beset with semantic inconsistencies. Changes in long-established terminology, therefore, require full justification. Recent electrophysiological studies have failed to confirm that the A.V. node is the most important subsidiary pacemaker in the heart. The term A.V. junctional or junctional must therefore be used instead of nodal for that type of extrasystole, escape rhythm or tachycardia believed to originate in the A.V. junction. This change in traditional terminology is fully justified on physiological grounds and has been adopted in this edition. I agree with Papp, however, that to substitute dysrhythmia for arrhythmia is false linguistic purism. The term arrhythmia has become hallowed by tradition and there is no sound physiological reasons for changing it, although the occasional use of the term dysrhythmia as an alternative is acceptable.

It is a pleasure to acknowledge my very sincere thanks to Dr A. Schott for his very helpful criticisms of the first edition and for his constant help and advice with the second.

I am grateful to Dr R. Gold for allowing me to use *Figure 10.7* and also to Dr Hudson for *Figure 10.3*.

Once again I must acknowledge my indebtedness to my secretary, Mrs O. Adams, for all her help in the preparation of the manuscript and index for the second edition.

INTRODUCTION TO THE FIRST EDITION

Disorders of cardiac rhythm have long been a source of great interest to physicians, but any appreciation of their underlying mechanism or significance had to await some understanding of cardiac physiology. Towards the end of the nineteenth century, the development of graphic methods for recording the activity of the different heart chambers, together with a recognition of the fundamental physiological properties of heart muscle, began to shed light on a subject which had been wrapped in mysticism and dogma.

At the beginning of this century, Sir James Mackenzie, when working as a general practitioner in Burnley, Lancashire, made perhaps the first major clinical contributions to our understanding of different forms of irregular heart action. He developed his 'polygraph' which recorded simultaneously the jugular venous pulse and an arterial pulse. By painstaking and inspired analysis of his polygraphic records, he was able to differentiate between several different forms of irregular pulse, such as sinus arrhythmia, extra-systoles and atrial fibrillation, and to recognize their widely varying clinical significance.

The development of the electrocardiograph by Einthoven provided a new instrument for the analysis of arrhythmias, for it enabled the electrical activity of the different heart chambers to be recorded on a single tracing. Today, the electrocardiograph remains largely unchallenged as the most informative method of studying clinical disorders of cardiac rhythm. More recently, in animal studies, the electrophysiologist has begun to shed new and fundamental light on the initiation and propagation of the cardiac impulse. There seems little doubt that disturbances of rhythm encountered clinically will eventually be explained in terms of changes in the flow of electrically charged ions across the cardiac cell membrane.

A relatively brief acquaintance with the subject of clinical arrhythmology soon reveals that it has two distinct sides. On the one hand, there is the essentially practical aspect which entails the rapid recognition, from the electrocardiogram, of the type of arrhythmia present and the institution of the appropriate therapy. On the other hand, there is the more academic aspect, in which the record of an unusual arrhythmia is carefully studied and analysed in the hope of understanding its underlying mechanism in terms of cardiac physiology.

The pragmatist may object that the leisurely study of an arrhythmia, treating its analysis as a proposition in logic, with no sense of urgency in reaching a solution, is a task better suited to the philosopher, for, he may argue, a belated solution can offer little practical help to the patient. Such a view is very short term. In the first place, its acceptance would close the door, to the physician, on a fascinating and intellectually rewarding study. In the second place, to acquire virtuosity in the essentially practical side of arrhythmias demands an apprenticeship on the academic side. In the past 20 years in Great Britain, interest in this side of arrhythmias has tended to lapse. This book has been written, firstly, in the hope that it may prove useful to those engaged in hospital practice who are called upon to deal with patients suffering from arrhythmias and, secondly, that it may re-awaken interest in the purely academic side of the subject.

It is now the established practice in recording an electrocardiogram to employ approximately twelve different leads from each patient; conse-quently, the length of the individual leads has tended to become shorter. When the patient is in normal sinus rhythm, short strips of individual leads are quite adequate, but many arrhythmias demand much longer records of at least one lead before an adequate analysis is possible. It is impossible to give any dogmatic guide as to the best lead to use or the optimum length to

INTRODUCTION

record. As a general rule, the lead for recording an arrhythmia, for analysis, should be that in which the P waves are most clearly discernible. This is most commonly lead II or VI, but the best lead may vary from patient to patient. The optimum length of the record depends on the arrhythmia; one lasting half a minute is usually adequate, but intermittent arrhythmias may demand much longer recordings.

TERMINOLOGY

It is unfortunate that during the past 50 years the subject of arrhythmias has become beset with semantic inconsistencies. There is still, for example, no general agreement about the terminology for the commonest disturbance of rhythm, the extrasystole. The terminology used in this book is, as far as possible, the one most generally accepted by writers on the subject.

No attempt has been made to provide a complete bibliography to the subject. Nevertheless it is hoped that the limited number of references given may prove useful to those seeking further information.

Most of the records given were recorded at the conventional paper speed of 25 mm per second, so that the large squares on the records represent one-fifth of a second. Some were recorded at a paper speed of 50 mm per second and this is indicated in the legend as 'time markings one-tenth of a second'.

I am deeply grateful to many colleagues and friends who have encouraged me in writing this book and who have helped by allowing me to use their illustrations. I am particularly grateful to Dr D. Scherf and Dr A. Schott for allowing me to use *Figure 5.20b* and to Dr Schott for *Figure 9.7*. I am very grateful to Professor R. Hudson for *Figure 1.1*, and to Dr L. Schamroth for *Figure 5.20a* and *Figure 7.4*. My thanks are also due to Dr Evan Fletcher, Dr Clifford Parsons, Dr A. Hudson and Dr R. Gibson for allowing me to reproduce some of their records. The photograph illustrated in *Figure 1.4* was taken by Mr E. Bailey of Imperial Chemical Industries.

My particular thanks are due to my secretary, Mrs O. Adams, not only for typing the manuscript, but also for her unfailing help in many onerous tasks associated with the preparation of this book.

J. P. P. STOCK

CHAPTER 1

ANATOMY AND PHYSIOLOGY IN RELATION TO ARRHYTHMIAS

ANATOMY OF THE 'SPECIALIZED' TISSUES OF THE HEART

In addition to the purely contractile muscle fibres composing the atria and ventricles, the heart possesses certain 'specialized' tissues, the primary functions of which are the genesis and conduction of impulses. These specialized tissues consist of the sino-atrial (S.A.) and atrioventricular (A.V.) nodes, the bundle of His, with its left and right main branches, and the Purkinje network of fibres in each ventricle. Although each of these structures is macroscopic in size, they are none of them readily identifiable by the naked eye, and histological or chemical techniques are necessary to demonstrate them. It is curious that historically these structures were discovered in the reverse order in which they are normally activated during the cardiac cycle. The terminal elements of the system, the conduction networks in the ventricles, were first described by Purkinje in 1845, although he did not appreciate their function. The A.V. bundle was identified and described by His, Jnr., in 1893. The A.V. node was first described by Tawara in 1906, although perhaps his most important contribution was the demonstration that the A.V. node, bundle of His and the Purkinje networks formed one continuous structure linking the atria to all parts of the ventricles. The sino-atrial node, the primary pacemaker of the heart, was the last of the specialized tissues to be identified by Keith and Flack in 1907. It is now well established that these specialized tissues are essentially muscle fibres, although they differ in histological detail from ordinary atrial and ventricular muscle cells.

Until comparatively recently, it was generally thought that no special pathways existed in the atrium, linking the sino-atrial and atrio-ventricular nodes. It was considered that the sinus impulse spread radially over the atrial myocardium to reach the atrio-ventricular node and the left atrium in a non-selective manner. However, in the past few years increasing evidence has accumulated that there are in fact three specialized pathways in the atria for rapid conduction of a sinus impulse, both to the left atrium and to the atrio-ventricular node. James (1963) has called these the internodal tracts.

The old controversy between the myogenic and the neurogenic views of the conduction of the cardiac impulse is now of only historical interest. Recent studies, both of morphology by the electron microscope and of electrophysiology by modern techniques, have established beyond doubt that the genesis and transmission of impulses in the heart are solely effected by muscular structures.

Although the specialized tissues are macroscopic in size, they are difficult to differentiate from the surrounding myocardium with the unaided eye. The most certain and consistent method of showing them is by taking histological sections of appropriate blocks of the myocardium. The histological appearance of both the sinus and A.V. nodes is closely similar. The muscle fibres are smaller than those of the neighbouring atrial musculature. They are striated, but the striations are difficult to see unless stained with silver preparations. The most characteristic feature of nodal tissue is that the fibres are branched and interwoven to form a complex three-dimensional network (*Figure 1.1*). In section, therefore, some of them are cut transversely and others at varying angles. At the periphery the fibres tend to run more vertically forming an incomplete border to the node. The sinus node is fairly clearly demarcated from the surrounding tissues by being embedded

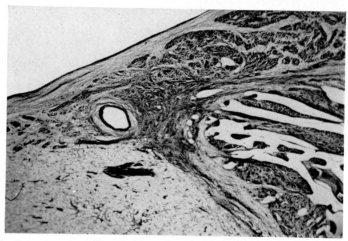

Figure 1.1—Low-power view of human sinus node, stained by Holme's silver method × 22. The sinus node is seen disposed round its nutrient artery. Reproduced from 'The Human Pacemaker and its Pathology' by R. E. B. Hudson by courtesy of Edward Arnold

in a matrix of fibro-elastic tissue. The A.V. node contains rather less collagenous tissue than the sino-atrial node. Both nodes are richly supplied with autonomic nerve fibres and blood vessels.

The muscle fibres of the bundle of His, its left and right branches, and the Purkinje network in the ventricles all show the same basic structure, although differing in minor details. The cells tend to be arranged in parallel with only occasional interconnecting branches. They are larger and paler staining than the cells of the common myocardium and are arranged in staggered fashion. The individual cells are approximately 100–200 μm in length. They tend to be arranged in groups to form fibres. Each fibre contains from two to seven cells, the membranes of which are in direct contact, the group being surrounded by a basement membrane which does not penetrate between the individual cells.

Until comparatively recently it had always been believed that there was protoplasmic continuity between myocardial cells, so that the whole heart could be regarded as a syncytium. Electron microscopic studies, however, have established that the intercalated discs are primarily formed by the cell membranes of two fibres in end-to-end contact, which separates the protoplasms of the two cells completely.

Gross Anatomy of Specialized Tissues

Sino-atrial Node

The sino-atrial node is the primary pacemaker of the heart. It is situated in the upper part of the right atrium, close to its junction with the superior vena cava and close to the sulcus terminalis. It is usually described as being about 25 mm in length, having a head, body and tail, and with its long axis running backwards, downwards and to the left. However, Hudson (1960) carefully examined the sino-atrial node histologically in 65 human hearts and gave a very clear description of its normal anatomy. On the antero-lateral aspect of the junction of the superior vena cava with the right atrium,

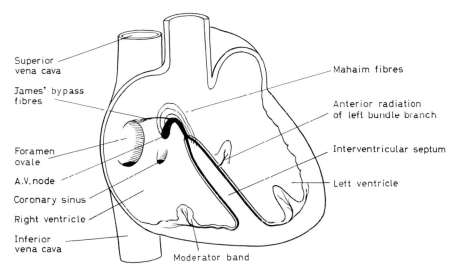

Figure 1.2—Diagram of A.V. conduction system of human heart

the latter rises to a well defined summit which is constantly present. This summit is the landmark for the node, the main part of which lies just below it, immediately beneath the epicardium. He describes the normal average human node as a crescentic structure, measuring 3–4 mm at its widest part and tapering medially and laterally to a point, the long axis lying virtually transversely. The nodal tissue is usually disposed round its central artery, and there is no overlying atrial muscle. Although it lies immediately beneath the epicardium, it is rarely discernible to the naked eye but readily demonstrated in histological sections.

The Internodal Tracts

The anatomy of the three internodal tracts in the atria was clearly described by James (1963) and his findings have been largely accepted by other workers. He called them the anterior, middle and posterior internodal tracts and pointed out that each had previously been described; the anterior tract was partially described by Bachmann (1916), the middle tract by Wenckebach (1907) and the posterior tract by Thorel (1910). The delay

3

in accepting the existence of these specific fast-conducting internodal pathways was probably largely due to the fact that although they contain numerous Purkinje fibres, they are not exclusively composed of such specialized cells. Nevertheless, a direct fibre-to-fibre connection has been established in all three pathways, between the sinus and A.V. nodes. The anterior internodal tract arises from the anterior part of the sinus node and passes to the left round the superior vena cava to enter the anterior interatrial

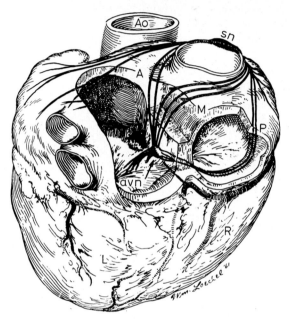

Figure 1.3—The internodal tracts. The anterior tract (marked A) is seen to divide into two. The upper fibres pass in the interatrial myocardial band to reach the left atrium. They are often referred to as Bachmann's bundle. The posterior internodal tract (marked P) is the longest of the three tracts and may bypass the major portion of the A.V. node (marked avn). The terminal portion of these fibres is often referred to as James' bypass tract. (After James, reproduced by courtesy of Dr T. James and 'Diseases of the Chest')

myocardial band which was first described by Bachmann. Bachmann was only interested in interatrial conduction and he did not note that his tract divided into two parts, the first going on to the left atrium and known as Bachmann's bundle, and the second group of fibres descending anteriorly in the interatrial septum to reach the A.V. node (*Figure 1.3*). The middle internodal tract originally described by Wenckebach also descends in the interatrial septum to reach the A.V. node. The posterior internodal tract originally described by Thorel terminates with most of its fibres bypassing the bulk of the A.V. node and joining the lower part of the node. The lower part of this tract is often referred to as James' bypass tract.

In the experimental animal hyperkalaemia may produce atrial paralysis yet sinus rhythm is maintained via the internodal tracts although no P waves appear in the electrocardiogram. Moreover, disturbances in atrial conduction with a change in the morphology of the P waves have been described by Hamilton and his colleagues (1968), following the surgical creation of an atrial septal defect by the Blalock–Hanlon technique.

The remaining 'specialized' tissues of the heart may be viewed as a single continuous structure linking the atria to all parts of the ventricles and containing the subsidiary pacemakers of the heart (*Figure 1.2*). It consists of the A.V. node which is continuous with the main bundle of His. This divides into left and right main branches, which ramify in their respective ventricles to form the peripheral conduction pathways, the ultimate twigs of which probably penetrate from endocardium to epicardium, terminating in the fibres of the common ventricular myocardium. In the normal heart, the atria and ventricles are otherwise completely separated from each other by the two fibrous A.V. rings and this specialized pathway forms the only link between them over which an impulse can pass from one to the other.

Atrioventricular Node

The A.V. node lies on the right side of the lower part of the interatrial septum, just in front of the opening of the coronary sinus and above the attachment of the septal cusp of the tricuspid valve to the right A.V. ring. Unlike the sinus node, it is possible, with practice, to dissect it macroscopically from the surrounding musculature, and its continuity with the main bundle of His can be demonstrated. The macroscopic appearance of the A.V. node has been compared to a flask, measuring approximately $6 \times 3 \times 2$ mm. The 'neck' of the flask is continuous with the bundle of His, which is narrow in comparison, having a diameter of only 2–4 mm.

In addition to these bypass fibres of James, Mahaim (1947) described fibres linking the A.V. node directly to the interventricular septum. He termed these 'preferential' or 'paraspecific' fibres. Their existence, at least in some hearts, has been confirmed by Lev and Lerner (1955). The precise function of these fibres is also uncertain, and they may be responsible for the delta wave in some cases of the Wolff–Parkinson–White syndrome (page 73).

Theory of Kent

In 1893 Kent first described direct muscular connections between the atria and ventricles in some newborn animals. In a later series of papers in 1913 and 1914 he suggested that conduction between the atria and ventricles was via a series of muscular bridges linking the lateral walls of the atria to the ventricles. Since that time many workers have searched for the muscular bridges described by Kent without success. It is possible that such connections occasionally exist and may explain some examples of ventricular preexcitation (Wolff–Parkinson–White syndrome), but it is now certain that in the vast majority of mammalian hearts, the A.V. node and bundle of His form the only link between the atria and ventricles.

Anatomy of Atrioventricular Conduction System

Rosenbaum and his colleagues (1968) have shown that the A.V. conduction system is not quite as conventionally pictured. The thin cylindrical bundle of His which is approximately 20 mm in length originates from the 'tail' of the A.V. node and is divisible into the 'penetrating' segment and a 'branching' segment. The penetrating segment runs through the central fibrous body where it has no contact with the common myocardium and is relatively immune from the cardiomyopathies and coronary artery disease. It is, however, susceptible to pathological processes arising from the surrounding fibrous structures. The branching portion of the bundle of His extends from the point where it begins to give off the most posterior fibres of the left bundle branch to where it divides into the right bundle branch and the anterior fibres of the left bundle branch. Rosenbaum and his colleagues point out that there is no true bifurcation of the bundle in man and refer to the separation of the right bundle branch and the anterior division of the left bundle branch as the 'pseudo-bifurcation'.

Thus the intraventricular conduction system consists of three fascicles: the right bundle branch and the anterior and posterior divisions of the left bundle branch. The most robust of these three fascicles is the posterior division of the left bundle branch (see Figure 5.4, page 95). A great advance in our knowledge of the clinical electrocardiogram has been the recognition that conduction block may occur in each of these three fascicles alone or in any combination of two or in all three simultaneously.

Bundle of His

The main bundle of His is approximately 20 mm in length and penetrates the central fibrous body reaching the top of the muscular interventricular septum, where it divides into its left and right main branches.

In the terminology of arrhythmias, it is convenient to refer to the A.V. node and the main bundle of His as the 'A.V. junction'.

Right Main Bundle

The right main bundle passes down the right ventricular side of the muscular septum towards the apex. It gives off few branches at first and lies rather more deeply beneath the endocardium than does the left main bundle. It then runs in the free edge of the moderator band to reach the base of the anterior papillary muscle where it breaks up into a network to supply all parts of the right ventricular musculature.

Left Main Bundle

The left main bundle emerges on the left ventricular side of the septum just below the posterior cusp of the aortic valve. As it passes down the septum, branches penetrate and ramify in the substance of the septum. At the junction of the upper and middle third of the septum, it divides into an anterior and a posterior branch, which pass to the bases of the corresponding papillary muscles. Each branch breaks up into a complex network, the fibres of which run in the trabeculae lining the ventricle, particularly the 'false tendons', and penetrating branches reach the subepicardial muscle fibres.

The A.V. node, the bundle of His and the Purkinje networks in the ventricles are often referred to collectively as the conduction system.

Blood Supply of Specialized Tissues

The blood supply to the S.A. node is by a special artery, which in 60 per cent of hearts is derived from the right coronary artery, and from the left main coronary in the remaining 40 per cent. There is a rich anastomosis with neighbouring vessels.

The blood supply to the A.V. node is generally from a specific artery, the ramus septi fibrosi, which is a branch of the right main coronary artery in 92 per cent of hearts, and from the left circumflex in the remaining 8 per cent.

Nerve Supply

Both the S.A. and the A.V. nodes are richly supplied with sympathetic and parasympathetic nerve fibres. The parasympathetic fibres to the sinus node are derived from the right vagus and those to the A.V. node from the left vagus.

Embryology

The S.A. node is derived from the right horn of the sinus venosus and the A.V. node from the left horn. Morphologically, therefore, the sinus node is a right-sided and the A.V. node a left-sided structure, which accounts for their different vagal supply.

Direct Visualization of the Peripheral Conduction System

Under certain circumstances, it is possible to visualize the peripheral conduction system in the left ventricle where the system lies immediately beneath the endocardium. In the sheep's heart, the conduction fibres are enclosed in a continuous sheath, and this arrangement enables them to be displayed by injecting indian ink into the sheath. No such sheath is present in human, canine or ox hearts. A characteristic feature of the conducting tissues is their high content of glycogen. This enables fresh specimens to be selectively stained by various techniques. The simplest method of demonstrating the Purkinje system in the left ventricle is to flood it with Lugol's iodine. *Figure 1.4* shows the left main bundle and its branches in the left ventricle of a dog's heart displayed in this way. Unfortunately, application of this technique is limited to fresh specimens, for glycogen rapidly undergoes post-mortem autolysis and ceases to stain after about two hours. Nevertheless, the human left main bundle and its branches has been demonstrated in this way when an autopsy has been possible $1\frac{1}{2}$ hours after death (Uhley and Rivkin, 1959, Spach and colleagues, 1963). The chance of success is much greater if death occurred suddenly; when death was more gradual, ante-mortem autolysis of glycogen may occur. It is possible that this accounts for the bizarre conduction anomalies seen in the electrocardiogram of the 'dying' heart. Although at first sight this technique looks promising, it clearly has very limited applications and would probably prove valueless for demonstrating pathological lesions.

The most refined and accurate technique for studying the specialized tissues of the heart is that evolved by Lev, Widron and Erickson (1951). The method is painstaking, laborious and time consuming, for it involves

7

the cutting and histological examination of over 3,000 serial sections from a single heart. The authors rightly point out that this is essential to determine the site and nature of any pathological lesions in the conduction system

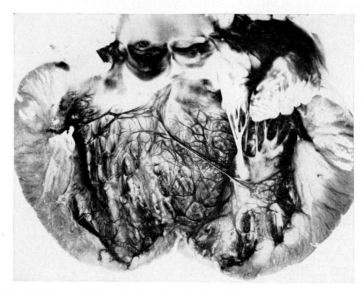

Figure 1.4—Distribution of left bundle branch in the dog, stained by Lugol's iodine. The division of the left main bundle into its two chief branches is clearly seen and takes place at a rather higher level on the septum than it does in the human heart

which may be correlated with the electrocardiographic findings in life. However, at present, this technique is necessarily restricted to the dedicated expert. Even so, it has already made significant contributions to our knowledge of the anatomy and functions of the specialized tissues.

CARDIAC PHYSIOLOGY IN RELATION TO ARRHYTHMIAS

The clinical electrocardiogram, which is recorded from the body surface, registers the electrical changes produced by the spread of the excitation wave over the heart. The genesis of these electrical changes will be considered later under the heading Electrophysiology. The excitation wave may be regarded as the trigger which releases the contractile forces of the heart, and therefore the onset of the electrocardiogram precedes the onset of contraction. *Figure 1.5* shows a simultaneous recording of the electrocardiogram and the left ventricular pressure pulse. The onset of the QRS complex precedes the rise in left ventricular pressure by 0·12 second. While part of this time interval is an artefact due to delay in transmission of the pressure wave down the catheter, accurate simultaneous recordings show that the electrical changes in the heart precede the mechanical changes. In fact, the electrocardiogram tells us nothing about the contractile events which follow. Occasionally, during angiography, the heart has been seen to stop while the electrocardiogram continued unchanged. On the other hand, careful analysis of the electrocardiogram almost always enables the site of origin of the excitation wave to be recognized and its pathway of conduction to be deduced. All disorders of cardiac rhythm are primarily due to disturbances either of the origin or conduction of the excitation wave, and for this reason the electrocardiogram reigns supreme in the analysis and interpretation of arrhythmias.

An appreciation of some of the fundamental physiological properties of

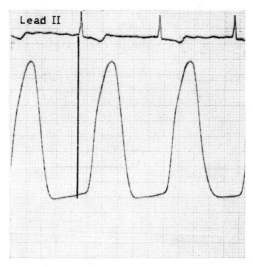

Figure 1.5—Simultaneous recording of left ventricular pressure trace and surface electrocardiogram. The onset of the QRS of the electrocardiogram precedes the commencement of left ventricular systole by 0·12 second. Part of this delay is an artefact

heart muscle is essential for an understanding of the mechanisms underlying many disorders of cardiac rhythm. The description of cardiac physiology which follows is in no sense intended to be comprehensive but will be mainly restricted to those properties of heart muscle concerned with the formation and propagation of impulses. It is conventional to describe five fundamental physiological properties of heart muscle, namely excitability, conductivity, refractoriness, rhythmicity and contractility. In addition, the intact heart possesses remarkable powers of adaptation to changing conditions. These powers, which are independent of nervous control, have been termed, by Sarnoff and his colleagues (1960), homeometric responses.

Excitability

Heart muscle is excitable in that it responds to a variety of natural and artificial stimuli by contracting. The response of the heart to artificial stimuli obeys the 'all or none' law. This was first observed in 1884 by Bowditch in the frog ventricle. Using induction shocks as stimuli, he found that once the strength of a stimulus reached threshold level, it immediately evoked from the ventricle the maximum response of which it was capable at that moment. Further increase in the strength of stimulus did not increase the strength of the resulting contraction. His findings have been fully confirmed in mammalian heart muscle. The degree of excitability of heart muscle may be assessed by the strength of stimulus necessary to produce a response. As will be seen when the refractory period is discussed, this varies throughout the cardiac cycle. Excitability is at its peak during the non-refractory period, but the level of this peak may vary under different conditions. It is increased by such factors as CO_2 retention, or by circulating catecholamines and by numerous drugs. The 'irritability' of the heart is also profoundly influenced by electrolyte disturbances, particularly of potassium.

Conductivity

Conductivity is that property of heart muscle whereby activation of any individual muscle fibre automatically initiates activity in neighbouring muscle cells. In consequence, if an adequate stimulus is applied at any point in cardiac tissue during its resting phase, an 'excitation wave', that is, a wave of electrical activity, will be propagated over the whole of the tissue without decrement. This property of conductivity is unique to cardiac muscle and visceral smooth muscle; it is not possessed by skeletal muscle. It used to be thought that the myocardium was a syncytium, so that the whole intact heart could be regarded as functioning as a single muscle cell. If this were true, it would of course explain conductivity; however, recent electron microscopic studies of the myocardium have established that the individual muscle fibres are separate anatomical units, each measuring approximately $100 \times 15 \times 15$ μm. The precise mechanism by which the excitation wave is propagated from fibre to fibre (without innervation) has not yet been firmly established. There appear to be two possible mechanisms; one is that propagation is mediated by local electrical currents from cell to cell. This would imply that the electrical resistance of the myocardial cell membrane is low. The alternative mechanism is that propagation of the impulse is chemical via synaptic junctions between individual fibres.

Conductivity is a property possessed by all types of heart muscle. Under 'normal' conditions, if a stimulus arises (or is induced) in any part of the heart, an excitation wave will spread over the whole heart, provided all parts are in the non-refractory phase. In principle, this is true wherever the stimulus originates. In normal sinus rhythm, the excitation wave originates in the sino-atrial node and is conducted over the heart to activate the various parts of its four chambers in a definite orderly sequence which is precisely repeated from beat to beat. The sequence and timing of activation of the individual parts of the heart is so arranged as to ensure that the maximum mechanical efficiency results from their ensuing contraction. This is largely achieved by the special conduction system already described. Although conductivity is a property possessed by all myocardial cells, the speed of conduction varies appreciably in different types of heart muscle.

In the mammalian heart, the speed of conduction in atrial muscle is 1,000 mm/second. In ventricular muscle, it is substantially slower, measuring only 400 mm/second. Conduction is fastest in the Purkinje network where it is 4,000 mm/second. It is slowest of all in the A.V. junction where it averages only 200 mm/second. There is an important teleological reason for this; one of the main functions of the A.V. junction in sinus rhythm is to delay the transmission of the excitation wave to the ventricles in order to ensure that atrial systole is complete before ventricular systole begins. Most of the P–R interval is occupied by this slow transmission of the impulse through the A.V. junction. The importance of the length of the P–R interval has recently been elegantly demonstrated by Gillespie and colleagues (1967). They devised a method for measuring the right ventricular stroke output of successive beats. Very briefly, the technique consists of enclosing a subject in a whole body plethysmograph while breathing a weak mixture of nitrous oxide in air. The plethysmograph records the volume of gas absorbed from

TABLE 1.1

Speed of Conduction in Mammalian Heart Muscle	*mm/second*
Atrial muscle	1,000
Ventricular muscle	400
Purkinje fibres	4,000
Atrioventricular junction	200

the lungs following each right ventricular systole and thus enables the volume of blood ejected at each systole to be calculated. They studied patients with congenital complete heart block, in whom the interval between atrial and ventricular systole was continuously varying. They found that when the P–R interval measured 0·2 second, the right ventricular stroke output was 30 per cent greater than when atrial and ventricular systole coincided, that is, when the P–R interval was zero. Similarly, during right heart catheterization, it is not uncommon for transient A.V. dissociation to be induced with the ventricles controlled by an A.V. junctional pacemaker. When right atrial and right ventricular systole coincide, there is always an abrupt fall in right ventricular systolic pressure compared with when the time relationship of the contraction of the two chambers is normal. This pressure change is more marked when the right ventricle is under an increased load, that is, in pulmonary hypertension or pulmonary stenosis. This contribution of atrial systole to ventricular efficiency is explained by Starling's law, namely that the strength of contraction depends on the preceding diastolic length of the myocardial fibres, atrial systole contributing the final 'stretch' to the ventricle. Atrial fibrillation, even when adequately controlled by digitalis, reduces the efficiency of the heart because of the loss of atrial systole.

The A.V. junction is normally capable of conducting an impulse in either direction. Conduction from atria to ventricles is termed 'orthograde'* and conduction in the opposite direction is termed 'retrograde'. It is possible to recognize in the electrocardiogram when retrograde activation of the atria has occurred, for the excitation wave then spreads over the atria in the opposite direction to normal. In consequence, the P waves in the electrocardiogram have an opposite contour to normal, being negative in leads II, III and AVF. Retrograde conduction in the A.V. junction is normally slower than orthograde conduction. The physiology of A.V. conduction will be discussed more fully under the heading Electrophysiology.

High-speed cinematography of the beating heart reveals that all parts of

* The term 'antegrade' can also be used.

the ventricles do not contract simultaneously. The inflow tracts of both ventricles contract before the outflow tracts, imparting a peristaltic action to ventricular systole. This will clearly improve the mechanical efficiency of the ventricles in propelling blood into the aorta and pulmonary artery. It is now known that ventricular depolarization begins in a cup-shaped area involving the apex and septum and spreads upwards to the base. The achievement of this orderly sequence of ventricular activation is a function of the A.V. conduction system. It is probably accomplished by the anatomical arrangement of the fast conducting Purkinje networks, though it is possible that some slowing of conduction occurs in the more peripheral parts of the system. The A.V. node, bundle of His and peripheral conduction system is thus analogous to the electric distributor of an internal combustion engine, the function of which is to trigger explosions in the different cylinders in orderly sequence. A fundamental concept of the A.V. node and bundle of His is that each part of the node is connected to a particular part of the ventricular musculature and that there is longitudinal dissociation between these individual units which are 'insulated' from each other. In this sense, the A.V. junction has been compared with the internal capsule of the brain. In effect, this concept implies that, if an impulse were conducted down one part of the A.V. junction, it would activate one particular region of the ventricles first. The free 'anastomosis' of the individual units of this system in the peripheral Purkinje network would enable such an impulse to reach all parts of the ventricular musculature by fast conduction pathways, so that, although the order of excitation of the ventricles might be changed compared with when the whole A.V. junction was involved, the QRS duration would not be increased, although its contour would be changed. This concept is of importance in explaining some features of A.V. junctional arrhythmias (page 64).

Although ordinary ventricular muscle fibres possess the property of conduction, in normal sinus rhythm (or A.V. junctional rhythm) the speed of conduction in the Purkinje system is ten times faster, so that ventricular activation occurs entirely through these pathways. In bundle branch block, however, the impulse has to spread from the unblocked to the blocked ventricle by the slower ventricular myocardial route. In consequence, the QRS complex of the electrocardiogram is widened. Similarly, in ectopic ventricular rhythms, for example, ventricular extrasystoles or ventricular tachycardia, when the impulse arises in a ventricular focus, the excitation wave has to reach the other ventricle by the slow myocardial route and the resulting QRS complexes are characteristically widened.

Synchronized Sinoventricular Conduction

Sherf and James (1969) have recently suggested that there is a highly organized integration between impulse formation and conduction which begins in the sinus node and ends at the ventricular Purkinje cell junction. They visualize that the sinus impulse is preferentially conducted over the anterior and middle internodal tracts (which are the shortest) to reach the crest of the A.V. node early. Stimuli arriving later along the posterior internodal tract may then find the A.V. node refractory. The wave front descending from the crest of the A.V. node reaches the bundle of His where it is fractionated into a number of parallel smaller depolarization fronts which are insulated from each other and will continue their passage to given destinations in the ventricular myocardium. Under physiological conditions, this synchronized sinoventricular conduction is precisely repeated from beat to beat, producing identical P waves and QRS complexes. They suggest that in pathological or unphysiological conditions, the sinus impulse might be preferentially conducted over, say, the posterior internodal tract and reach the lateral margin of the node early and thus the wave front of excitation in the A.V. node would be distorted. This would result in simultaneous changes in the contour of both the P wave and the QRS complex. They publish several records in which this occurs and suggest that disturbance of the normal synchronized sinoventricular conduction may explain many features of the Wolff–Parkinson–White syndrome (*see* page 172).

Refractoriness

Refractoriness is a property possessed by all types of cardiac muscle. During its period of contraction, heart muscle is absolutely refractory and will not respond at all to external stimuli. This means that any contraction must be completed and recovered from before another can occur. It is obviously important that this should be so, for if the heart did not possess refractoriness it could conceivably develop tetanus which would be disastrous to its function as a pump.

The refractory period is divisible into two parts: the absolute refractory

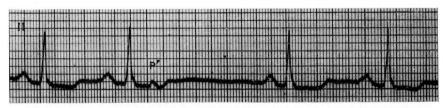

Figure 1.6—Blocked atrial extrasystole. An atrial extrasystole marked P′ falls in the S–T segment of the second QRS complex. It prematurely discharges the sinus node but is not conducted to the ventricles and a pause in the ventricular rhythm results (time markings $\frac{1}{10}$ second)

period, during which heart muscle shows no response to external stimuli, however strong they may be, followed by the relative refractory period, during which the excitability of the heart gradually returns to normal. During this latter phase, the heart will respond to a stronger stimulus than is normally required, and the force of the resulting contraction is weaker than normal. The operation of the relative refractory phase is best seen from its effect on the rate of conduction, particularly in the A.V. junction. The effect of the refractory phase on conduction is of considerable importance in arrhythmias. If an impulse reaches the A.V. junction during its absolute refractory phase, it will be blocked. *Figure 1.6* shows an atrial extrasystole which has reached the A.V. junction during the absolute refractory phase. It is not followed by a QRS complex and therefore was blocked. *Figure 1.7* shows an atrial extrasystole which has reached the A.V. junction during its relative refractory phase. This is followed by a QRS complex, but the P–R interval is longer than that of the sinus beat preceding it. Conduction has occurred, but conduction time is prolonged. During the relative refractory period there is a progressive return to normal, both of excitability and conduction time. There is no way in which the recovery curve of excitability can be plotted from the clinical electrocardiogram. In some records, however, it is occasionally possible to plot the recovery curve of conduction time during the relative refractory period, and this will be described later. The absolute refractory period of the ventricles extends from the commencement of the QRS complex of the electrocardiogram to approximately the peak of the T wave. The relative refractory period then lasts till about the end of the U wave.

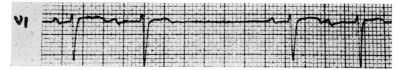

Figure 1.7—The first and third beats of this record are sinus beats. Each is followed by an atrial extrasystole, both of which reach the A.V. junction during its relative refractory phase, so that the P–R intervals of the extrasystoles are prolonged

Trendelenberg (1903) first showed that the duration of the refractory period varies with heart rate. He found that if the frequency of artificial stimulation of the heart were slowly increased, the response of the heart would remain 1:1 up to a rate which, if started abruptly, would only evoke a 2:1 response. He found the converse also to be true; when a rapid rate of stimulation was started abruptly, evoking a 2:1 response, gradual slowing of the frequency of stimulation continued to result in a 2:1 response down to a rate which would ordinarily have produced a 1:1 response. These experiments showed that the duration of the absolute refractory period shortens with increasing heart rates, but the change is gradual, taking several cycles. A similar lengthening of the refractory period occurs as the heart rate slows. In the clinical electrocardiogram, this is approximately paralleled by the change in the Q–T interval with changes in rate, this interval varying with the square root of the cycle length.

In clinical practice changes in cycle length most commonly occur in atrial fibrillation. In this condition a long cycle length may be followed by a short cycle. The long cycle lengthens the refractory period and the beat terminating the succeeding short cycle may show aberrant conduction because of the lengthened refractory period.

Rhythmicity

Rhythmicity or automaticity is that property of heart muscle which enables it to initiate its own impulses without the intervention of external agencies. It used to be taught that rhythmicity was common to all forms of heart muscle, but it is now believed that this property is confined to the specialized tissues (De Haan, 1961). Erlanger in 1910 found that excised strips of the left atrium of the cat might or might not show spontaneous activity. Some strips frequently remained quiescent, whereas strips of either the right or left atrium, which included parts of the interatrial septum, usually showed spontaneous automaticity. It is now known that the parts of the atria which Erlanger found it necessary to include in his strips, in order to obtain spontaneous activity, were those which contained specialized fibres. Although final proof is lacking, the evidence is highly suggestive that pacemaker activity in the heart is a property confined to the specialized tissues.

The normal pacemaker of the heart is, of course, the sino-atrial node. The heart, however, is protected against failure of the sinus node by the presence of numerous subsidiary pacemakers in the remaining specialized tissues. The inherent rate of discharge of these subsidiary pacemakers is slower than that of the sinus node and becomes slower the more peripheral the site of the pacemaker. It is a fundamental rule of the heart that it is controlled by the pacemaker with the fastest rate, for the excitation wave, as it spreads over the heart, automatically extinguishes all immature impulses which are forming in other pacemakers. If, for any reason, the sinus node should fail to produce an impulse for one or more beats, the pacemaker with the next faster inherent rate of discharge will take over.

This will normally be pacemaking cells in the lower part of the A.V. node or in the bundle of His which usually have a rate between approximately 40 to 60 per minute. (The old view that the A.V. node possessed upper, middle and lower pacemaking cells is no longer tenable, *see* page 67.) Pacemaker cells with still slower rates are present in the left and right main branches of the bundle of His and these may have to assume control of the ventricles when complete A.V. block results from bilateral bundle branch block. These 'idioventricular' pacemakers are often very slow, having rates between 20 and 40 per minute, and they often tend to be very unstable.

Contractility

Contractility is the fifth main property of heart muscle. The physiology of cardiac contraction forms a very large subject and no attempt will be made to review it here, since it has little relevance to the analysis of disorders of rhythm. The haemodynamic effects of some arrhythmias are best discussed in the appropriate sections.

One of the homeometric responses of the intact heart is the increased force of contraction of the next normal beat following an extrasystole. In the past this was attributed to the increased filling of the heart which occurred during the pause following the ectopic beat. However, it is now known that this post-extrasystolic potentiation of contraction occurs after an interpolated extrasystole when there is no pause following the ectopic beat.

ELECTROPHYSIOLOGY OF THE HEART

During the past two decades our knowledge of the electrophysiology of cardiac excitation has been greatly extended by direct intracellular recording. This was first achieved in skeletal muscle by Ling and Gerard in 1949 and was soon afterwards applied to the heart. In this technique a micro-capillary electrode is made to penetrate the cell membrane of a single myocardial fibre and is paired with an extracellular electrode. This enables the difference in electric potential between the inside and outside of the fibre to be measured, at rest, and the changes in potential which occur during activity to be recorded. The difference in potential is termed the 'transmembrane potential', and the changes during activity are termed the 'action current'.

Figure 1.8a shows the action current recorded in this way from a single ventricular muscle fibre. During the resting phase, when the fibre is said to be polarized, the inside is electrically negative compared with the outside. The resting transmembrane potential is surprisingly large, measuring

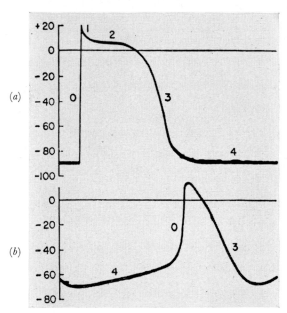

Figure 1.8—Diagram of action currents recorded by intracellular electrodes: (a) shows the action current recorded from a ventricular muscle fibre; (b) shows the action current recorded from a pacemaker fibre

90 mV. During the first phase of the action current the transmembrane potential falls rapidly to zero and transiently 'overshoots', so that the inside of the fibre at the peak becomes approximately 30 mV positive to the outside. This transient overshoot is followed by a plateau and then the more gradual downstroke of repolarization.

The ionic concentration of the intracellular fluid of cardiac muscle fibres, like that of all living cells, is markedly different from that of the extracellular fluid. All ions by definition carry electric charges, and the resting transmembrane potential largely results from the high concentration of positively charged sodium ions in the extracellular fluid. Since the cell membrane is ordinarily permeable to all simple ions, it is necessary to explain how the ionic composition of the intracellular fluid is maintained. The generally accepted view is that the cells contain metabolic sodium 'pumps' which continually eject sodium ions from the cell. Since this is achieved in the face of both electrical and chemical gradients, active metabolic work is involved. The electrical changes represented by the action current are brought about by rapid fluxes of ions across the cell membrane. It is believed that both depolarization and repolarization are 'passive' events resulting from abrupt changes in the permeability of the cell membrane to different ionic species. When suitably stimulated, the permeability of the cell membranes to sodium ions suddenly increases. Sodium ions then rapidly enter the cell as a result of the electrochemical gradient, and the upstroke of the action current is written. Repolarization is initially achieved by an increase in potassium permeability, so that a rapid egress of positive charged potassium ions from the cell occurs and the transmembrane potential is restored. This egress of potassium ions from the cell is facilitated by the large chemical gradient and the disappearance of the electrical gradient following depolarization. At the end of the action current, the inside of the fibres will have gained sodium ions and lost potassium ions. Following activity, the original differential ionic concentrations are restored by the metabolic sodium pump. As sodium ions are ejected, potassium ions re-enter the cell (owing to the electrical gradient), until the original state is restored. Detailed accounts of the experimental proof of these events in cardiac excitation, with appropriate references, are given by Hoffman and Cranefield (1960).

A characteristic feature of the action currents of atrial and ventricular muscle fibres is that the transmembrane potential remains constant during diastole. On the other hand, the action current of pacemaker fibres is characterized by slow spontaneous depolarization during diastole (*Figure 1.8b*). For reasons which are not entirely clear, once the transmembrane potential has fallen to threshold value, which is approximately 40 mV, rapid depolarization follows, and this automatically fires off a propagated response which will be conducted over the heart. Clearly, therefore, the inherent rate of discharge of a pacemaker fibre is determined by the angle which its slope of spontaneous diastolic depolarization makes with the threshold line. It also becomes obvious that the pacemaker with the steepest slope of diastolic depolarization will control the heart, for the excitation wave originating from it will depolarize all other pacemakers before they are ready to fire.

Electrophysiology of Atrioventricular Conduction

Electrical activity generated in the A.V. node, bundle of His and peripheral Purkinje fibres is not apparent in the electrocardiogram recorded from the body surface. Although a great deal of information about normal and abnormal A.V. conduction has been deduced from clinical electrocardiograms, the evidence is necessarily indirect. More precise knowledge of the physiology of A.V. conduction in the canine heart has now been obtained by electrophysiological techniques. Two methods have been employed. In one, small electrodes are attached to the endocardium, at different sites in the A.V. conduction system, during total cardiopulmonary bypass. The activity recorded by these electrodes are termed electrograms and they accurately record the time of onset of electrical activity in the structures they overlie. Sometimes these observations have been acute, and at other times records have been made from 'healthy' dogs who had had such electrodes implanted previously. This technique reveals the exact time sequence of activation of various parts of the conduction system. These studies have revealed that the A.V. node is activated early during the P wave of the surface electrocardiogram. The main delay in A.V. transmission occurs at the atrial margin of the A.V. node, where conduction velocity has the very low value of 50 mm per second. Within the node, conduction velocity progressively increases to reach 1,000 to 1,500 mm per second in the bundle of His. In the free-running Purkinje fibres in the ventricles, conduction reaches a velocity of 4,000 mm per second and then slows again in the fine terminal ramifications of the system. During retrograde transmission from ventricles to atria, the same conduction velocities occur, except at the atrial margin of the node where retrograde conduction is even slower than orthograde.

The second technique has made use of intracellular recordings from the conduction system. Intracellular electrode recordings reveal that conduction velocity is materially influenced by the rate of rise and the amplitude of the action current. The faster the rate of rise and the greater the amplitude of the action current, the faster is conduction velocity. In A.V. nodal fibres the rate of rise of the action current and its overshoot are both relatively reduced. These characteristics are most marked in fibres at the atrial margin of the node and become less evident in the lower portion of the node. The reduced amplitude and slow rise of the action potential at the atrial margin of the node would conduce to a low conduction velocity. The A.V. nodal fibres at this site are small (about 6 micrometres or less in diameter), and this would also contribute to a slow conduction velocity because of increased electrical resistance. In contrast, the resting transmembrane potentials in the larger fibres of the bundle of His and Purkinje fibres are larger, and the upstroke of the action potential is much faster and the amplitude larger. This is associated with a much faster conduction velocity.

Experimental Atrioventricular Block with Acetylcholine

Experimental A.V. block may be produced by high concentrations of acetylcholine. This has been shown to result from failure of the fibres at the atrial margin of the node to develop an action potential. A possible cause for this is the known capacity of acetylcholine to increase the membrane permeability to potassium. This results in a greatly enhanced potassium efflux which will tend to cancel depolarization due to the inward sodium current.

Decremental Conduction

If a stimulus reaches any part of the conduction system early in diastole, before repolarization is complete, the transmembrane potential will necessarily be lower than after full repolarization has taken place. Conduction, however, can still occur, provided the transmembrane potential has reached two-thirds of the normal resting level, but the amplitude and rate of rise of the ensuing action potential will be reduced. Conduction will in consequence be slowed. This is termed decremental conduction. Under certain conditions decremental conduction results in a progressive reduction in both the amplitude and the rate of rise of the action current as the stimulus passes from fibre to fibre until they become too small to propagate further and the impulse is blocked. When decremental conduction leads to block, it will not be recorded directly on the electrocardiogram but its occurrence may be deduced since it leaves refractory tissue in its wake which may affect the transmission of a subsequent impulse. This is called 'concealed conduction' and will be discussed further in Chapter 2.

Note on Excitation–Contraction Coupling

This brief review of electrophysiology would be incomplete without some reference to recent work on the link between excitation and contraction. The basic chemistry of muscle contraction is now well established. The protein actomyosin is contractile, the energy source being adenosine-triphosphate (A.T.P.). If A.T.P. is added to a protein suspension of actomyosin in a test tube, shortening of the actomyosin occurs, provided that calcium and magnesium ions are present. The calcium must be in ionized form. Skeletal muscle contains 'relaxing factor vesicles' which sequester calcium. It is at present believed that excitation of skeletal muscle releases calcium ions from these vesicles, which then initiate contraction. Relaxation is effected by active transfer of calcium ions back into the vesicles. Although myocardial cells contain these 'relaxing factor vesicles', cardiac contraction appears to be dependent on extracellular calcium ions entering the cell. If calcium is excluded from the perfusing fluid, contractions cease, although electrical activity continues unchanged. Thus, the calcium ion seems the vital link in excitation–contraction coupling. The extracellular concentration of calcium ions is over 1,000 times greater than intracellular concentration, so that a large chemical gradient is present. The resting cell membrane, however, is relatively impermeable to calcium, but permeability has been shown to increase during depolarization, with a rapid influx of calcium ions into the cell.

CHAPTER 2

SOME GENERAL CONCEPTS OF ARRHYTHMIAS

Before proceeding to a description of individual arrhythmias, it will be useful to consider first some broad concepts about the physiological disturbances which underlie them. In health, the activity of the whole heart is controlled by the sinus node. Variations in cardiac output which are required to meet varying metabolic needs are largely achieved by varying the rate of discharge of the node, which is brought about by both nervous and humoral influences. The parasympathetic nerves decelerate, and the sympathetic nerves accelerate, the rate of the heart. Continuous nervous action on heart rate is demonstrated by receptor blocking drugs. The intact heart may be 'medically' denervated by giving both atropine, and a beta receptor blocking drug, intravenously. The heart rate is then independent of nervous tone and the resulting rate is termed the 'intrinsic heart rate', and in health this is always faster than before, indicating that parasympathetic tone is dominant (Jose, 1966). Recent studies using continuous monitoring of the electrocardiogram on a portable tape recorder have shown that the heart rate of a normal sedentary worker may vary between 70 and 132 beats per minute in the course of daily activities.

In some forms of arrhythmia, variations in heart rate are effected by variations of the refractory period of the A.V. junction. For example, in digitalized patients with atrial fibrillation, increase in ventricular rate on exertion is achieved by the shortening of the refractory period of the A.V. junction, thus enabling more impulses from the atria to reach the ventricles. A similar effect on ventricular rate can be achieved by atropine.

Virtually all disorders of rhythm result either from disturbances of impulse formation in the heart, or from disturbances of conduction or from both.

Disturbances of Impulse Formation

Ectopic Beats and Ectopic Rhythms

In many forms of arrhythmia, the whole heart, or part of the heart, is activated for one or more beats by a pacemaker other than the sinus node. These are called ectopic beats and ectopic rhythms, to indicate that the excitation wave originated from an abnormal site, and they fall into two main groups. First, there are escape beats and escape rhythms and, secondly, there are extrasystoles and ectopic tachycardias. An escape beat occurs when, for any reason, there is a pause in the dominant rhythm, and it is therefore late in occurrence, terminating a pause. This may only be for a single beat; on the other hand, if the sinus node fails for longer periods, an escape rhythm occurs, and its rate is characteristically slow. Escape beats and escape rhythms originate in the subsidiary pacemakers of the heart. They may be regarded as 'passive' phenomena. If the sinus impulse is sufficiently late, the delay permits an impulse forming in a subsidiary pacemaker to reach maturity and fire off a propagated impulse. The A.V. junction is the commonest site of origin of escape beats and rhythms, since its inherent rate of discharge is faster than that of lower pacemakers. Extrasystoles and ectopic tachycardias, on the other hand, are 'active' phenomena. The mechanism of origin of extrasystoles will be discussed in greater detail in Chapter 6. Ectopic tachycardias, which are generally regarded as a continuous succession of extrasystoles, originate in pacemaking cells in some part of the specialized tissues of the heart which have, for some reason, acquired a fast rate of discharge. In order to maintain control of the heart, this rate must clearly be faster than the sinus rate. Such abnormal pacemakers are referred to as 'ectopic foci', and the excitation waves arising from them are referred to as 'ectopic stimuli'. It is probable that ectopic foci only develop in the specialized tissues. There are islands of such tissue in the atria (in the internodal tracts) which may develop fast pacemaking activity resulting in atrial tachycardias. Similarly, fast pacemaking activity may develop in the A.V. junction or any part of the A.V. conduction system. When the ectopic focus is situated above the bifurcation of the bundle of His, the resulting tachycardia is termed A.V. junctional, particularly if inverted P waves are visible. It is sometimes difficult to decide from the electrocardiogram whether the focus is atrial or A.V. junctional, and then the less specific term 'supraventricular tachycardia' is employed. When the focus is below the division of the bundle, the resulting tachycardia is called ventricular, and the QRS complex, like that of ventricular extrasystoles, is characteristically widened. However, as will be seen later, widening of the QRS, although suggestive of a ventricular tachycardia, is not a reliable diagnostic feature.

In the majority of instances the onset of an ectopic tachycardia is abrupt, the rapid rate being present from the outset, and the termination is similarly sudden. In some forms of junctional tachycardia the onset is gradual, the rate increasing slowly, and the termination is likewise gradual. This variety has been termed non-paroxysmal nodal tachycardia (Pick and Dominguez, 1957).

It is rare for normal sinus rhythm to be absolutely regular; particularly in the young and in elderly subjects there is a phasic variation with respiration, the rate accelerating with inspiration and slowing down with expiration. Marked sinus arrhythmia, unrelated to respiration, is not infrequent. Even when the sinus rate appears to be perfectly regular, careful measurement frequently reveals variation in the length of individual cycles. This is presumably because autonomic nervous tone is not absolutely constant. On the other hand, ectopic pacemakers tend to be absolutely regular whether they are passive escape rhythms or ectopic tachycardias. This statement needs some qualification, for escape rhythms often show some initial acceleration before settling to a steady rate, and ventricular tachycardias frequently show some irregularity of cycle length. Atrial and A.V. junctional tachycardias, on the other hand, are commonly absolutely regular, even over periods of days or even weeks. Supraventricular tachycardias can be influenced by the parasympathetic, for increased vagal tone, elicited by carotid sinus stimulation, eyeball pressure or abrupt raising of the blood pressure with pressor drugs may terminate the arrhythmia. When such

21

techniques are successful, the tachycardia usually terminates abruptly without preliminary slowing down. Ventricular tachycardias cannot be influenced in this way.

Re-entrant Tachycardias

On the other hand, much evidence has recently been put forward that many paroxysmal supraventricular tachycardias are due to a re-entry mechanism. In the Wolff–Parkinson–White syndrome (*see* Chapter 11) in which a characteristic clinical feature is recurrent attacks of supraventricular tachycardia there is good evidence that these are due to a 're-entry' mechanism. In this condition, two pathways are known to connect the atria and ventricles: the normal pathway through the A.V. node and bundle of His and a separate accessory pathway, most often a bundle of Kent, which is a muscular bridge which may connect the atria and ventricles in the right or left atrioventricular groove. There is good evidence that the supraventricular tachycardias in this condition are due to a disturbance of conduction rather than a rapid impulse formation in an ectopic focus; the impulse having travelled down the normal pathway may find the accessory pathway in a non-refractory state and then return to the atria. From here it may then again travel down the normal pathway and in this way set up a circus movement known as a reciprocating tachycardia. As long ago as 1923, Iliescu and Sebastiani suggested that a similar mechanism might operate in paroxysmal tachycardia in patients without the Wolff–Parkinson–White syndrome. This view at first gained little credence since only one pathway was known to connect the atria and ventricles in normal subjects. However, in 1956, Moe and his colleagues produced experimental evidence in animals for the presence of a dual pathway in the A.V. junction. They showed that the A.V. junction is split longitudinally in its upper part, the pathways uniting lower down to form a final common pathway. In order to become manifest these pathways must clearly have different physiological properties and it is simplest to envisage them as having different refractory periods. If then an atrial extrasystole should occur it might well find one pathway absolutely refractory and the other still in the relative refractory state. The impulse having then been slowly conducted along the relative refractory pathway may reach the final common pathway at a time when the second pathway has recovered excitability. The excitation wave would then divide into two fronts, one travelling on to the ventricle down the final common pathway and the other returning to the atria. Such an event occurring once is termed an atrial echo. Alternatively a circus movement might be set up, known as a reciprocating tachycardia, which would be initiated by an atrial extrasystole with a prolonged P–R interval. This mechanism will be further discussed on page 109. A similar mechanism has also recently been shown to operate in at least some ventricular tachycardias (Wellens and colleagues, 1972) (*see* page 138).

Although in most instances an ectopic focus gains control of the whole or part of the heart in virtue of its rapid rate, there is an important group of arrhythmias in which pacemakers with a slower manifest rate than the sinus node may continue to discharge independently and their impulses invade the surrounding myocardium, when they discharge outside its refractory period. This situation is termed parasystole (*see* page 101). In order to explain how an ectopic pacemaker with a relatively slow manifest rate can continue to maintain its own rhythm, it is necessary to postulate that it is 'protected' from discharge by the faster impulses of the dominant rhythm by what is termed 'entrance block'. The nature of entrance block is not yet fully understood, but it is almost certainly a physiological rather than an anatomical barrier. Similarly, ectopic foci can also develop exit block, so that, although they continue to discharge independently, their impulses do not always invade the surrounding myocardium, even when it is outside its refractory period. Although the evidence for the occurrence of entrance block and exit block around an ectopic focus is mainly indirect, it is wholly convincing and will be considered in the appropriate chapters.

A final characteristic common to all pacemakers, both sinus and ectopic, deserves mention here. When any pacemaker is depolarized (or discharged) by an excitation wave which has originated from another focus, its rhythmicity is quite commonly transiently depressed. In consequence, the next impulse to arise from that focus may be unexpectedly delayed. This is why the 'escape interval' before an escape rhythm begins may be longer than the subsequent cycle length of the rhythm. Numerous examples of this temporary depression of pacemakers following discharge will be encountered in later chapters.

Disturbances of Impulse Conduction

It should be emphasized that disturbances of impulse conduction may be entirely physiological. For example, in rapid atrial tachycardias, with atrial rates in excess of 200 per minute, the refractory period of the A.V. junction rarely shortens sufficiently to permit 1:1 A.V. conduction. Quite often, alternate atrial impulses will encounter normally refractory tissues in the

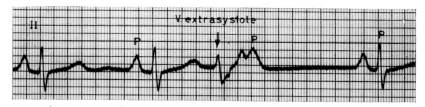

Figure 2.1—The third beat of the record is a ventricular extrasystole. A blocked sinus P wave is clearly seen deforming the T wave of the extrasystole (time markings $\frac{1}{10}$ second)

conducting system, so that they are blocked, and A.V. response will be in the ratio of 2:1. Similarly, following a ventricular extrasystole (which may, of course, occur in an otherwise normal heart), the next sinus impulse, although activating the atria, may be blocked in the A.V. junction. This is simply because the sinus impulse has encountered tissue which has been rendered refractory by the ectopic ventricular impulse. *Figure 2.1* shows a typical example. It is obvious that when two pacemakers in different parts of the heart discharge more or less simultaneously, and their excitation waves travel towards each other, the impulses are likely to meet somewhere in the conduction system and undergo mutual extinction. In the example shown in *Figure 2.1*, the sinus impulse fails to reach the ventricles and the ectopic ventricular impulse fails to reach the atria. When an impulse is blocked because it has encountered tissue which is in a normal refractory phase, the phenomenon has often been termed 'interference' in recent American literature. The use of the term 'interference' in this connotation is unfortunate, for it had previously been used in a quite different sense in arrhythmias. Much acrimonious discussion has centred round the use of the term 'inter-

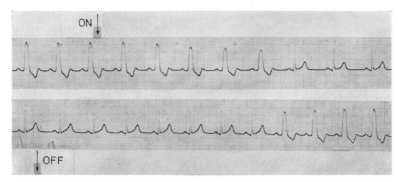

Figure 2.2—Left bundle branch block disappears when rate is slowed by carotid sinus massage

ference', and it would probably be in the best interests of accurate terminology not to use it at all. As a possible alternative 'physiological block' would perhaps be more acceptable. In 'pathological block' an impulse is either stopped or is conducted with delay, in tissues which should normally have been in the non-refractory phase. Pathological block may be due to an anatomical lesion interrupting some part of the conduction pathways. At other times it is a manifestation of disturbed function with prolongation of

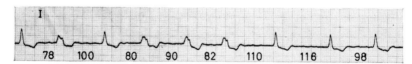

Figure 2.3—The record shows atrial fibrillation. The second, fourth, fifth and sixth beats show the pattern of left bundle branch block. In each case the preceding diastolic pause measures 0·9 second or less. With longer diastolic pauses, intraventricular conduction is normal

the absolute or relatively refractory phase of the region of the conduction pathway involved. For example, it is well known that left bundle branch block will sometimes transiently disappear when the heart rate is slowed by some manoeuvre, like carotid sinus stimulation (*Figure 2.2*). This implies that the refractory period of the left bundle is prolonged and that increasing the duration of diastole allows it to recover. *Figure 2.3* shows an example of left bundle branch block in a patient with atrial fibrillation. Following the longer diastolic pauses, the QRS complexes show normal intraventricular conduction.

The most familiar site for disturbances of conduction is the A.V. junction. It is customary and convenient to classify impaired A.V. conduction into three grades: first-degree block, second-degree or partial block, and complete A.V. block. In first-degree block, conduction of each impulse occurs but conduction time is prolonged. In some circumstances this may be physiological; when pathological, it implies prolongation of the relative refractory period, and in A.V. block it is recognized in the electrocardiogram by prolongation of the P–R interval.

In second-degree or partial A.V. block, one or more of a succession of impulses fail to pass the area of depressed conduction. The severity of second-degree block is generally expressed as the ratio of the number of impulses arriving at the A.V. junction to the number of impulses conducted. For example, one speaks of 5:4 A.V. block, when every fifth atrial impulse fails to yield a ventricular response, or of 2:1 A.V. block, when only alternate impulses arriving at the A.V. junction are conducted to the ventricles. In higher degrees of partial block only one in three or one in four impulses may be conducted, giving conduction ratios of 3:1 or 4:1. In a given case, the conduction ratio may vary with rate and this will be discussed more fully in the chapter on A.V. block. A special variety of second-degree heart block is the Wenckebach phenomenon which will be discussed in detail below.

In complete heart block no impulses are able to pass the area of depressed conduction. Thus, in complete A.V. block, no atrial impulses are transmitted to the ventricles, and a continued circulation is then dependent on the latter being activated by a subsidiary pacemaker. Since the rate of subsidiary pacemakers is slow, complete A.V. block is ordinarily characterized in the electrocardiogram by an atrial rate which is faster than the ventricular rate, and the P waves show a constantly varying time relationship to the QRS complexes.

Wenckebach Type of Partial Heart Block

In 1899 Wenckebach described a form of irregularity of the pulse characterized by progressive lengthening of the A.V. conduction time of successive beats until an atrial impulse was blocked. Following the ensuing pause, the same cycle is again repeated. *Figure 2.4* is a line drawing of the electrocardio-

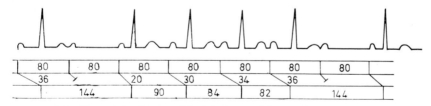

Figure 2.4—Time relationships in a Wenckebach type of A.V. conduction anomaly (see text)

gram in Wenckebach's type of partial A.V. block. The group of beats up to and including the blocked impulse is commonly referred to as a Wenckebach period. Before analysing the Wenckebach type of conduction anomaly further, it is convenient here to explain a useful device commonly used in electrocardiography to demonstrate the mechanism of arrhythmias. This device consists in putting a key below the record to show the origin, path of conduction and conduction times of the impulses responsible for the deflections of the electrocardiogram. These are sometimes referred to as Laddergrams. A conventional key of this type is shown below the line drawing of a Wenckebach period in *Figure 2.4*. The 'key' consists of four horizontal lines. The three spaces between the lines represent, from the top downwards, the atria, the A.V. junction and the ventricles. Vertical lines drawn in the upper and lower spaces indicate the onset of atrial and ventricular activation, respectively. The sloping lines in the middle space represent the passage of an impulse through the A.V. junction. Lines terminating in a bar indicate that the impulse encountered absolutely refractory tissue and became blocked at that point. The figures show the time intervals expressed in hundredths of a second. In clinical arrhythmology it is customary to use a hundredth of a second as the most convenient unit of time.

Experimental electrophysiologists usually work with faster paper speeds than are employed in clinical tracings and this enables them to use a shorter

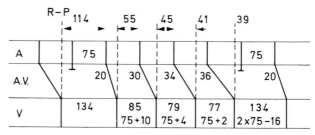

Figure 2.5—Idealized diagram of a Wenckebach type of A.V. conduction disturbance (see text)

time interval with accuracy and they express their findings in milliseconds. The millisecond unit is now often used in clinical work, particularly in recordings made directly from the bundle of His (*see* page 34).

The key below the record in *Figure 2.4* illustrates a number of important features of Wenckebach periods. The A.V. conduction ratio is 5 : 4. It will be seen that although the P–R intervals of successive conducted beats show progressive lengthening, each increment in the P–R interval becomes smaller. A curious result of this is that the ventricular rate accelerates during a Wenckebach period up to the pause. This is evident in the key which shows that the ventricular cycle lengths become progressively shorter up to the blocked beat. It is important to appreciate this, for it enables a Wenckebach type of conduction anomaly to be recognized elsewhere in the heart. such as in sino-atrial block, where conduction times cannot be measured directly on the record. In *Figure 2.4* the electrocardiogram has been drawn with an absolutely regular sinus cycle length of 0·8 second (rate 75 per minute).

Figure 2.5 shows an idealized diagram of a Wenckebach period in A.V. block to demonstrate its structure. (This figure demonstrates another application of the conventional 'key'; it can be used to show the mechanism of an arrhythmia without illustrating the electrocardiogram itself.) In this diagram a completely regular sinus rate is again assumed, this time with a cycle length of 0·75 second. The diagram illustrates the mechanism of a

Wenckebach period and demonstrates the 'rules' which enable this type of conduction anomaly to be recognized wherever it may occur in the heart. These 'rules' were first enunciated by Winton (1948) for diagnosing Wenckebach conduction in sino-atrial block. They are (1) short ventricular cycle lengths are separated by pauses, (2) successive short cycles show progressive shortening in length, (3) the length of the pause never equals the sum of any two short cycles and (4) the first cycle length following a pause is always longer than the last cycle length preceding it.

It will be seen that each short ventricular cycle length following a pause equals the atrial cycle length plus the increment of the second P–R interval of the cycle over the first. Since successive increments become smaller, successive cycle lengths become shorter. In this case, the first increment in the P–R interval is 10 (hundredths of a second), the second 4, and the third 3. Thus, successive ventricular cycle lengths measure $85(= 75 + 10)$, $79(= 75 + 4)$ and $77(= 75 + 2)$. Following the pause, the first P–R interval is again normal (in this case 20), so the ventricular cycle length of the pause is shortened. When the sinus rhythm is completely regular, the pause following the blocked beat should equal two sinus cycles *minus* the total increments in the P–R interval of the last beat preceding it. In this case, it is $134(= 75 \times 2 - 16)$. Although the electrophysiologist has shown that in the canine heart the sinus impulse arrives at the A.V. junction after approximately half of the P wave of the surface electrocardiogram has been written (page 17), we have no means of knowing when it does so in human records. In studying A.V. conduction in clinical electrocardiograms, it is useful to have some measure of the time interval available for the junction to recover from the passage of an impulse before the next one arrives. Since this cannot be measured directly, it is customary to take the interval from the commencement of the QRS to the commencement of the next P wave as an approximate measure of the time available for recovery. This is termed the R–P interval. In *Figure 2.5* the R–P intervals are shown in the upper part of the diagram. In records where the P–R interval varies, it will normally be found to have an inverse relation to the preceding R–P interval. As can be readily seen in the diagram, the longest R–P interval of a period occurs when a P wave is blocked. It is therefore followed by the shortest P–R interval, but since this P is conducted, the next R–P interval is substantially shorter so that the second P–R interval of the period is prolonged. When the sinus rate is regular, prolongation of the P–R interval necessarily shortens the next R–P interval. It thus automatically follows that, in Wenckebach periods, successive sinus impulses reach the A.V. junction earlier and earlier in its relatively refractory phase until finally one arrives in the absolute refractory phase and is blocked. The cycle will then be repeated. Thus, Wenckebach periods are an automatic result of prolongation of the relative refractory period.

In clinical electrocardiograms, Wenckebach periods, particularly those involving the A.V. junction, commonly show minor departures from these 'rules'. For example, the number of conducted beats in each period often shows considerable variation, and the last cycle length before a pause is by no means invariably the shortest. There are two main causes for these variations. First, the sinus cycle is seldom, if ever, completely regular, so that

27

the length of successive R–P intervals is determined to some extent by variations in cycle length. Secondly, the degree of depressed conduction in the A.V. junction is not necessarily constant but may vary with fluctuations in autonomic tone. Nevertheless, it is important to be familiar with these 'idealized' rules, since they may enable Wenckebach conduction to be identified in parts of the heart where conduction times cannot be measured directly on the record.

Exceptions to the Wenckebach Type of A.V. Conduction

On the other hand, Watanabe and Dreifus (1967) have shown in the isolated rabbit heart poisoned by lanatoside C or quinidine with or without lowering of potassium concentration that they were able to produce varying types of second-degree A.V. block. While in the majority of instances the Wenckebach type of A.V. block obeyed the rules described above, on rare occasions the increments in P–R interval may progressively increase so that the ventricular cycle lengths actually become longer before the pause. In consequence at first sight the dropped beat may not be apparent. This paper includes an illustration of this phenomenon occurring in a clinical electrocardiogram.

A second, less common, type of partial A.V. block in which intermittent impulses are blocked, without preliminary lengthening of the P–R intervals, will be described in the chapter on A.V. block (*see* Chapter 14).

Impaired Conduction at other Sites

The same three grades of impaired conduction are applicable at most other sites in the heart. It is not, of course, possible to recognize in the electrocardiogram the occurrence of first-degree sino-atrial block. Second-degree sino-atrial block can be recognized when there is, say, a 2:1 conduction ratio. It is also possible to recognize a Wenckebach type of sino-atrial block from the grouping of the sinus cycles, using the rules given above (*see* Chapter 14).

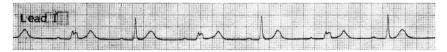

Figure 2.6—2 : 1 left bundle branch block

First-degree block of one or other main branch of the bundle of His is manifested in the electrocardiogram by the so-called incomplete or partial forms of left or right bundle branch block. Second-degree block of one or other main bundle usually takes the form of a 2:1 conduction ratio, so that alternate beats show normal conduction and a bundle branch block pattern (*Figure 2.6*). Recently Rosenbaum and colleagues (1969) have published two convincing examples of Wenckebach periods occurring in the main bundle branches.

Depressed conduction in more peripheral parts of the conduction system may be recognized in the clinical electrocardiogram. First-degree block of uniform distribution occurs in such conditions as quinidine intoxication and is manifested in the electrocardiogram by widening of the QRS complexes without other changes in contour. Varying degrees of isolated block confined to the anterior or posterior divisions of the left bundle branch is a fairly common clinical finding which produces characteristic changes in the electrocardiogram. These are known as left anterior and left posterior hemi-block respectively. They can readily be identified in the electrocardiogram. Left anterior hemi-block is far the commoner lesion of the two; isolated left posterior hemi-block is relatively uncommon for the posterior division of the left bundle is a more robust structure than the anterior, with a richer blood supply. The whole subject of the hemi-blocks will be discussed in greater detail in Chapter 14.

It has already been mentioned that ectopic foci may develop both entrance block and exit block. Varying degrees of entrance block have not, so far as we are aware, been described. First-degree exit block from an ectopic focus could not be recognized in the electrocardiogram. Second-degree exit block is relatively common and may be recognized by a varying conduction ratio or by Wenckebach conduction periods. The latter can be diagnosed from the characteristic grouping of ectopic cycle lengths already described.

A knowledge of certain other anomalies of impulse conduction is essential for the understanding of some arrhythmias.

Concealed Conduction

Our knowledge of concealed conduction mainly relates to its occurrence in the A.V. junction. The concept of concealed conduction implies that an impulse can penetrate for varying distances into the A.V. junction and then

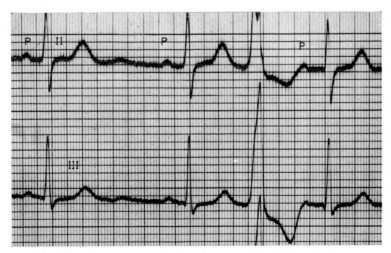

Figure 2.7—Interpolated ventricular extrasystole with concealed conduction. This is manifested by prolongation of the P–R interval of the first sinus beat following the extrasystole (time markings $\frac{1}{10}$ second)

become blocked before it has completely traversed it. In doing so, it leaves in its wake a path of refractory tissue which will require time to recover. Such an event will not, of course, be recorded directly by the clinical electrocardiogram, but its occurrence may be deduced from its effect on a subsequent impulse, and it is for this reason that it is called 'concealed'. The phenomenon of concealed conduction was first deduced by elegant analyses of clinical electrocardiograms. Incontrovertible evidence of its occurrence now rests on a firm experimental basis. *Figure 2.7* shows a simple example of concealed conduction from a clinical record of an interpolated ventricular extrasystole. The P–R interval of the first sinus beat following the extrasystole is prolonged. From this it may be deduced that the ventricular ectopic impulse penetrated the A.V. junction in a retrograde direction, but became blocked, since it did not activate the atria. However, it rendered the lower part of the A.V. junction refractory and in consequence the conduction time of the next sinus impulse was prolonged.

In general, concealed conduction is often responsible for unexplained delay or block of a subsequent impulse. It may also affect impulse formation. Sometimes in A.V. dissociation, when the atria are controlled by the sinus node and the ventricles by the A.V. junction concealed conduction of a sinus impulse may penetrate into the A.V. junction pacemaker, before becoming blocked, and depolarize it. The timing of the next junctional impulse will then be unexpectedly delayed.

Supernormal Phase of Conduction

From time to time, clinical records are encountered in which an impulse has been unexpectedly conducted or has been conducted with less delay than would have been anticipated from the predicted state of recovery of the tissues involved following the preceding impulse. Although relatively uncommon, such records have led to the concept of a supernormal phase of recovery during the cardiac cycle, which usually occurs during the critical transition between the absolute and relative refractory phases. In the experimental animal, both a supernormal phase of excitability and a supernormal phase of conductivity have been demonstrated. There is no evidence that a supernormal phase of conductivity occurs in the normal human heart, but it undoubtedly occurs occasionally when there is a region of depressed conductivity. It may, for example, result in paradoxical shortening of a P–R interval during the course of a Wenckebach period or in an alternation in length of the P–R interval. In the past, it was thought that a supernormal phase of recovery was a rare occurrence. Pick, Langendorf and Katz in a comprehensive review of the subject in 1961 were only able to find 48 cases previously reported in the literature and they added 18 further cases of their own. However, Moe, Childers and Merideth (1968) in a critical review of the supernormal phase of conduction have pointed out that alternative explanations for the apparent supernormality can often be given. Yet cases have been described in the literature which would appear to admit of no alternative explanation except for a supernormal phase of conduction, and a convincing example was recently described by one of the authors of this volume (Williams, 1973).

Unidirectional Block

The A.V. junction is normally capable of conducting a stimulus in either direction. In junctional escape rhythm or junctional tachycardia, therefore, the atria are usually activated from below by the junctional impulse. Some-times, however, unidirectional block may develop and the A.V. junction is then only capable of conducting impulses in one direction. Usually the block is retrograde so that junctional impulses are prevented from reaching the atria. The combination of retrograde (unidirectional) A.V. block and a junctional tachycardia which is faster than the sinus rate results in A.V. dissociation, with a ventricular rate faster than the atrial rate. Antegrade conduction is usually unimpaired, so that when a sinus impulse reaches the A.V. junction outside its absolute refractory period, it will be conducted to and 'capture' the ventricles. This interesting disturbance of rhythm is relatively common in active rheumatic carditis, recent myocardial infarction and digitalis intoxication. It will be discussed in more detail in Chapter 10.

Rarely, unidirectional block is confined to only a part of the A.V. junction, a longitudinal strip of the junctional tissues remaining capable of conduction in both directions. When this occurs during junctional rhythm, a junctional impulse, which has been retrogradely conducted to the atria, may re-enter the part of the A.V. junction in which unidirectional block is present and be conducted to the ventricles and elicit a second ventricular contraction. This second contraction is called either a 'return extrasystole' or a 'reciprocal beat'. A full account of reciprocal beats is included in the chapter on extrasystoles (Chapter 6).

Aberrant Conduction

Supraventricular impulses, when premature in time, may find one or other of the main bundle branches of His still in the refractory phase from the preceding beat. In consequence, intraventricular conduction of the impulse will be disturbed and the QRS complex will resemble that of bundle branch block. This is called 'aberrant conduction' and the phenomenon is known as aberration. It is commonly seen in supraventricular extrasystoles or tachycardias and is important, for it may lead to a mistaken diagnosis of the site of origin of the aberrant beat. It is generally said that 85 per cent of supraventricular beats with aberrant QRS complexes show the pattern of right bundle branch block. This is because the refractory period of the right bundle is usually slightly longer than that of the left. In a supraventricular tachycardia with aberrant conduction and right bundle branch block, one might have expected that shortening of the refractory period with the rapid rate would soon result in normal intraventricular conduction. This however does not often occur for the impulse travelling down the left bundle and its branches spreads over the septum and enters the blocked right bundle from below to activate that bundle branch in a retrograde direction. The re-fractory periods of the two bundles are thus put out of phase with each other, the right bundle being always refractory when a supraventricular impulse arrives at the division of the bundle of His. Theoretically, a right ventricular extrasystole, if appropriately timed, could prevent this retrograde invasion of the right bundle by the impulse coming down the left bundle and subsequent impulses would have normal intraventricular conduction.

Wellens and Durrer (1968) have reported a corresponding change of left aberrant ventricular conduction in a case of supraventricular tachy-cardia to normal conduction following a ventricular premature beat. The

31

tachycardia continued at its previous rate but with normal intraventricular conduction. Schamroth and Chesler in 1963 proposed that the term 'aberrant conduction' should be limited to rhythms in which all QRS complexes were aberrantly conducted. When aberration involves some QRS complexes but not others, as for example with supraventricular extrasystoles conducted with aberration and mimicking ventricular ectopic beats, they suggest the term 'phasic aberrant ventricular conduction'.

Fusion Beats

It has already been mentioned that ectopic foci may develop entrance block and will then continue to produce rhythmic stimuli which are independent of the dominant rhythm. Sometimes the timing of the discharges of the dominant and ectopic pacemakers will result in two excitation waves invading part of the heart from different routes, simultaneously. The resulting complex in the electrocardiogram will then have a contour intermediate between that which would have been produced by either pacemaker alone. Such complexes are called either fusion beats or combination beats. This phenomenon forms one of the diagnostic criteria for parasystole (page 102). Fusion complexes may be either atrial or ventricular according to which chambers have been invaded simultaneously by two excitation waves.

This brief survey of some of the mechanisms involved in disorders of cardiac rhythm is intended as a general introduction to a complex subject. Most mechanisms will require more detailed review in the appropriate sections of later chapters.

Classification of Arrhythmias

It is difficult to formulate a satisfactory classification of arrhythmias either for descriptive or indexing purposes. A classification based on aetiology is impractical since apparently identical disorders of rhythm may result from widely varying causes. It has already been pointed out that virtually all arrhythmias result either from disturbances of impulse formation or of impulse conduction, or both. This provides only three categories for a classification based on disturbed physiology, each of which would be inconveniently broad. Subdivision could be conveniently made on anatomical grounds, according to the main site of disordered function. For example, it is useful to classify extrasystoles or ectopic tachycardias into atrial, junctional and ventricular, according to the site of origin of the abnormal impulses. At times, however, anatomical subdivision tends to become cumbersome when there are multiple sites of disordered function. No formal, detailed classification of disorders of rhythm will therefore be followed, and the grouping of arrhythmias in the chapters which follow has sometimes been made on a physiological, sometimes on an anatomical and sometimes on an aetiological basis. The individual choice has been governed by convenience of presentation.

Aetiology of Arrhythmias

Little purpose would be served by attempting to give a comprehensive list of all possible causes for disturbance of cardiac rhythm at this stage. In the following chapters the aetiology of the individual arrhythmias described will be discussed in some detail. In the past it was commonly taught that the three main causes of arrhythmias were acute myocardial infarction, active rheumatic carditis, and digitalis intoxication. With the rapid advances in medicine and surgery this list must now be considerably extended. Many modern drugs carry potential arrhythmogenic hazards; for example, some of the newer anaesthetic agents like cyclopropane or halothane may be arrhythmogenic and psychotropic drugs, particularly the tricyclic anti-depressants, have now been shown to be responsible for sudden deaths apparently from arrhythmias when patients on these drugs are given a general anaesthetic. In recent years the cardiac surgeon has assumed an important role in the genesis of arrhythmias occurring either during surgery or in the immediate post-operative phase. There are of course many other causes, such as endocrine disorders and electrolyte disturbances. In some common arrhythmias, as, for example, paroxysmal tachycardia occurring in otherwise healthy hearts, no aetiological cause may be found and in the present state of our knowledge they must be termed 'idiopathic'.

CHAPTER 3

HIS BUNDLE ELECTROGRAPHY

RECORDING EQUIPMENT AND TECHNIQUE

The potential clinical application of intracardiac recording techniques was considerably enhanced when in 1958 Alanis, Gonzalez and Lopez were able to demonstrate activity within the bundle of His by recording from needle electrodes positioned along the A.V. groove in the isolated perfused dog heart. It was clearly necessary to determine that the recorded potential did not represent part of the adjacent atrial or ventricular activity and this was achieved by a variety of experiments. Crushing the sino-atrial node abolished atrial depolarization but ventricular activity continued and was always preceded by the His deflection. Similarly, inducing complete heart block below the level of the recording dissociated this deflection from the QRS, whilst it still retained its constant relationship to the P wave. Increasing the rate of atrial pacing and slowing it by vagal stimulation and the administration of acetylcholine consistently modified the P–H interval, whereas the H–V interval remained remarkably stable. This work was soon followed by open and closed heart investigation in animals, and culminated in 1969 with the report from Scherlag and colleagues of its safe and reliable application for human investigation. In 29 of the 30 patients reported, His bundle activity was successfully recorded from an electrode catheter which had been inserted into the femoral vein using the Seldinger technique and advanced to the right ventricle close to the tricuspid valve at the base of the atrial septum. Since this time His bundle electrography has become established as a valuable diagnostic aid and is increasingly used in many cardiac investigative centres. This technique now permits electrocardiographic analysis to be based on more definitive evidence and has reduced the number of possible interpretations of complex arrhythmias for which direct proof was previously lacking.

When combined with programmed cardiac stimulation, His bundle electrography has considerably advanced our knowledge of disorders of rhythm and conduction, but in view of the nature of the equipment required, it is probable that such advanced methods of investigations will be confined to specialized centres where they will be undertaken by those with specific interest and training in basic electrophysiological principles.

Recording Equipment

Most conventional ECG machines in use on the hospital wards are unsuitable for recording His bundle electrograms due to their frequency characteristics. The frequency of the bundle of His potential is of the order of 90–200 Hz and is therefore much higher than those recorded on the standard 12-lead electrocardiogram. These machines are limited by the mechanical inertia of the writing system. Ink jet and mirror galvanometer recorders do not have this limitation and are therefore suitable.

For the purpose of the research described here the apparatus used in the laboratory was designed and built at a low cost to provide specified requirements for electrophysiological analysis, and to incorporate a 12-channel mirror galvanometer already in use in the department. The basic principles do not significantly differ from those used in commercially produced equipment. The bundle of His signal is delivered through an isolating amplifier for pre-amplification. Further amplification and filtering permit the visual dynamic display of the signal. Driving amplifiers control the input to the mirror galvanometers and a permanent photographic record at variable speed is obtained on Linagraph 1930 paper (Kodak) which can be developed in the x-ray department. Output to a storage oscilloscope allows immediate analysis when required during the investigation.

Filtering is essential to provide records suitable for reliable analysis. In this laboratory, 40–800 Hz has been selected to obtain maximum information with minimum distortion due to low frequency signals. *Figure 3.1* illustrates recordings with and without these filtering characteristics. At the same gain setting (*Figure 3.1a*) the His potential is identical but the excess low frequency produces a record so large as to be impracticable and prohibits accurate interval measurement. At a reduced gain (*Figure 3.1b*) the His potential is almost lost.

The frequency characteristics of this apparatus are compared in *Figure 3.2* with those of a Mingograf 34B and a conventional pen recorder at the limits of its filtering range. It can be seen that with the pen recorder the His signal frequency has such a relationship that only a small percentage of the potential will be recorded, whereas the conventional Mingograf has a satisfactory high frequency scan but with no low frequency filtering. Mingograf recording machines with suitable filtering characteristics are now available and produce excellent records which are available for immediate analysis.

At present the apparatus provides the facilities to record simultaneously two intracavitary electrograms, three surface leads and an event marker. Pacing circuits have been incorporated to provide asynchronous pacing from 30 to 330 per minute, paired pacing and programmed extrastimulus sequences at variable rates.

Technique

The patient should be resting flat in the supine position with the legs separated and the feet slightly externally rotated. This will tend to separate the femoral vein from the artery in those patients in whom it lies close and somewhat posterior to it. The right femoral vein is usually preferred as the electrode within the heart is under more direct control with easier manipulation into the desired position. Local venous disorders in the right leg, such as recent thrombosis, may however make this site unsuitable and a successful investigation may be achieved from the left side. The inguinal region should then be prepared by skin cleansing and towelled in the usual way. The electrode can be introduced into the vein in one of two ways: either by the Seldinger technique using a vessel dilator and sheath, or by puncture with a cannula of sufficient diameter to permit direct entry of the electrode through it. Care should be taken to localize accurately femoral arterial pulsation and

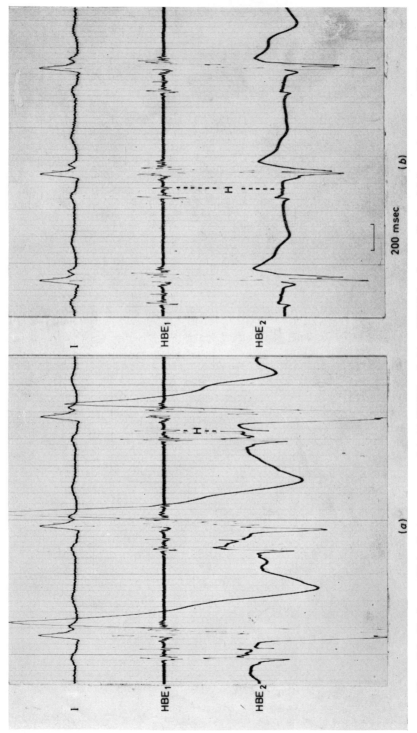

Figure 3.1—Simultaneous His bundle electrograms recorded with (HBE₁) and without (HBE₂) low frequency filtering. (a) Same gain setting on HBE₁ and HBE₂. (b) Reduced gain on HBE₂

to select the site for puncture medial to it. Accidental arterial puncture sometimes occurs even in most experienced hands. If this should occur, external pressure should be applied for sufficient time to ensure that extravasation has been controlled, before venous puncture is attempted again. The

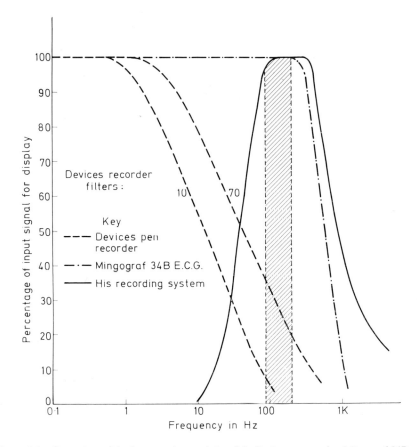

Figure 3.2—Comparison of the frequency characteristics of the Devices pen recorder, Mingograf 34B and the His recording system used in this laboratory. Frequency range of the His potential is indicated by the vertical hatched area

presence of a haematoma makes successful puncture more difficult and increases the complications of the procedure.

The catheter is advanced under x-ray control into the inferior vena cava (I.V.C.). Frequently venous tributaries are entered in the pelvis but these can be invariably avoided by careful rotation and manipulation of the electrode catheter. The passage of the electrode should be quite free and if any resistance is encountered this invariably means that the electrode has entered a venous branch. This may not always be radiologically apparent when screening in one plane if a posterior vessel is entered. If there is any doubt, the electrode should be withdrawn slightly and another attempt

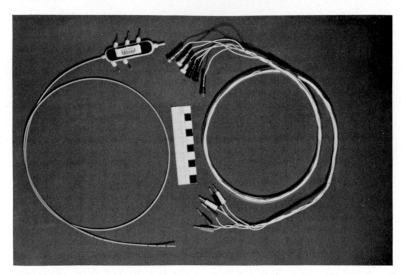

Figure 3.3—Multipolar electrode. Designed to individual specification by Vygon (Kimal Scientific Products Ltd., Hillingdon, Middx.)

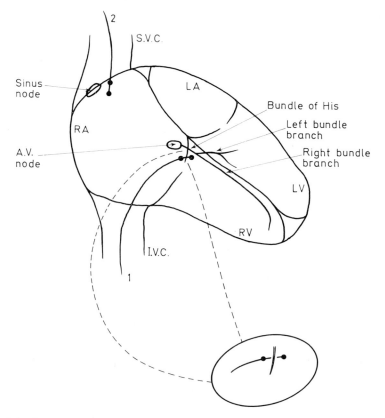

Figure 3.4—Diagram to illustrate position of electrode to record His bundle electrogram (1). Note proximity to right bundle branch. Electrode 2 used for atrial pacing and recording high right atrial electrogram

made. This annoying complication is more common in elderly patients, presumably due to vascular tortuosity and it is often helpful to withdraw the electrode and inject a small quantity of contrast medium to identify the venous anatomy and select the correct route. In the majority, however, the electrode can be easily advanced into the right atrium.

If the electrode has been precurved, rotation of the tip towards the midline and advancing the electrode often results in immediate entry into the right ventricle. This may be associated with a few ventricular extrasystoles which are a useful guide to its position. This will be confirmed by connecting the electrode to the visual display system when the ventricular electrogram will be seen to dominate the tracing. If the electrode remains in the atrium, the intracavitary atrial deflection will be large and the QRS small. If the ventricle is not easily entered in this way, manipulation within the atrium will be necessary to accentuate the loop, and catheter rotation usually enables it to pass through the tricuspid valve. Provided care is taken, it is of little importance where the electrode tip is impinged when making the loop, but, if possible, the right atrial appendage should be avoided as perforation may occur at this point. The free right atrial wall or the atrial septum are safer and to be preferred. Occasionally an intra-atrial communication may be passed and the left atrium entered; this is of value in some electrophysiological studies, but may be confusing if it is not expected or appreciated. When the ventricle is entered by the loop technique, the tip of the electrode usually rests deeper into the apex of the ventricle and points downwards. It is then necessary to withdraw the electrode slowly under ECG control to a position in which His activity is seen to separate the P waves and QRS complexes. The most satisfactory records are obtained by rotating the electrode so that it is directed laterally upwards towards the infundibular region and observing the slow withdrawal. When the best recording position has been found, it may be necessary to maintain some torque on it from the groin to achieve a stable position; this minimizes the variation in the signal due to catheter movement. Occasionally the electrode has to be withdrawn so far from the ventricle to achieve a good His signal that the position is not stable and it may flick back into the atrium. Under these circumstances, a multipolar electrode (*Figure 3.3*) is invaluable as it may be advanced well into the ventricular cavity and the appropriate bipole along its length selected for recording. Although electrode position is critical to obtain good records (*Figure 3.4*), it is wise to spend some time making minor adjustments to avoid ventricular extrasystoles and this can usually be achieved without loss of the His signal. Under certain circumstances extrasystoles can be informative but they may interfere with programmed pacing sequences and cause difficulty in interpretation. With practice in uncomplicated cases, a satisfactory position can be achieved within a few minutes of entry into the femoral vein.

Bundle of His Electrogram

The P–R interval recorded from a surface lead represents the time taken for the stimulating impulse to traverse the atrium, the A.V. node and the intraventricular pathways before the ventricular myocardium is depolarized from the Purkinje network. It is impossible to subdivide this interval from the surface electrocardiogram. Identification of the bundle of His signal therefore enables the supraventricular and ventricular contribution to the total transmission time to be established.

A typical His bundle electrogram (HBE) is shown in *Figure 3.5*. There is simultaneous display of leads I, II and III and a recording from within the right atrium close to the S.A. node. The P wave is clearly seen in the three standard leads. Atrial depolarization recorded from the high right atrial position (HRA) occurs at the onset of the P wave. The first deflection of the His bundle electrogram (A) represents atrial depolarization occurring around the region of the A.V. node. This is followed by the bundle of His deflection (H) which falls within the P–R interval of the standard limb lead, and finally the deflection (V) representing local ventricular depolarization.

The P–R interval can therefore be accurately broken down into three separate components:

(1) Intra-atrial conduction time—this is measured from the onset of the P wave to the onset of the A deflection in the His bundle electrogram. Difficulty is sometimes encountered in identifying the onset of the P waves when they are of low amplitude and this difficulty is exaggerated at fast recording speeds. Under these circumstances a more accurate estimate can be made by measuring the interval between atrial activity recorded from the S.A. region and that recorded on the His bundle electrogram. It is important to appreciate that this interval only represents conduction time between these two points and is not a measure of the total atrial activation time.

(2) A.V. nodal conduction time—this is measured from the onset of the A deflection to the onset of the H deflection. In effect, this is not an exact index of A.V. nodal transmission time as it also includes time taken for the impulse to be conducted from the low atrial recording site into the A.V. node and from the node to the bundle of His.

(3) Intraventricular conduction time—this is measured from the onset of the H deflection to the earliest evidence of ventricular depolarization, whether it be seen on the electrogram or in the surface recordings. With normal QRS complexes the earliest onset is usually evident on the His bundle electrogram. However, when intraventricular conduction is abnormal and the pattern of activation altered, the surface recordings may more clearly indicate the onset of depolarization. In the experience of Scherlag and colleagues (1972) the use of more than one surface lead increases the accuracy of this measurement.

Validity of Recording

It is now established that A.V. nodal and right bundle branch activity can also be recorded by this technique and it is therefore important that the origin of the deflection recorded within the P–R interval should be identified. Proof that the deflection represented His bundle activity was not difficult in isolated perfused animal hearts (Alanis, Gonzalez and Lopez, 1958) but less direct means of validation are clearly necessary during investigation in man. The bundle of His deflection is biphasic or triphasic, sharp and rapid, with a duration of 15–20 msec. Provided the P–R interval in the standard electrocardiogram remains constant, the P–His duration should not significantly vary from beat to beat. The potential should also retain its biphasic or

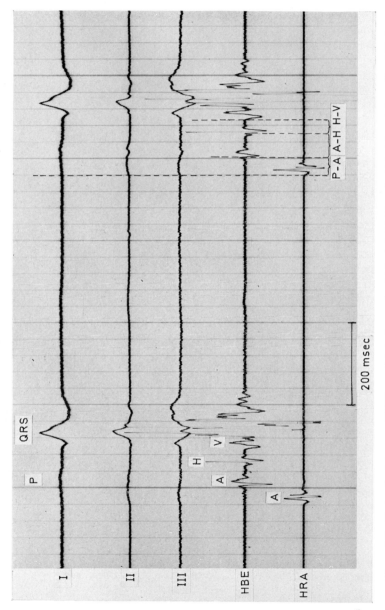

Figure 3.5—His bundle electrogram (HBE) recorded simultaneously with leads I, II, III and a high right atrial recording (HRA)

triphasic configuration, but the degree of positivity or negativity may gradually vary during consecutive cycles.

If the A.V. nodal, bundle of His and right bundle branch potentials are recorded at the same time, either on the same electrogram or simultaneously from different sites, their differentiation is not difficult. The A.V. nodal potential is closer to the P wave, slow and of lower amplitude with a longer duration of up to 50 msec. The right bundle branch potential is closer to the QRS complex and of a similar configuration to that of the bundle of His though with a slightly shorter duration. The usual situation, however, is to record only one signal within the P–R interval and it would appear that the only definite way to distinguish between bundle of His and right bundle branch activity is by pacing at the site of the electrical activity (Narula and colleagues, 1970).

His Bundle Pacing

This is a safe and usually easy procedure. When the electrode has been positioned to record the optimal His bundle signal, it is disconnected from the recording apparatus and the leads are attached to a pacemaker. Stimuli are delivered at a rate slightly faster than that of the sinus rate, preferably in the demand mode, to eliminate the dangers of competitive pacing. If successful His bundle pacing is achieved (*Figure 3.6*), it will be seen that the QRS configuration does not change. This will apply whether the QRS complexes in sinus rhythm are normal or abnormal, and it is the direct result of stimulation of the bundle of His, with physiological delivery to both bundle branches. If any QRS abnormality is present, due to pre-existing disease within the intraventricular conduction system, it will therefore be retained. It can also be seen (*Figure 3.6*) that the interval from the pacing stimulus to the onset of ventricular depolarization is the same as that from the His deflection to ventricular depolarization when measured in the same surface lead during sinus rhythm. If the electrode has been positioned so as to record the right bundle branch potential, pacing stimuli delivered at this site will produce a left bundle branch block pattern. This is due to the altered sequence of ventricular activation with preferential early depolarization of the right ventricle.

Right bundle branch block does not necessarily validate the bundle of His origin of a deflection occurring within the P–R interval. When this occurs as a transient functional event during stimulation sequences with the simultaneous disappearance of the deflection on the His electrogram, it is strong evidence that the deflection represents the right bundle branch potential. However, if the electrode was positioned proximal to the level of block, the potential may still be recorded. It is wise, therefore, not to assume that the deflection must be from the bundle of His because it persists during right bundle branch block, without confirmation by pacing.

Normal Values

Despite the increasing volume of literature involving analysis of His bundle recordings, there have been relatively few reports primarily concerned with the range of normal values for the individual conduction times which together comprise the P–R interval. This undoubtedly reflects the ethical

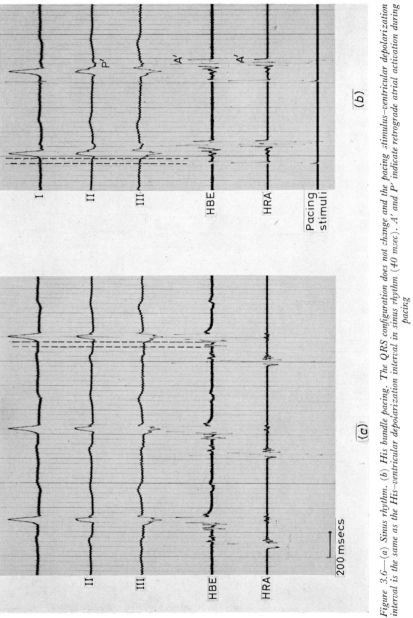

Figure 3.6——(a) *Sinus rhythm.* (b) *His bundle pacing. The QRS configuration does not change and the pacing stimulus–ventricular depolarization interval is the same as the His–ventricular depolarization interval in sinus rhythm (40 msec).* A' *and* P' *indicate retrograde atrial activation during pacing*

43

considerations of an invasive procedure in patients with no overt conduction abnormalities. To investigate a patient in whom some abnormality is suspected, and to include the patient in the control group if none is found, is to some extent preselection. The main error of this is that the range of values which are presumed to be normal are widened by the inclusion of those which in fact represent minor abnormalities. However, the analysis of large enough numbers will minimize this inaccuracy provided the limitations of interpretation in individual borderline cases are appreciated. When invasive cardiac investigation is justified on other grounds, the recording of a His bundle electrogram does not significantly increase the risk nor duration of the investigation. This particularly applies when it is necessary to enter the femoral vein, for example during trans-septal left heart catheterization or when arm veins are unsuitable. However, it must still be appreciated that cardiac disease exists and that it may be difficult to evaluate the effect it has on cardiac conduction. Nevertheless, this is probably the closest acceptable compromise towards establishing the normal range.

Narula and colleagues (1970) published the following mean values ($\pm$SD) from patients with normal P–R intervals:

$$P\text{–}A\ 43\ \pm 14\ msec \quad A\text{–}H\ 88\ \pm 21\ msec \quad H\text{–}V\ 41\ \pm 4\ msec$$

Subsequent reports have not seriously questioned these values. It now appears to be generally accepted that the normal range of intra-atrial conduction time is 20–40 msec, A.V. nodal conduction time 50–120 msec and intra-ventricular conduction time 35–55 msec.

Bundle Branch Block

In patients with right or left bundle branch block, the H–V interval represents conduction time along the remaining branch. When bundle branch block is rate dependent and is produced by incremental atrial pacing, the H–V interval will not change provided the remaining pathway is functionally normal. This indicates that the conduction time is not significantly related to the pattern of ventricular activation. Thus left bundle branch block with a normal H–V interval indicates normal conduction along the right bundle branch, but with a prolonged H–V interval it signifies associated first-degree right bundle branch block. Rosen, Ehsani and Rahimtoola (1972) studied 57 patients with left bundle branch block and defined three groups; those with normal H–V (less than 50 msec), intermediate H–V (50–60 msec) and prolonged H–V (greater than 60 msec). The association of left bundle branch block, normal H–V and arteriosclerotic heart disease suggested isolated ischaemic disease of the left bundle branch, whereas left bundle branch block, prolonged H–V and the absence of arteriosclerotic heart disease was felt to indicate sclerodegenerative bilateral bundle branch disease.

CARDIAC PACING IN ASSOCIATION WITH HIS BUNDLE ELECTROGRAPHY

Recording His bundle activity during resting sinus rhythm provides useful information about conduction at various sites in the heart. The combination of atrial pacing and His electrography enables observations to be made at increasing heart rates. In many respects these can be considered unphysiological as the chronotropic drive is artificial and the intrinsic effect of sympathetic activity upon conduction tissue is minimized or lost. Although the

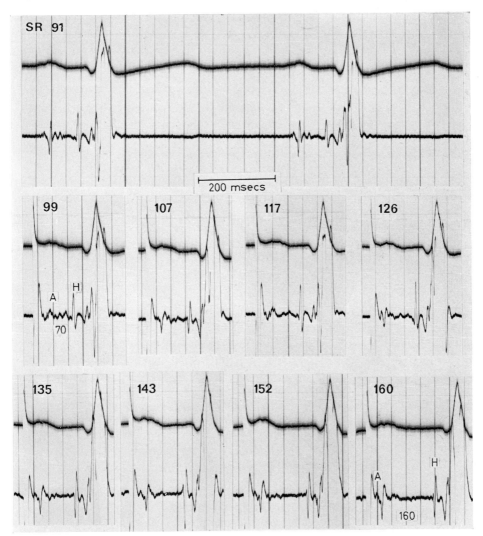

Figure 3.7—Effect of atrial pacing on conduction times. As rate increases from 99 per minute to 160 per minute, the A–H intervals progressively lengthen from 70 msec to 160 msec

results should be applied with caution to the exercise situation, it does provide a method which can give independent evaluation of the effects of heart rate and drugs upon conduction intervals.

The normal response to accelerating the heart rate by atrial pacing is to progressively prolong the P–R interval. It can be seen (*Figure 3.7*) that this is due entirely to an increase in the A–H interval, representing A.V. nodal delay. It appears that intraventricular conduction is not significantly affected in this way. A more reliable method of measuring the refractory periods is to combine His bundle electrography with programmed atrial stimulation. The extra stimulus technique or variations of it are most frequently used. The pacemaker delivers a series of driving stimuli to the atrium at a rate slightly in excess of the basic sinus rate to achieve regular capture. This series is followed by a premature testing stimulus. The degree of prematurity can be adjusted so that it can be delivered at any instant during and after the electrical recovery phase of the atrium. The pacing sequence is then inhibited to prevent further stimulation, thus permitting the effect of the testing stimulus to be observed. The series of driving impulses stabilizes the heart rate and thus eliminates the fluctuations in the refractory periods that occur with sinus arrhythmia. Stimulation after full recovery will result in normal conduction, whereas delivery in the relative refractory period will delay conduction. When the absolute refractory period is entered propagation will fail. The simultaneous recording of a His bundle electrogram permits the identification of the site of delay or block and enables the individual refractory periods to be calculated. Illustrative examples are presented in *Figures 3.8–3.11*. The last pacing stimulus of the driving sequence (S_1) and the premature testing stimulus (S_2) are shown. The atrial, His bundle and ventricular responses to these stimuli are designated A_1, H_1, V_1 and A_2, H_2, V_2 respectively.

Figure 3.8 demonstrates a normal response after full recovery. The conduction times have not altered. *Figure 3.9* illustrates entry into the relative refractory period of the A.V. node with prolongation of the A_2–H_2 interval. H_2–V_2 interval is not changed. The intraventricular conducting system is to some extent protected by the A.V. nodal delay since the depolarizing wave will reach it later than it would have done if A.V. nodal conduction had been normal. Thus it is not directly the S_1–S_2 interval that stresses ventricular conduction but the H_1–H_2 interval resulting from this stimulation. The longest H_1–H_2 interval that fails to produce a ventricular response indicates, therefore, the effective refractory period of the intraventricular conducting system. This is illustrated in *Figure 3.10* where block has been induced distal to the bundle of His. The site of block in such a situation could be either in the peripheral His–Purkinje network or in the refractory ventricular muscle itself. Gallagher and colleagues (1972) have demonstrated by direct ventricular pacing that the muscle is capable of depolarization at this time thus concluding that the impulse was extinguished in the peripheral conducting system and never in fact reached the myocardium.

Block may also be induced within the atrium. As the prematurity of the testing stimulus is increased, so also does the interval from the stimulus to atrial depolarization (S_2–A_2) increase. At S_1–S_2 interval of 360 msec (*Figure 3.11*) S_2–A_2 has increased from 35 msec to 80 msec and at S_1–S_2 of 290 msec (*Figure 3.12*) atrial depolarization fails. Under such circumstances the investigation is limited by the refractory period of the atrium itself. During investigations of this type a separate simultaneous atrial recording can be of considerable value. At short interstimulus intervals atrial depolarization will occur during the inscription of ventricular activity and may be difficult

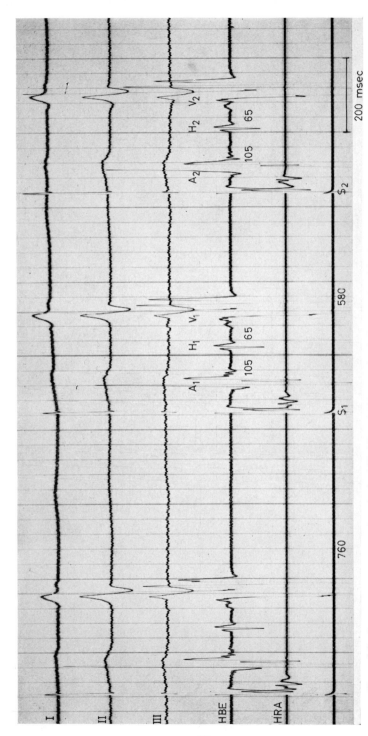

Figure 3.8—Response to premature testing stimulus (S_2) delivered 580 msec after the last stimulus (S_1) of the driving sequence (cycle length 760 msec). No alteration in conduction times indicates full recovery

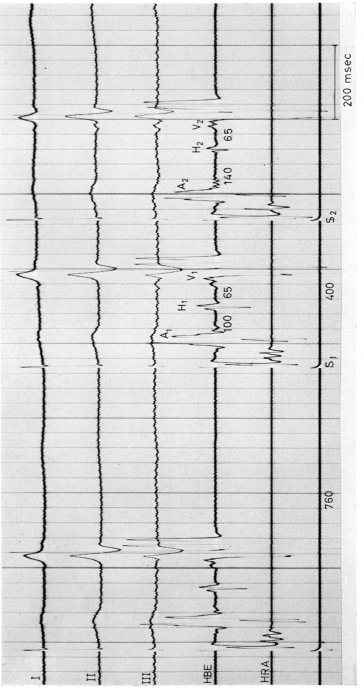

Figure 3.9—Response to premature testing stimulus (S_2) delivered 400 msec after the last stimulus (S_1) of the driving sequence (cycle length 760 msec). A_2–H_2 has increased to 140 msec, indicating entry into the refractory period of the A.V. node

to identify in the surface leads and His electrogram. If block is induced proximal to the bundle of His as evidenced by absence of H_2, it may be at atrial or A.V. nodal level and clear identification of atrial activity is essential

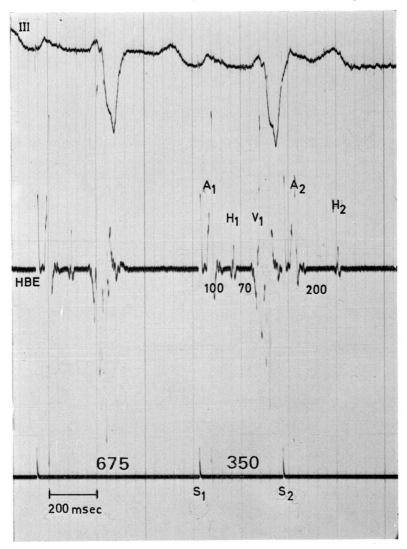

Figure 3.10—Response to premature testing stimulus (S_2) delivered 350 msec after the last stimulus (S_1) of the driving sequence (cycle length 675 msec). A_2–H_2 has increased to 200 msec and the impulse is blocked distal to the bundle of His. H_1–H_2 is 440 msec (see text)

for their differentiation. A separate atrial electrogram permits this distinction to be easily made.

The importance of His bundle pacing has already been discussed. If a right atrial electrogram is recorded simultaneously, retrograde conduction can be identified (*Figure 3.6b*) and retrograde conduction time across the A.V. node

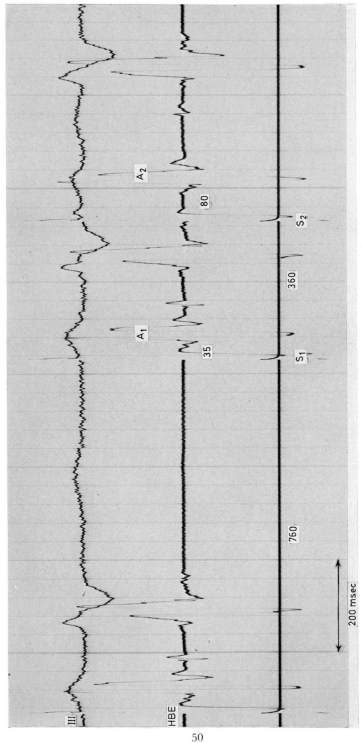

Figure 3.11—Relative refractory period of atrium. Interval from pacing stimulus to onset of atrial depolarization has increased (S_1–A_1 is 35 msec, S_2–A_2 is 80 msec) with S_1–S_2 interval of 360 msec

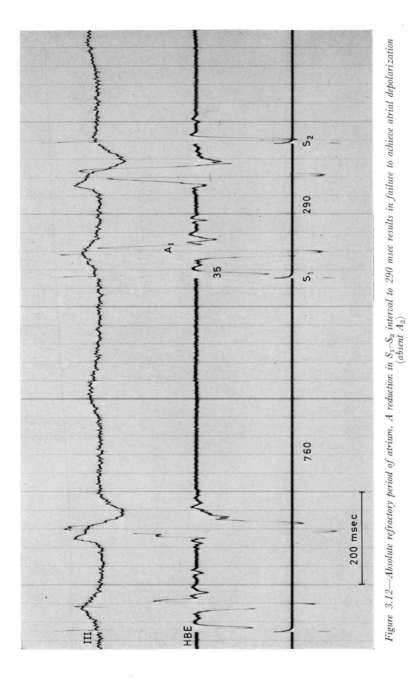

Figure 3.12—Absolute refractory period of atrium. A reduction in S_1–S_2 interval to 290 msec results in failure to achieve atrial depolarization (absent A_2)

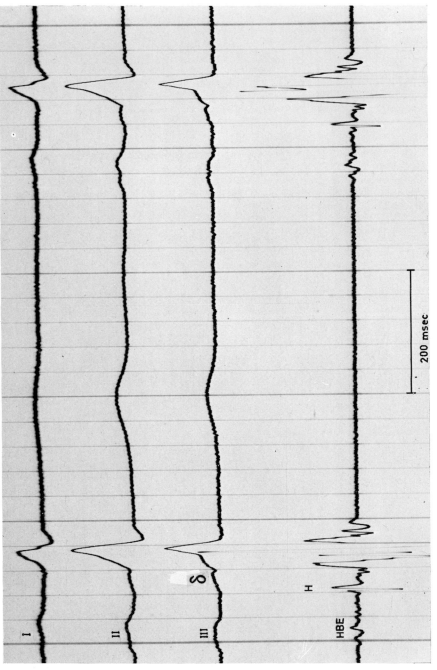

Figure 3.13—Wolff–Parkinson–White syndrome in sinus rhythm. The His deflection occurs almost simultaneously with the delta (δ) wave

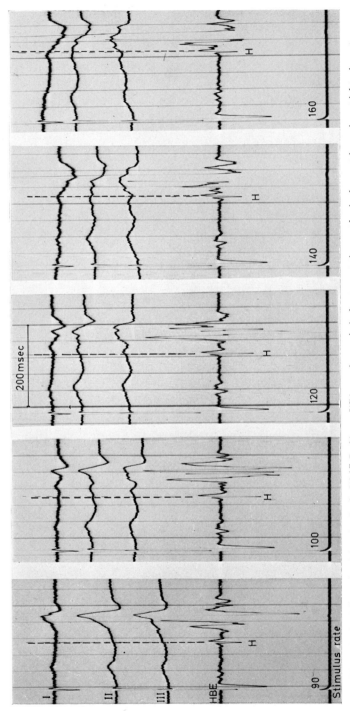

Figure 3.14—Effects of atrial pacing in the Wolff–Parkinson–White syndrome. A single representative complex is shown at increasing atrial pacing rates (90–160 per minute). Note the His deflection is progressively delayed and merges with the QRS complexes at faster rates. Also the QRS morphology alters as the contribution of the anomalous pathway to total ventricular depolarization increases

measured. In many patients with impaired conduction, antegrade and retrograde transmission are not equally affected. The demonstration of the ability of the A.V. node to conduct in a retrograde direction is an essential prerequisite for the diagnosis of some reciprocating arrhythmias.

His bundle electrography combined with atrial pacing has considerably increased our knowledge of the electrophysiology of the Wolff–Parkinson–White syndrome. This will be discussed in detail in Chapter 11. Basically, the stimulating wavefront divides to enter both the anomalous pathway and the His–Purkinje system and the ventricles are therefore activated from two routes. The anomalous pathway does not slow conduction and permits part of the ventricle to be depolarized before those impulses, which have been delayed in the A.V. node, reach the periphery of the His–Purkinje network. Consequently, the interval between the inscription of the His deflection and the earliest outset of ventricular depolarization (H–V) is shortened (*Figure 3.13*). Increasing the heart rate by atrial pacing progressively shortens this interval until the His deflection disappears into the QRS (*Figure 3.14*). Under these circumstances the rate-dependent A.V. nodal delay has slowed conduction to such an extent that ventricular depolarization has occurred via the anomalous pathway before the other impulses have emerged to reach the bundle of His. The degree of pre-excitation varies from patient to patient and at different times in the same individual. The standard electrocardiogram may not therefore be totally reliable and minor degrees may be missed. This characteristic response to atrial pacing provides clear evidence of a dual conducting mechanism and allows a definite diagnosis to be established.

The contribution of His bundle electrography in various disturbances of cardiac rhythm and its clinical application will be considered in the following appropriate chapters.

CHAPTER 4

NORMAL SINUS RHYTHM

Normal sinus rhythm is characterized in the electrocardiogram by a regular succession of P waves of normal contour, each succeeded by a QRST complex. The P–R interval is constant for a given rate and measures from 0·12

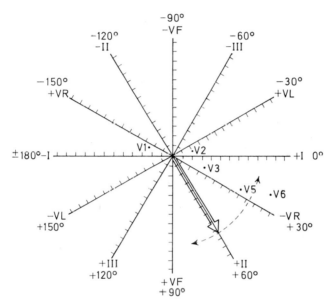

Figure 4.1—Normal range of direction of the mean electrical axis of the P forces in the frontal plane

to 0·2 second. It is rare for sinus rhythm to be completely regular when all P–P cycles are carefully measured. By an entirely arbitrary definition, variations of cycle length up to 0·16 second are accepted as 'regular' sinus rhythm. If the cycle lengths alter by more than 0·16 second, sinus arrhythmia is said to be present.

In normal sinus rhythm the mean electrical axis of the P waves is generally around +60 degrees, with a range of from +15 to +75 degrees. For clinical purposes, the direction of the mean electrical axis of the P forces can be determined with sufficient accuracy by simple inspection of the usual six limb leads using the method described by Grant (1957). *Figure 4.1* shows the hexaxial reference system with the normal range for the mean electrical axis of the P waves. When, as is usual, the P axis is around +60 degrees, the P waves will have a positive contour in all the limb leads, except VR, where it will be negative. Since the direction of the P forces is along the axis of lead II, this lead will show the largest P wave. If the reference system is pictured in relation to the atria, it will be seen that with an axis of +60 degrees the P forces are pointing approximately from the sinus node to the A.V. node. Since the normal P axis may be directed as far 'leftwards' as +15 degrees, sinus P waves may show a negative deflection in lead III.

In many normal subjects, successive QRS complexes often show minor variations in size, corresponding to the different phases of respiration. This is because the anatomical axis of the heart alters with respiration. The main ventricular muscle mass swings in pendulum fashion, so that the mean electrical axis of the QRS complexes may vary by 7–10 degrees during the respiratory cycle. The atria, on the other hand, are relatively fixed so that there is much less respiratory variation in the P axis.

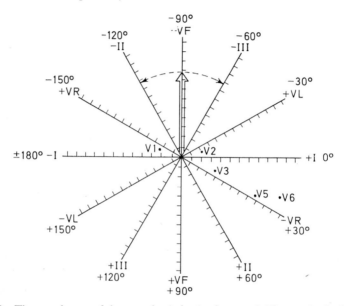

Figure 4.2—The normal range of the mean electrical axis of retrograde P′ waves in the frontal plane

It is clearly important to be able to recognize when the atria have been activated by an ectopic pacemaker. The direction of the P axis is of little help when the ectopic pacemaker is situated close to the sinus node. On the other hand, when the atria have been activated in a retrograde direction as, for example, in A.V. junction rhythm, or from a pacemaker located in the lower atrial septum, the mean electrical axis of the P waves will be in the opposite direction to normal. The mean P axis is then generally around −90 degrees. *Figure 4.2* shows the hexaxial reference system with the usual range of the P axis when the atria are activated in a retrograde direction. It is clear that the P waves will be small or absent in lead I and will be inverted in leads II, III and AVF. Such P waves are termed 'retrograde' and it is conventional to designate them with the symbol P′. The symbol P′ is also used to denote P waves arising from any ectopic site in the atria.

The presence of a normally directed P axis does not necessarily imply that the atria are activated by the sinus node. The P waves generated by an ectopic atrial focus lying close to the sinus node may be normally directed, and there are times when it may be difficult to differentiate between a sinus tachycardia and an ectopic tachycardia of atrial origin. A diagnosis of sinus tachycardia would be favoured by the presence of even slight variations in cycle length. A confident differentiation may only be possible if a previous record of the patient in known sinus rhythm is available, for the P waves of an atrial tachycardia always show minor, but distinct, variations in contour from those of sinus rhythm.

Normal Resting Sinus Rate

The sinus rate of most normal human adults lies between 72 and 80 per minute. The resting rate varies with age, and the following ranges for different ages are given by Katz and Pick (1956):

At birth	110–150
Aged 2 years	85–125
Aged 4 years	75–115
Aged 6 years	65–105
Over 6 years	60–100

Variants of Normal Sinus Rhythm

Sinus Bradycardia

In a resting adult, a heart rate of less than 60 per minute is arbitrarily defined as sinus bradycardia. The rate is rarely slower than 45 per minute. The condition is symptomless and is common in well trained athletes in whom it is sometimes associated with a prolonged P–R interval. The rate promptly increases on exercise, when the P–R interval, if prolonged, becomes normal. It is presumably a manifestation of increased vagal tone. It is important to appreciate that a slow heart rate is necessarily associated with an increased stroke volume and, in consequence, radiological increase in heart size. Subjects with sinus bradycardia often have cardiothoracic ratios of over 50 per cent and may be misdiagnosed as suffering from heart disease. Intravenous atropine promptly increases the heart rate, and this is associated with an immediate reduction in the radiological size of the heart.

Occasionally sinus bradycardia may be a manifestation of some systemic disease, such as jaundice, myxoedema or hypopituitarism, or it may occur in raised intracranial pressure. In some subjects, a transient sinus bradycardia may result from emotional stress and lead to 'fainting'. Episodes of sinus bradycardia, or even sinus standstill, occur in the carotid sinus syndrome, producing symptoms of transient cerebral ischaemia.

A fairly common cause of sinus bradycardia today is the use of beta-adrenergic receptor drugs, particularly propranolol, and, to a lesser extent, practolol.

It is important to differentiate between simple benign sinus bradycardia which is physiological and a pathological disorder of the sinus node itself or the atrial tissue surrounding it. This condition has become increasingly recognized in recent years and has been variously termed the 'sick sinus syndrome', the 'lazy sinus syndrome' or sino-atrial disorder, including the brady-tachycardia syndrome. The whole subject will be discussed in greater detail in Chapter 14.

Sinus Tachycardia

Sinus tachycardia occurs normally in response to exertion (or emotion) and is one of the most important mechanisms for increasing cardiac output. Rates as high as 190 per minute may be reached during violent effort. Although the Q–T interval of the electrocardiogram shortens with rate, diastole becomes so short that the P wave may become buried in the preceding T wave and may be difficult to define.

When the heart rate exceeds 100 per minute at rest, it is arbitrarily defined as a sinus tachycardia. Sinus tachycardia at rest is frequent in many conditions which have in common an increased demand of the tissues for oxygen and therefore an increased cardiac output. Such conditions include fevers and thyrotoxicosis. A persistent resting sinus tachycardia may be due to certain drugs, such as belladonna or its derivatives and sympathomimetic amines (including dextro-amphetamine).

The commonest cause of a persistent sinus tachycardia is an anxiety state. In chronic anxiety states, the rate may be consistently as high as 120 or even 140 per minute and may be associated in the electrocardiogram with S–T segment and T-wave changes not due to heart disease. Sinus tachycardia of nervous origin may be paroxysmal and may superficially mimic a true paroxysmal arrhythmia. Differentiation is usually simple from the history, for the onset of paroxysmal sinus tachycardia is gradual and rarely reaches the rates which occur in true ectopic tachycardias. Since paroxysmal sinus tachycardia is catecholamine induced, it is usually associated with forcible cardiac contractions, so that the patient is acutely aware of his rapidly beating heart.

Sinus Arrhythmias

When sinus cycles in a resting subject vary in length by more than 0·16 second, sinus arrhythmia is said to be present. Three distinct forms of sinus arrhythmia can be identified. The commonest form, most frequently encountered in children and elderly subjects, is respiratory sinus arrhythmia. This results from reflex variations in vagal tone on the sinus node so that the rate accelerates during inspiration and slows during expiration. The transitions in rate are gradual and phasic, 3–4 beats showing progressive shortening in cycle length followed by 2–3 with lengthening cycles. It is, of course, an entirely benign finding with no clinical significance. The diagnosis can readily be established, for the irregularity disappears when the breath is held. It is worth noting, however, that respiratory sinus arrhythmia never occurs in children with atrial septal defects when the left to right shunt is large. When it is present in atrial septal defects, it clearly indicates that the shunt is trivial.

In the other two forms of sinus arrhythmia, changes in sinus rate are unrelated to the respiratory cycle. In one, the contour of the P waves remains constant for all cycle lengths. The intervals between series of short or long cycles tends to be longer than in the respiratory form, the phases lasting 10–15 seconds instead of 2 or 3 seconds. This variety of sinus arrhythmia is commonly induced by digitalis or morphine administration.

The second form of non-respiratory sinus arrhythmia is believed to be due to 'wandering' or 'shifting' of the site of pacemaking in the sinus node itself. There is evidence that the rate of impulse formation varies in different parts of the sinus node. On first principles it would be expected that the region of the sinus node with the highest rate of impulse formation would retain control of the heart. Occasionally, however, regions of the node with a slower inherent rate of discharge may take over control, though the mechanism is

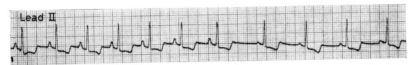

Figure 4.3—Shifting pacemaker in the sinus node. The site of the pacemaker changes abruptly during the record. The shorter cycle lengths have tall P waves with a P–R interval of 0·16 second. The longer cycle lengths show greatly reduced P waves with a P–R interval of 0·14 second

unknown. When a change occurs in the site from which an impulse emerges from the sinus node, there is often a change in the direction of the mean P axis. Arrhythmia due to a wandering of the pacemaker in the sinus node is therefore associated with a mean electrical axis of the P waves, which changes with differing cycle lengths. In practice, this change in the contour of the P wave is most obvious in lead II where larger P waves are associated with short cycles and vice versa. *Figure 4.3* shows an example. This change in P-wave contour is sometimes associated with a change in P–R interval, the shorter cycles having slightly longer P–R intervals, as well as taller P waves.

Sinus Rhythm with Short P–R Interval

It is sometimes asserted that one of the criteria for diagnosing sinus rhythm in the electrocardiogram is that the P–R interval must measure 0·12 second or more. Records are occasionally encountered in which a normally directed P axis, giving positive P waves in leads II and VF, is associated with a P–R interval of less than 0·12 second. It is asserted that the pacemaker in these cases is ectopic and is situated low in the atrial septum close to the coronary sinus, and such records are called 'coronary sinus rhythm'. It is clear that this interpretation must be incorrect. The P waves generated by a focus situated in the lower part of the atria would necessarily have an axis directed superiorly, with negative P waves in leads II, III and AVF. It is probable that most records with a normally directed P axis and a short P–R interval (less than 0·12 second) are examples of the Wolff–Parkinson–White syndrome without obvious QRS widening. This is known as the 'Lown–Ganong–Levine Syndrome' (*see* Chapter 11). The term 'coronary sinus rhythm' should be reserved for records with inverted P waves in leads II, III and VF. The subject is further discussed in the next chapter.

Note on Measurement of Time Intervals

In analysing arrhythmias, accurate measurement of time intervals on the cardiographic record is often of considerable importance. Gross irregularities of rhythm or marked variation in the duration of certain parameters, such as the P–R interval, may be immediately apparent to the unaided eye, and less evident irregularities may be spotted at a glance with practice. The time markings on electrocardiographic paper provide a simple method for making reasonably accurate measurements of time intervals. In this country and in America it is customary to record electrocardiograms at a paper speed of 25 mm per second. Modern direct writing machines use paper which is already ruled by vertical and horizontal lines forming squares. The small squares are 1 mm apart, and every 5 mm both the vertical and horizontal lines are more heavily marked, forming 5 mm squares. At a paper speed of 25 mm per second, the small squares represent 0·04 second and the large squares 0·2 second. It is possible to use the vertical lines to measure time intervals to the nearest ½ mm or 0·02 second. Such measurements are facilitated by the use of dividers or calipers. The type provided with a screw

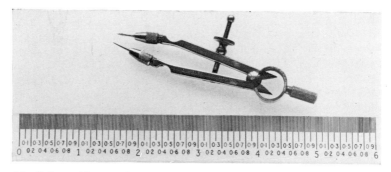

Figure 4.4—Calipers with screw adjustment for measurement of short time intervals and transparent ruler graduated in time intervals for a paper speed of 25 mm per second*

adjustment as illustrated in *Figure 4.4* are very useful for measuring short time intervals. Having adjusted the points to the interval to be measured, the left hand point should be placed on a vertical line marking a large square and the interval is measured by counting the number of small squares between the points. It is possible to make measurements with greater speed and accuracy by using a transparent ruler graduated in time intervals. *Figure 4.4* illustrates a useful ruler of this type. The finer divisions are ½ mm apart and it is calibrated for a paper speed of 25 mm per second, so that the finer divisions represent intervals of 0·02 second. With the aid of a hand lens, it is possible to measure time intervals to the nearest hundredth of a second. It has already been stated that for accurate electrophysiological measurements, fast paper speeds of 100 mm/sec or more should be used and the basic unit of measurement becomes the millisecond rather than a hundredth of a second.

Sources of Fallacy in Measurements

Since the paper used by direct writing machines already has time markings on it, it is clear that their accuracy must depend on the accuracy of the paper drive. In mains operated equipment, the paper is driven by a synchronous motor which is likely to be consistently accurate. This is not of course true of battery operated models and the paper speed should be frequently checked.

* This ruler is obtainable from the British Engraving & Nameplate Co , 196 Old Shoreham Road, Hove 4, Sussex.

This is most readily done by deliberately introducing a.c. interference, for example, by disconnecting the earth electrode lead. At a paper speed of 25 mm per second there should be 10 interference lines in each large square (that is, 0·2 second).

When the base line of the recording is drifting, it is important to orientate the measuring device, whether a ruler or calipers are used, so that it is parallel to a horizontal line on the paper. If this is not done, considerable errors in measurements will occur.

CHAPTER 5

ESCAPE BEATS AND ESCAPE RHYTHMS

It has already been pointed out that when, for any reason, the sinus node fails to produce an impulse, the heart is protected from asystole by the presence of subsidiary pacemakers. An escape beat occurs when a pause in the sinus rhythm equals the escape interval of the fastest subsidiary pacemaker. The Germans have a picturesque term for escape beats; they are called ersatz-systole, that is, a substitute systole. Escape beats may be either A.V. junctional, or ventricular in origin. In the vast majority of instances a pause in sinus rhythm is terminated by a junctional escape beat.

Three electrocardiographic criteria serve to identify an A.V. junctional escape beat occurring in sinus rhythm. First, it is late in occurrence, the

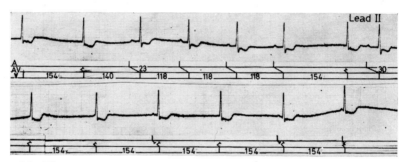

Figure 5.1—The two rows are continuous: they show intermittent S.A. arrest with a junctional escape rhythm. Although in the second row, the third, fifth and sixth beats are preceded by P waves, these are not conducted and all QRS complexes in this row are junctional in origin

interval between the last sinus beat and the escape beat being always longer than the longest sinus cycle. This immediately differentiates an escape beat from an extrasystole which is invariably premature. A second criterion is that the QRS complex is not preceded by a sinus P wave or, if it is, the P–R interval is shorter than normal, indicating that the ventricular complex could not have been conducted. The third criterion is that the QRS complex is normal in duration; it may be aberrant (q.v.), but otherwise it has all the characteristics of a supraventricular beat. The average escape interval of A.V. junctional beats varies from 1·5 to 1·0 seconds, corresponding to rates between 40 and 60 per minute.

A.V. junctional escape beats occur when, for any reason, there is transient sinus slowing or arrest. They are common in sinus bradycardia with sinus arrhythmia, when they may terminate the longer sinus pauses. *Figure 5.1* illustrates junctional escape beats and runs of junctional rhythm occurring as a result of sinus bradycardia with sinus arrhythmia, due to digitalis intoxication. A conventional key below the record illustrates the mechanism of the arrhythmia. All six QRS complexes in the lower strip are junctional in origin, although four of them are preceded by sinus P waves with a short P–R interval, the sinus excitation wave having reached the A.V. junction too late in each case to capture the ventricles before the A.V. junctional pacemaker had discharged.

Retrograde conduction of the impulse from A.V. junctional escape beats may or may not occur. Long records made from the patient whose record is illustrated in *Figure 5.1* never showed retrograde conduction of junctional impulses to the atria.

A.V. junctional escapes may also follow atrial extrasystoles which discharge the sinus node. Premature discharge of the sinus node often temporarily depresses its automaticity, resulting in a prolonged sinus pause. A similar

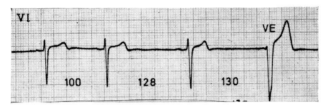

Figure 5.2—Ventricular escape beat terminating a pause in sinus rhythm. The first three beats of the record are sinus in origin. The fourth beat is a ventricular escape beat occurring with an escape interval of 1·3 seconds. This occurred many times throughout a long record and clearly the ventricular escape interval was shorter than the A.V. junctional escape interval

sinus pause may follow ventricular extrasystoles if the ectopic impulse is conducted to the atria and reaches the sinus node before its next normal discharge.

Far less often a sinus pause is terminated by a ventricular escape beat. A ventricular escape beat is recognized by its bizarre QRST complex, the QRS duration being at least 0·12 second. The escape interval is usually appreciably longer than that of a junctional beat and may measure as much as two or three seconds. There are two circumstances in which ventricular escapes may occur in sinus rhythm. Occasionally the inherent rate of an idioventricular pacemaker below the division of the bundle of His may be faster than that of the A.V. junction. Such a pacemaker would necessarily escape before the A.V. junction was ready to discharge (*Figure 5.2* shows an example). A second mechanism leading to ventricular escape in sinus rhythm is the virtually simultaneous discharge of both the sinus and A.V. junctional pacemaker by an ectopic impulse. This may be due to a blocked atrial extrasystole which discharges the sinus node and also reaches and discharges the A.V. junction before becoming blocked. The ensuing pause is now terminated by the escape of an idioventricular pacemaker.

Aberrant Contour of the QRST Complexes of A.V. Junctional Beats

One would have expected that the QRST complexes of A.V. junctional escape beats would be identical with those of sinus origin, differing only by the absence of a preceding P wave with the appropriate P–R interval. While this is commonly the case it is by no means unusual for the QRS complexes (and the T waves) of junctional beats to show distinct differences in contour compared with the sinus beats of the same subject. An example is shown in *Figure 5.3.* The first two beats are sinus in origin; the third QRS complex is a

63

junctional escape beat for although it is preceded by a P wave the P–R interval is too short for it to have been conducted. The QRS complex of this and the subsequent five beats differ obviously in contour from the first two sinus beats of the record. It will be noted that the duration is normal (0·08 second). The difference in the contour is usually much more evident in some

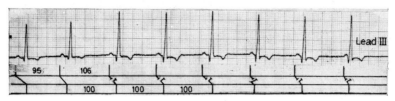

Figure 5.3—A.V. junctional beats with a different QRS contour from sinus beats. A junctional escape rhythm occurs when the sinus rate falls below that of the junctional rate. The first two complexes of the record are sinus in origin. The last six are junctional in origin. The junctional beats have more prominent Q waves and R waves, 23 mm in amplitude compared with 18 mm of the sinus beats

leads than others. Many explanations have been put forward for this phenomenon. The difference in contour represents a change in the order of spread of excitation to different parts of the ventricle.

Pick (1956) has suggested that this aberrant ventricular conduction of A.V. junctional beats may be due to an eccentric location of the junctional pacemaker, the impulses of which reach the ventricles by the 'paraspecific' or 'preferential' pathways of Mahaim instead of by the normal conduction system. The presence of such alternative pathways has been demonstrated in some normal foetal, newborn and young adult hearts by Lev, Widron and Erickson (1951).

Narrow Ventricular Ectopic Beats

Rosenbaum and colleagues in Buenos Aires have recently put forward the suggestion that these apparently aberrantly conducted supraventricular beats are in fact ventricular in origin. They point out that Pick's explanation of eccentric location of the A.V. nodal pacemaker is unsatisfactory since no active pacemaking cells are demonstrable in the A.V. node. Rosenbaum and colleagues (1970) have suggested that in fact the aberrant beats are actually ventricular in origin and that they arise from the proximal part of the three main conducting fascicles. In support of this hypothesis they point out that such aberrant beats show a relatively small constant and well-defined group of QRS complexes which appear either to be incomplete left bundle branch block or else incomplete right bundle branch block with either left anterior hemi-block or left posterior hemi-block. *Figure 5.4* indicates the sites from which such ectopic beats may arise. Since they will be using fast conduction pathways the QRS complexes will be little if at all widened but the usual order of excitation of the ventricles will be altered and the resulting beats will appear aberrant. The frequent occurrence of fusion beats strongly supports the view that such ectopic beats are ventricular in origin and while the hypothesis awaits final experimental proof it does seem the most intellectually satisfying explanation for this common electrocardiographic finding.

It can sometimes be very helpful in analysing complex arrhythmias when the QRS complexes of A.V. junctional and atrial beats are different in contour.

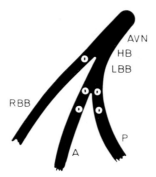

Figure 5.4—Diagram of the atrioventricular conduction system of the human heart: AVN, atrioventricular node; HB, bundle of His; RBB, right bundle branch; LBB, left bundle branch; A, anterior division of LBB; P, posterior division of LBB. The open circles represent the probable sites of origin of narrow ventricular ectopic beats. (After Rosenbaum and colleagues, 1969)

Escape Beats in Atrial Fibrillation

In atrial fibrillation, particularly when A.V. conduction has been depressed by digitalis therapy, escape beats are relatively common. It has in fact been stated that optimum digitalization in atrial fibrillation may be judged by the occurrence of a resting ventricular rate of approximately 70 per minute and the occasional occurrence of A.V. junctional escape beats. The latter are easy to recognize if they happen to have a different contour from those of atrial origin (*Figure 5.5*). They will be found terminating the

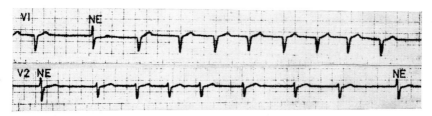

Figure 5.5—Leads V1 and V2 are shown. There is atrial fibrillation and the longer diastolic pauses are terminated by A.V. junctional escape beats which have a different contour from the conducted beats. The A.V. junctional escape beats are marked NE

longer cycles with roughly constant escape intervals of 1–1·5 seconds. It is less easy to recognize junctional escapes when their QRS complexes have the same contour as the atrial beats. However, occasional long cycles measuring 1–1·5 seconds can safely be assumed to be terminated by junctional escapes, particularly if the 'escape intervals' are closely identical in length.

It is probable that in atrial fibrillation something of the order of 600 impulses a minute reach the A.V. junction. While many of these are blocked at the atrionodal junction, many others undergo concealed conduction, penetrating for varying distances into the A.V. junction before becoming blocked. In consequence of this concealed conduction, the A.V. junction is in a constantly varying state of absolute or relative refractoriness and, as will be seen later (page 113), this probably largely accounts for the irregularity of the ventricular rhythm. Some impulses undergoing concealed conduction may penetrate to, and discharge, the A.V. junctional pacemaker but then fail to reach the ventricles. This will necessarily alter the timing of the next A.V. junctional impulse, so that the apparent escape intervals may show

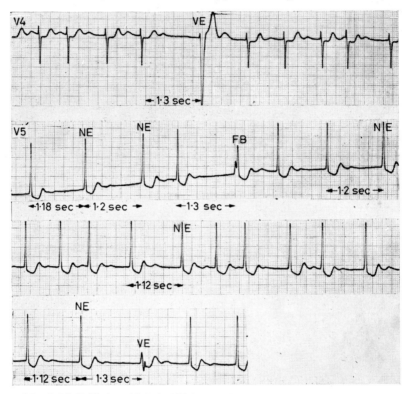

Figure 5.6—Atrial fibrillation with both A.V. junctional and ventricular escape beats. The upper row is lead V4; the lower three rows are a continuous extract from lead V5. A.V. junctional escape beats are marked NE and ventricular escape beats VE. The fifth complex in V5 is probably a fusion between an A.V. junctional and a ventricular escape beat and is marked FB

minor variations. An example of this is shown in *Figure 5.6*. This record illustrates well the occurrence in atrial fibrillation of both A.V. junctional and ventricular escape beats, the phenomenon of concealed conduction and also the occurrence of fusion beats. The occurrence of concealed conduction in this record is proved by the occasional appearance of ventricular escape beats (marked VE). The escape interval of the idioventricular beats is always 1·3 seconds. Obviously an idioventricular pacemaker is immune from concealed conduction. It can only be discharged by manifest conduction of an impulse. The ventricular origin of these beats is shown from their bizarre, wide QRS complexes. Their occurrence is only possible because escape of the A.V. junctional pacemaker has been prevented by its premature discharge by concealed conduction of an atrial impulse following the last conducted beat. Other long cycle lengths in the record, terminating in normal QRS complexes, all measure less than 1·3 seconds (the ventricular escape interval). It is probably safe to assume that all cycle lengths measuring between 1·1 and 1·23 seconds are terminated by A.V. junctional escape beats, the minor variations in the escape interval resulting from chance variations in the time of concealed discharge of the A.V. junctional pacemaker early in diastole. The bizarre complex, marked FB in lead V5, is intermediate in contour between a normal QRS complex and a ventricular escape beat. It occurs after an escape interval of 1·24 seconds and is a fusion beat resulting from nearly simultaneous invasion of the ventricles by A.V. junctional and ventricular escape impulses.

ESCAPE RHYTHMS

When arrest of the sinus node is of longer duration, an escape rhythm takes over control of the heart. This is simply a succession of escape beats and, in the majority of instances of sinus arrest, the escaping pacemaker is junctional. All escape rhythms are characteristically slow, although, once established, the cycle lengths are usually a little shorter than the escape interval of the pacemaker.

Until comparatively recently, the atrio-ventricular node was generally accepted as being the most important subsidiary pacemaker in the heart. It was regarded as being responsible for those forms of escape rhythm in which the duration of the QRS complex was normal and the P′ wave, if visible, was retrograde in contour. Such records were called 'nodal rhythm' and on electrocardiographic grounds were divided into upper, middle and lower nodal rhythm, according to the position of the P′ wave. In upper nodal rhythm, the P′ preceded the QRS complex with a P–R interval of 0·12 second or less. In middle nodal rhythm the P′ wave coincided with the QRS complex and was generally invisible whereas in 'lower nodal rhythm' the P′ wave was present in the ST segment (*Figure 5.8*). At one time it was thought that the A.V. node contained three groups of pacemaking cells, the upper, middle and lower, but later the difference in the site of the P wave was attributed to differences in the time for retrograde conduction or for conduction from the node to the ventricles. These concepts have now had to be changed since careful electro-physiological studies have failed to demonstrate pacemaking cells in the A.V. node except perhaps in that part adjoining the bundle of His and referred to as the H–N portion of the node. It is therefore now clear that the term 'nodal rhythm' is inappropriate. Damato and colleagues (1969) claim to have demonstrated by bundle of His recordings in the human subject that 'lower' and 'middle' rhythms originate in the bundle of His and they suggest the term 'bundle of His rhythm'. Until these claims are substantiated it is probably best to use the non-specific term 'A.V. junctional rhythm' and to drop the term 'nodal rhythm' completely. In the past, if the P′ wave preceded the QRS complex it was regarded as 'upper nodal' rhythm if the P–R interval was 0·12 second or less. If the P–R interval was greater than 0·12 second, the pacemaker was thought to lie on the atrial side of the node close to the orifice of the coronary sinus and was called 'coronary sinus rhythm'. An example of coronary sinus rhythm is shown in *Figure 5.7*. It would now seem sensible to call all rhythms with a retrograde P′ wave preceding the QRS complex coronary sinus rhythm and to call those rhythms with normal QRS complexes and either

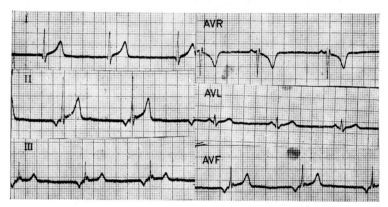

Figure 5.7—Coronary sinus rhythm. The P′ waves are retrograde in contour, being negative in II, III and AVF, and positive in AVR. The P–R interval measures 0·14 second, excluding a junctional origin of the rhythm

no visible P′ waves or retrograde P′ waves in the ST segments, A.V. junctional rhythm.

A.V. junctional rhythm, once established, is usually perfectly regular, with rates varying between 40 and 60 per minute. The commonest form

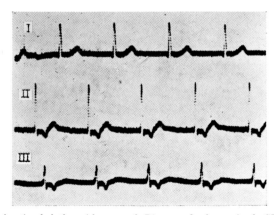

Figure 5.8—A.V. junctional rhythm with retrograde P′ waves clearly seen in the ST segments of leads II and III

encountered clinically is that variety in which a retrograde P′ wave is seen in the ST segments of the QRST complexes. The P′ waves are usually most evident in leads II, III and AVF, where they have a sharply inverted contour (*Figure 5.8*).

Clinically, A.V. junctional rhythm is encountered in sino-atrial block from any cause, the most common aetiologies being digitalis intoxication, recent myocardial infarction and chronic degenerative forms of heart disease, involving the sinus node. Sometimes A.V. junctional rhythm or coronary sinus rhythm is found in otherwise healthy hearts. In complete A.V. block the ventricles may be controlled by an A.V. junctional pacemaker. Activation of the atria and ventricles is then dissociated, the atrial rate being faster than the ventricular.

In that variety of A.V. junctional rhythm which used to be called 'middle nodal rhythm' there is usually no evidence of atrial activity in the conventional leads since the retrograde P' waves are buried and hidden in the QRS complexes.

Wandering or Shifting Pacemaker between the Sinus and the A.V. Junction

A fairly common and usually quite benign finding is abrupt changes in the site of the pacemaker between the sinus node and the A.V. junction. This occurs when the rates of the two pacemakers are closely similar so that a slight slowing of the sinus rate results in transient A.V. junctional escape rhythm. The site of the pacemaker may change several times during the

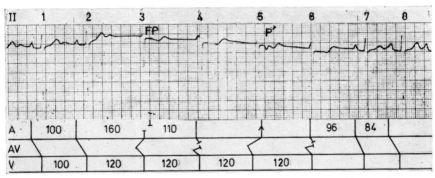

Figure 5.9—Shifting pacemaker between sinus node and A.V. junction (lead II). The record commences with two sinus beats followed by a pause, which is terminated after 1·2 seconds by a junctional escape beat with a slightly different QRS contour. The sinus node discharges just as the junctional impulse reaches the atria and an atrial fusion beat (marked FP) results. The fifth beat of the record is junctional in origin with a retrograde P' wave in its S–T segment. Acceleration of the sinus rate restores sinus rhythm in the seventh and eighth beats of the record. By courtesy of C. Parsons

recording of a routine electrocardiogram. The phenomenon is usually simply a manifestation of variations in autonomic tone. A typical example, which includes an atrial fusion beat is shown in *Figure 5.9*.

An example of a junctional escape rhythm with 2:1 retrograde block is shown in *Figure 5.10*. A retrograde P' wave is only present in alternate ST segments of the QRS complexes.

Ventricular Escape Rhythms

In rare instances the inherent rate of an idioventricular pacemaker may be faster than the A.V. junctional rate; in these circumstances a ventricular escape rhythm may occur instead of an A.V. junctional escape rhythm in sino-atrial inhibition or block. The ventricular rate is then relatively fast. The commonest form of ventricular escape rhythm occurs in complete A.V.

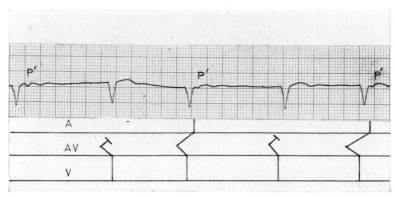

Figure 5.10—Junctional rhythm with 2:1 retrograde block. Retrograde P′ waves are present in alternate ST segments of the QRS complexes

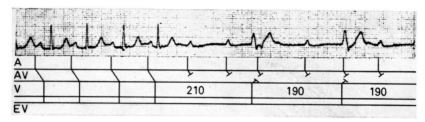

Figure 5.11—Ventricular escape rhythm developing when complete A.V. block occurs suddenly

block when the site of the conduction defect lies below the division of the bundle of His. *Figure 5.11* shows an idioventricular escape rhythm occurring when A.V. block develops suddenly. As in most escape rhythms, the escape interval is usually longer than the subsequent cycle length, the subsidiary pacemaker gradually 'warming up'.

CHAPTER 6

EXTRASYSTOLES AND PARASYSTOLE

EXTRASYSTOLES

Extrasystoles are by far the most common cause of disturbance of the normal heart rhythm. While they not infrequently occur in subjects with normal hearts, given equal numbers, their incidence is greater in patients with organic heart disease. Although in general their occurrence has no ominous significance, they may herald the onset of more serious arrhythmias, such as atrial fibrillation or ventricular tachycardia, or they may provide evidence of serious digitalis intoxication.

Despite their familiar incidence in clinical practice, it is difficult to define extrasystoles precisely. This difficulty is reflected by the varied nomenclature that has been used to describe them. The term extrasystole was originally used by Engelman (1896). This term has been objected to on the grounds that an 'extra' beat only occurs when extrasystoles are interpolated. Some authorities have preferred the term ectopic beats, indicating that the abnormal stimulus responsible has arisen in some part of the heart other than the sinus node. There are, however, two objections to the term ectopic beat. In the first place, all escape beats are necessarily ectopic in origin, but their mechanism of production is quite different from that of extrasystoles. In the second place, extrasystoles may occasionally arise in the sinus node itself (*vide infra*) and such sinus extrasystoles are not, of course, ectopic. A third term which has often been used is premature beats. If the dominant rhythm of the heart is regular, then certainly prematurity is characteristic of extrasystoles, but if the rhythm of the heart is completely irregular, as in atrial fibrillation, there is no means of defining when a beat is premature. There are, moreover, other arrhythmias where a regular rhythm may be disturbed by premature beats, for example, ventricular captures occurring in A.V. dissociation (*see* Chapter 10). In a thoughtful discussion of these semantic difficulties, Scherf and Schott (1953) concluded that the term extrasystoles was the most acceptable, although the terms 'premature' and 'ectopic' beats could be used in the appropriate context. Much of the difficulty in defining extrasystoles stems from the present uncertainty and controversy about the mechanism of their production. Until this mechanism is clearly established, they are best defined by those features which enable them to be recognized in the electrocardiogram. In addition to their premature occurrence and their almost universal ectopic origin, extrasystoles are characterized by the fact that the time interval between them and the preceding beat is virtually constant in any individual case. This constant interval is referred to as the coupling time. The coupling time of extrasystoles is in a sense analogous to the escape interval of escape beats. In both cases these time intervals are constant, but the coupling time of extrasystoles is always shorter than the cycle length of the dominant rhythm so they are premature; the escape interval of escape beats, on the other hand, is always longer than the cycle

71

length of the dominant rhythm so they are late in occurrence and terminate a pause. It is difficult to improve on the definition of extrasystoles given by Scherf and Schott (1953). They define extrasystoles as 'contractions of the whole heart, or parts of the heart, due to impulses which are abnormal, either regarding their site or origin—ectopic—or their time of occurrence— premature—or both, interfering with or replacing a dominant rhythm, whereby in the electrocardiogram the abnormal beats are accurately coupled to the preceding beat and in many, though by no means all, cases have constant shape'.

If the dominant rhythm is regular, their timing can be seen to be premature and, in the vast majority of cases, the origin of the stimulus is ectopic. The contour of extrasystoles in the electrocardiogram will vary according to the site of origin of the abnormal stimulus.

Extrasystoles are subdivided according to their site of origin into sinus, atrial, A.V. junctional and ventricular. Ventricular extrasystoles are the commonest, atrial the next most common. In comparison, A.V. junctional extrasystoles are relatively infrequent and sinus extrasystoles are rare. There is a fifth variety which Scherf and Schott have called return extrasystoles; alternative names are reciprocal beats or echoes.

Ventricular Extrasystoles

These are recognized in the electrocardiogram by the wide contour of their QRS complexes which are often of considerable amplitude. The T waves of ventricular extrasystoles are usually written in the opposite direction to the QRS, with no intervening ST segment. Their time of occurrence is premature and there is no preceding P wave. There are good grounds for believing that the site of origin of ventricular extrasystoles is always in some part of the conduction system of the ventricles. The contour of individual

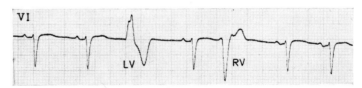

Figure 6.1—Ventricular extrasystoles arising in the left and right main branches of the bundle of His. That arising in the left main bundle is marked LV and shows the pattern of right bundle branch block, whereas that arising in the right main bundle, marked RV, shows the pattern of left bundle branch block

ventricular extrasystoles will therefore vary according to the precise site in the conduction system from which they originate. When the focus is situated in either the left or right main branch of the bundle of His, the contour of the extrasystole will be identical with that of bundle branch block of the opposite ventricle. *Figure 6.1* shows examples of ventricular extrasystoles arising from the left and right main branches of the bundle of His as recorded in lead V1. The more distal the site of the focus in the conduction system, the less resemblance does the contour of the extrasystole bear to a typical bundle branch block pattern, except in the width and amplitude of the QRS complex and the opposite direction of the T wave. However, in a recent paper

Swanick, La Camera and Marriott (1972) have described subtle differences between the morphological features of right ventricular ectopic beats and the pattern of left bundle branch block. They summarize three main differences: (1) a wider (more than 0·04 second in duration) wave in lead V1, (2) a QS or RS complex deeper in V4 than V1 and (3) right axis deviation in the frontal plane is common in right ventricular ectopic beats but rare in left bundle

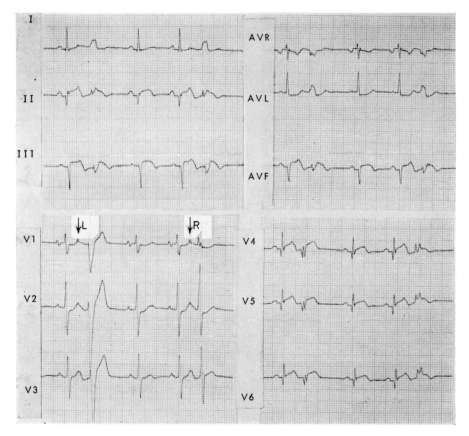

Figure 6.2—Aberrant ventricular conduction. The atrial extrasystoles (arrowed) are evident and are conducted with left (L) and right (R) bundle branch block patterns

branch block. These findings may be helpful in differentiating right ventricular ectopic beats from left bundle branch block aberration (*vide infra*).

Aberrant ventricular conduction is much less common with a left bundle branch block pattern but certainly occurs. An example is shown in *Figure 6.2* in which the ectopic P waves are clearly seen. In this patient aberrant conduction occurred with both right and left bundle branch block pattern.

73

Electrocardiographic Diagnosis of Ventricular Extrasystoles

The diagnosis of ventricular extrasystoles in the electrocardiogram is sometimes very difficult. It is very important to differentiate them from supraventricular extrasystoles with aberrant conduction. The latter, if atrial in origin, are preceded by an ectopic P' wave, but this may be hidden in the T wave of the preceding beat. Sandler and Marriott (1965) in a careful study of this problem stressed the following points. Eighty-five per cent of supraventricular beats with aberrant conduction show the pattern of right bundle branch block. If, therefore, the ectopic beat has a left bundle branch block pattern, it is much more likely to be ventricular in origin. Moreover, only 6 per cent of ventricular extrasystoles show a triphasic (RSR) QRS complex in lead V1, whereas 70 per cent of supraventricular beats with aberrant

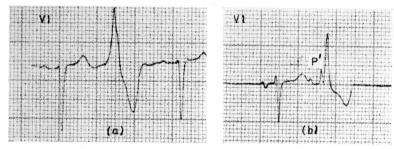

Figure 6.3—Showing two extrasystoles recorded in lead V1. (a) Shows what is almost certainly a ventricular extrasystole. It has the pattern of right bundle branch block but shows a monophasic upward deflection. (b) Shows an atrial extrasystole conducted with aberration. It is preceded by a P' wave and has an RSR complex. Although superficially this resembles a ventricular extrasystole it clearly is an atrial extrasystole with aberrant intraventricular conduction

contour show this complex. In lead V1, ventricular extrasystoles with a right bundle branch block pattern usually show a monophasic R wave or a QR pattern. Sandler and Marriott also point out that only 4 per cent of ventricular extrasystoles show the same initial deflection in lead V1, as do the flanking sinus beats. Since aberrant conduction of the right bundle branch block type would not be expected to alter the initial conduction of the impulse (across the septum from left to right), they anticipated that supraventricular beats with aberrant conduction would usually show the same initial deflection as the flanking sinus beats. Surprisingly they found that only 44 per cent of aberrant beats showed the same initial deflection. Thus, the electrocardiographic diagnosis of ventricular extrasystoles remains a matter of assessing probabilities; it is important to appreciate that complete certainty is rarely possible, but the criteria laid down by Sandler and Marriott are frequently helpful (*Figure 6.3*).

Marriott's recent criteria for differentiating between ventricular ectopic beats and those of supraventricular origin conducted with aberration include the finding of a right bundle branch block pattern with an RSR complex in lead V1; also a qRS pattern in lead V6 similarly strongly favours aberrant conduction for it is extremely uncommon to get even a small q wave in left ventricular ectopic beats. In favour of left ventricular ectopy is the occurrence of a right bundle branch block pattern in lead V1 which has two peaks on it which he refers to as 'rabbit's ears'. If the left 'rabbit ear' is taller than the right this strongly favours a left ventricular ectopic origin (*Figure 6.4*). On the other hand, if the right 'rabbit ear' is taller than the left this does not favour either aberration or ectopy (*Figure 6.4*). A QS complex of an ectopic beat in

Ventricular aberration v. ectopy : morphological clues

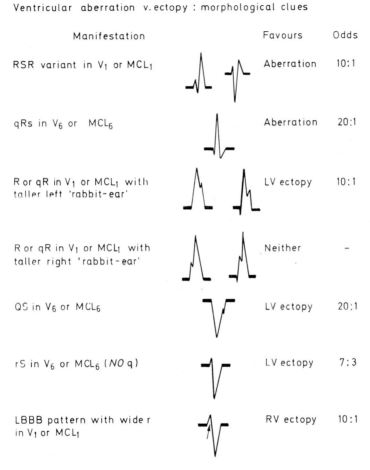

Manifestation	Favours	Odds
RSR variant in V₁ or MCL₁	Aberration	10:1
qRs in V₆ or MCL₆	Aberration	20:1
R or qR in V₁ or MCL₁ with taller left 'rabbit-ear'	LV ectopy	10:1
R or qR in V₁ or MCL₁ with taller right 'rabbit-ear'	Neither	–
QS in V₆ or MCL₆	LV ectopy	20:1
rS in V₆ or MCL₆ (*NO* q)	LV ectopy	7:3
LBBB pattern with wide r in V₁ or MCL₁	RV ectopy	10:1

Figure 6.4—This diagram illustrates points in the morphology of QRS complexes which help to differentiate between beats of supraventricular origin which have been conducted with aberration and those of ventricular ectopic origin. (Reproduced from 'Workshop in Electrocardiography', by H. J. L. Marriott by courtesy of the Author and the Publishers, Tampa Tracings)

lead V6 strongly favours a left ventricular ectopic origin. So also does an rS in lead V6, particularly if the R wave is broad. A similar pattern in lead V1 strongly favours a right ventricular ectopic origin (*Figure 6.4*). Finally, if the initial vector of an ectopic beat is the same as that of the flanking sinus beats, this should immediately suggest aberrant conduction of a beat of supraventricular origin. While it is possible by following these rules to be reasonably certain of differentiating beats of ventricular origin from supraventricular beats conducted with aberration there is no final certainty. Absolute distinction could always be obtained by recording a His bundle electrogram. For beats of supraventricular origin would always be preceded by an H deflection, whereas in ventricular ectopic beats the H deflection would either follow or be embedded in the QRS complex. However, it would rarely be necessary in clinical practice to use this technique for their differentiation.

Occasionally extrasystoles arise from the main stem of the bundle of His above its bifurcation. Anatomically such ectopic beats are ventricular, but since the impulse reaches the ventricles via normal conduction pathways, the resulting QRS complexes may be indistinguishable from those of sinus beats. Such 'stem' extrasystoles will be considered separately below.

In individual patients, both the contour of ventricular extrasystoles and their coupling times to the preceding normal beats usually remain absolutely constant in serial records over periods of years.

Coupling Time of Ventricular Extrasystoles

The coupling time of ventricular extrasystoles is measured from the commencement of the QRS complex of the preceding beat to the commencement of the extrasystole. In the vast majority of instances (91·6 per cent according to Schellong, 1924) this time interval remains accurate and constant, irrespective of whether the dominant rhythm is regular or irregular. In the majority of ventricular extrasystoles, the coupling time measures somewhere between 0·45 and 0·56 second, but is occasionally shorter and rarely much longer. When a variable coupling time is present, it should immediately raise the suspicion of parasystole (*vide infra*). Variation in coupling time is generally obvious from simple inspection of the record, for the eye can readily appreciate quite minor differences in the interval between the end of the T wave of the preceding beat and the commencement of the extrasystole. Variations of as much as 0·08 second do occasionally occur in records where a parasystolic mechanism cannot be demonstrated. Rare cases have been published (Scherf and Schott, 1953) in which ventricular extrasystoles occur regularly after each sinus beat, but show progressive lengthening of the coupling time until one is missed out. The cycle is then repeated.

Effect of Ventricular Extrasystoles on Cardiac Rhythm

Although occasionally ventricular extrasystoles are interpolated, in the majority of instances, single extrasystoles replace one beat of the dominant rhythm. Since the ectopic beat is premature, if the dominant rhythm is regular, the extrasystole is followed by a pause. When the interval between the last beat before the extrasystole and the first beat following it is equal to two cycle lengths of the dominant rhythm, the pause is said to be compensatory. This is illustrated in *Figure 6.5*. It has often been stated that the pause following single ventricular extrasystoles is always compensatory. However, this is by no means invariably true. It clearly cannot be true when ventricular extrasystoles occur in atrial fibrillation, since individual cycle lengths are unpredictable. Similarly, in the presence of sinus arrhythmia, the post-extrasystolic pauses will vary in length. When there is absolutely regular sinus rhythm, the pause will be compensatory, provided the sinus node is not disturbed by the ectopic impulse. In *Figure 6.5* the sinus P wave can clearly be seen deforming the T portion of the extrasystole. This sinus impulse is, of course, blocked, since the ventricles are refractory. It used to be thought that retrograde conduction to the atria of the ectopic impulse of ventricular extrasystoles seldom occurred. However, Kistin and Landowne (1951) were

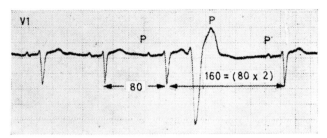

Figure 6.5—Ventricular extrasystole with compensatory pause

able to show by means of an oesophageal lead that retrograde conduction of ventricular extrasystoles occurred in 15 out of 33 unselected subjects, and it is now well established that this is a common occurrence in the human heart, although retrograde P waves are rarely seen in conventional leads. Very commonly the retrograde stimulus reaches the sinus node about the time it is due to discharge. Under these circumstances, measurement of the post-extrasystolic pause may show it to be 'compensatory', but this is fortuitous.

Interpolated Ventricular Extrasystoles

Interpolated ventricular extrasystoles, while uncommon, are by no means rare. The ventricular ectopic beat falls between two successive conducted sinus beats and, in this sense, are the only form of true 'extrasystole'. Their occurrence is favoured by a slow sinus rate and an extrasystole occurring early in diastole, that is with a short coupling time. Interpolated atrial or

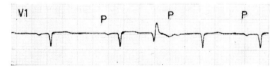

Figure 6.6—Interpolated ventricular extrasystole followed by a prolonged P–R interval of the next sinus beat

A.V. junctional extrasystoles rarely occur in the human heart. Following an interpolated ventricular extrasystole, it is extremely common for the P–R interval of the next sinus beat to be prolonged (*Figure 6.6* shows an example). This delay in A.V. conduction following an interpolated extrasystole is due to concealed conduction of the ectopic ventricular impulse which penetrates the A.V. junction for a short distance leaving it partially refractory to the next sinus impulse. *Figure 6.7* shows an even more pronounced example from a patient with first degree A.V. block. There is marked sinus bradycardia, the P–P cycle lengths ranging from 1·18 to 1·32 seconds. The P–R interval of the sinus beat before the extrasystole measures 0·23 second. The next P wave falls just after the T wave of the extrasystole and is conducted to the ventricles with the greatly prolonged P–R interval of 0·58 second. The following sinus beat has a P–R interval of 0·26 second, and it is not until the third sinus beat following the extrasystole that the P–R interval has returned to its original duration of 0·23 second. In analysing this short record, two questions require to be answered. First, how can it be established that the P wave immediately following the extrasystole is conducted, and that the QRS following it is not an A.V. junctional escape beat? Secondly, why is the P–R interval of the second sinus beat after the extrasystole still longer than 0·23 second? The answer to the first point is that an escape interval must always be longer than the longest cycle length of the dominant rhythm. The

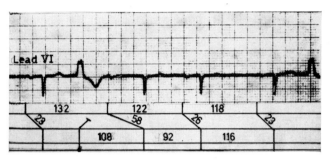

Figure 6.7—Interpolated extrasystole follows the first sinus beat of the record. The next 2 sinus beats following the extrasystole show lengthening of the P–R interval

interval between the extrasystole and the next QRS complex here is only 1·08 seconds, compared with a sinus cycle of up to 1·32 seconds. Thus, this QRS cannot be an escape beat and must have been conducted. The answer to the second point is that the very long P–R interval following the extra-systole necessarily shortens the next R–P interval, so the sinus impulse reaches the A.V. junction while it is still just in its relative refractory phase.

This short strip has been described in some detail, since it illustrates well the type of reasoning used in the analysis of arrhythmias. The occurrence of interpolated ventricular extrasystoles has no particular significance. They may occur both in patients with and without organic heart disease; the determining factor is usually a dominant rhythm with a relatively slow rate.

Kistin (1965) has shown that in some apparently interpolated ventricular extrasystoles the first post-extrasystolic beat is in fact a reciprocal beat. This will be further discussed later under reciprocal beats.

Changes in the First Post-extrasystolic Beat

It is not uncommon for the first beat following an extrasystole to show some minor variation in contour compared with the normal beats preceding it. The most frequent change observed is in the T wave of the first beat following the extrasystole. The T wave may be lowered in amplitude or even written in the opposite direction to the T waves of the other normal beats. *Figure 6.8a, b* shows two typical examples of post-extrasystolic T-wave changes in the first sinus beat following ventricular extrasystoles. The mechanism responsible for this phenomenon is at present obscure; nor is there complete unanimity of opinion about its significance. Scherf (1944) considered that post-extrasystolic inversion of the T wave, even in an otherwise normal electro-cardiogram, was always suggestive of the presence of structural heart disease, and others have concurred with this view. Certainly, in practice,

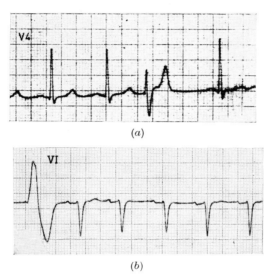

(a)

(b)

Figure 6.8—(*a*) *Post-extrasystolic T-wave changes. The last beat of the record following a ventricular extrasystole shows shallow T-wave inversion not present in the two sinus beats before the extrasystole, (b) The record commences with an extrasystole and the T wave of the first sinus beat following it is positive whereas it is quite flat in the remaining sinus beats*

post-extrasystolic T-wave changes seem to occur far more frequently in patients with myocardial disease, but this has been denied by some authors.

Occasionally, in patients with ischaemic heart disease, an injury current

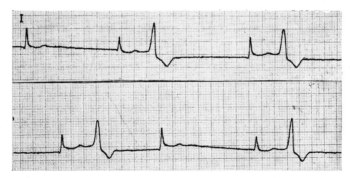

Figure 6.9—*Post-extrasystolic S–T segment shift. The two rows are continuous (see text)*

may appear following an extrasystole and be manifested as an S–T segment shift. *Figure 6.9* was recorded from a woman aged 70 years suffering from frequent anginal attacks. There is atrial fibrillation and, following extra-systoles, there is a considerable shift in the 'take-off' point of the S–T segment of the next conducted beat, whereas the S–T segment is normal if there is no preceding extrasystole.

Far less often the first post-extrasystolic beat may show a change in the contour of the QRS complex. For example, occasionally in patients with left or right bundle branch block, the first post-extrasystolic beat may show normal intraventricular conduction. This is most probably due to the longer period of recovery allowed by the compensatory pause following the ectopic beat.

Multiple Ventricular Extrasystoles

Ventricular extrasystoles usually occur singly, but two or more in succession are by no means uncommon. By an entirely arbitrary definition, three or more ventricular extrasystoles in succession are said to constitute a run of ventricular tachycardia.

Two successive ventricular extrasystoles usually replace only one beat of the dominant rhythm, but this is not invariable. Nearly always they have identical contours and the interval between them is constant in different parts of the record. Not infrequently the second ventricular extrasystole of a pair differs in contour from the first. There are two possible causes for this variation in contour. Either the second extrasystole has arisen from a different focus, for it is well recognized that the stimulus from one extrasystolic focus can awaken another, or, alternatively, the excitation wave of the second extrasystole may find part of the ventricular muscle mass still refractory from the first, so that it has to pursue a different path through the ventricular myocardium. It is often difficult to be sure which explanation is correct in any given case.

Multifocal Ventricular Extrasystoles

In the majority of instances, ventricular extrasystoles arise from a single focus in any individual case. In some cases, particularly with myocardial disease, more than one ectopic ventricular focus may be present. Two

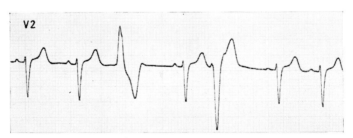

Figure 6.10—Multifocal ventricular extrasystoles. The first extrasystole has the pattern of right bundle branch block and a coupling time of 0·55 second to the preceding beat. The second extrasystole has the pattern of left bundle branch block and has a coupling time of 0·38 second to the preceding beat

criteria must be fulfilled to justify a diagnosis of multifocal ventricular extrasystoles. First, the extrasystoles must have different contours in any one lead; secondly, the ectopics with different contours must also have different coupling times to the initiating beat. *Figure 6.10* shows an example of two ventricular extrasystoles recorded in the same lead. The second ectopic differs from the first, both in contour and in coupling time. Sometimes ventricular extrasystoles may show quite wide variations in contour in any one lead but have the same coupling times. These probably originate in the same focus, and the difference in contour simply reflects variations in the path of conduction of the ectopic stimulus.

'Multiform ventricular extrasystoles' is probably a more appropriate term for this variety. Multiform ventricular extrasystoles are always highly suggestive of digitalis intoxication (page 279), though they are occasionally seen in undigitalized patients. True multifocal ventricular extrasystoles are always strongly indicative of underlying heart disease, but again exceptions occur.

Significance of Ventricular Extrasystoles

Ventricular extrasystoles may be entirely benign, or they may be the only manifestation of serious myocardial disease. There are no completely reliable criteria which enable the clinical significance of ventricular extra-systoles to be assessed in an individual record. There are, however, a number of useful guides which may enable a fairly confident opinion to be formed. Claims are sometimes made that the contour of the ectopic beats may help to differentiate between benign extrasystoles and those with more ominous import. In my experience, the contour of the extrasystoles is of no value in assessing their significance. Likewise, the frequency of their occurrence and whether they are single or multiple is of little help. For example, in repetitive paroxysmal ventricular tachycardia (see page 150), the majority of the QRS complexes in the record may be ventricular ectopics and yet the condition may be symptomless and benign. In the vast majority of instances, the presence of unifocal ventricular extrasystoles in an otherwise normal electro-cardiogram is an entirely benign finding, however numerous they may be. It has already been mentioned that the occurrence of post-extrasystolic T-wave changes may be the only indication of underlying myocardial disease, and the T wave of the first sinus beat following an extrasystole should always be carefully compared with the other T waves in the same lead. The presence of true multifocal ventricular extrasystoles should always be regarded seriously, although they may occasionally occur in otherwise normal hearts.

Perhaps the most useful guide to the significance of ventricular extra-systoles is the clinical circumstances in which they occur. In otherwise symptomless patients, with no clinical or radiological evidence of heart disease, their benignancy may be safely assumed. On the other hand, their appearance following acute myocardial infarction should always be viewed with apprehension, since they may presage the onset of ventricular tachy-cardia or ventricular fibrillation. It has been claimed that ventricular ectopics with a short coupling time are particularly dangerous in these circumstances. These have been referred to as 'R on T' ventricular extra-systoles, since the QRS commences on the downstroke of the preceding T wave. The importance of ectopic ventricular extrasystoles with a short coupling time in myocardial infarction will be further discussed in Chapter 16.

The significance of ventricular extrasystoles occurring during digitalis medication will be discussed in the chapter on Digitalis Intoxication (page 279).

Distribution of Ventricular Extrasystoles

Sometimes a ventricular extrasystole follows each beat of the dominant rhythm, resulting in one form of ventricular bigeminy. The term 'bigeminy' literally means 'twin beats' and refers to rhythms in which short ventricular pauses alternate with long ones. As will be seen, the term is applicable in other instances where extrasystoles are not the underlying mechanism. Scherf and Schott prefer to restrict the term 'trigeminal rhythm' to instances where each beat of the dominant rhythm is followed by two successive extrasystoles. However, the term would seem equally appropriate for the more common circumstance in which a single ventricular extrasystole follows every second beat of the dominant rhythm, although the mechanism should perhaps be stated. It is far less common for ventricular extrasystoles to fall regularly after more than two sinus beats and in the past it has always been considered that, apart from the forms of bigeminal or trigeminal

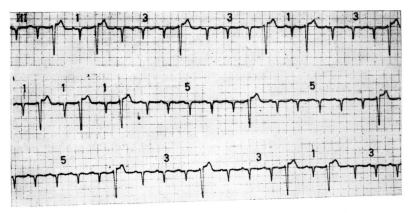

Figure 6.11—Ventricular extrasystoles showing the pattern of manifest and concealed bigeminy. The number of sinus beats between each ectopic is always an odd number

rhythm just mentioned, ventricular extrasystoles tend to be scattered at random in the record. However, in 1961 Schamroth and Marriott described a case whose record at times showed bigeminal rhythm with a ventricular extrasystole following every sinus beat, while at other times the extrasystoles appeared to become scattered at random. They made the remarkable observation that, when the ectopic beats appeared to have a random distribution, the interectopic intervals always contained an odd number of sinus beats. To confirm that this was not just fortuitous, a record was made over a period of twenty minutes, and all interectopic intervals were found to contain only odd numbers of sinus beats, the number varying from 1 to 43 beats. The statistical odds against such a distribution being due to chance are, of course, astronomical, and this pattern, which is by no means uncommon, must have some explanation (*Figure 6.11* shows an example). The mechanism postulated by Schamroth and Marriott is that ventricular extrasystoles continue to occur after every (alternate) sinus beat, but that from time to time they fail to appear owing to exit block developing around the ectopic focus. *Figure 6.12* illustrates this mechanism diagrammatically using the conventional key (after Schamroth). The first sinus beat, marked 1, is normally conducted to the ventricles and is followed by a (manifest) ventricular extrasystole. The latter prevents the second sinus impulse, marked 2, from reaching the ventricles. The third sinus beat is again followed by a ventricular extrasystole, but this fails to invade the ventricular myocardium owing to

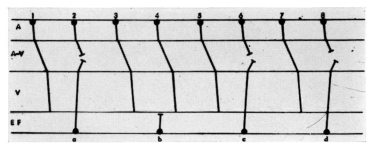

Figure 6.12—Explanation for concealed bigeminy (after Schamroth) (see text)

exit block round the ectopic focus, so the fourth sinus beat descends normally. It is not followed by an extrasystole, because the next one is not due until after the sinus beat numbered five. The authors refer to the extrasystoles which appear in the record as 'manifest', and to those which fail to appear as 'concealed'. They term the pattern of distribution of ventricular extrasystoles

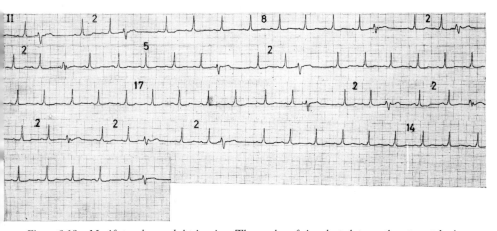

Figure 6.13—Manifest and concealed trigeminy. The number of sinus beats between the extrasystoles is either 2 or a multiple of 3 plus 2; that is, 5, 8, 14 or 17. When an extrasystole is concealed, the sinus beat descends normally but 2 sinus beats must then occur before another extrasystole is due

in which only odd numbers of sinus beats are seen in the interectopic intervals as 'concealed bigeminy'.

This mechanism is strongly supported by some cases of trigeminal rhythm in which a ventricular extrasystole follows every second sinus beat. When the extrasystoles appear to become scattered at random, the number of sinus beats in the interectopic intervals is now found to be a multiple of 3 plus 2, that is, 5, 8, 11, 14 and so on. *Figure 6.13* shows an example. This pattern is referred to as 'concealed trigeminy'. The same authors have also published a case (Schamroth and Marriott, 1964) in which the ventricular extrasystoles were interpolated. When these appeared to become scattered at random, the interectopic intervals always contained an extra sinus beat, so that the number of sinus beats is always either even, or a multiple of three.

When longish records containing ventricular extrasystoles are carefully examined, the patterns of manifest and concealed bigeminy and trigeminy will be found in approximately a quarter of the cases, particularly in sinus rhythm. These particular distributions of ventricular ectopic beats are less often seen in atrial fibrillation.

The occurrence of concealed ventricular extrasystoles is of considerable theoretical interest and must have some relevance to our knowledge of the underlying mechanism of ventricular extrasystoles. This will be further discussed in the later section on mechanism. Concealed extrasystoles have little clinical importance, except possibly that they indicate a greater degree of myocardial irritability than is immediately apparent from the record.

Ventricular Extrasystoles in Atrial Fibrillation

Langendorf, Pick and Winternitz (1955) pointed out that in atrial fibrillation there is a tendency for ventricular extrasystoles to follow the beats which terminate longer diastolic pauses. They termed this the 'rule of bigeminy' and, although there are often exceptions, in general it is found to

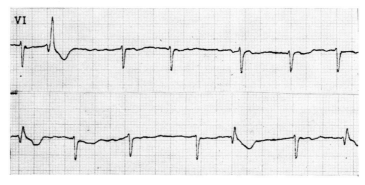

Figure 6.14—The two rows are continuous. There is atrial fibrillation and occasional beats show a right bundle branch block contour and mimic ventricular extrasystoles. For fuller explanation see text

be true. In atrial fibrillation, however, it is extremely important to differentiate between ventricular extrasystoles and conducted beats with aberration which can closely simulate them. Since the refractory phase of the conducting tissues varies with the heart rate, a long diastolic interval will result in a lengthened refractory phase and if the next diastole is short, this will favour aberration, which may mimic ventricular ectopy. *Figure 6.14* shows an example of apparent ventricular extrasystoles occurring in lead VI in atrial fibrillation. The apparent ectopic beats, however, show the pattern of right bundle branch block with an rSR pattern which strongly suggests aberrant conduction. Moreover, their coupling times to the preceding beats show wide variation from 0·34 to 0·65 second; measurement of the intervals between these anomalous beats excludes parasystole (*vide infra*) and it is therefore virtually certain that they are conducted beats with aberration and not ventricular extrasystoles.

Ventricular Extrasystoles in Complete A.V. Block

When ventricular extrasystoles occur in the presence of complete A.V. block, the ectopic impulse originates in the same region of the heart as the dominant pacemaker and will, therefore, almost inevitably enter the dominant pacemaker and extinguish its immature impulse. The post-extrasystolic pause cannot therefore be compensatory. In the majority of cases it approximates closely to one cycle length of the dominant rhythm, as would be expected. It is rarely shorter than this but is often longer, owing to transient depression of the dominant pacemaker following its premature discharge, so that its next impulse is delayed. On rare occasions, depression of the idioventricular pacemaker, following a ventricular extrasystole, may result in a pause of sufficient length for consciousness to be lost. This is more common if several extrasystoles occur in succession. This constitutes an occasional cause of Stokes–Adams attacks in complete A.V. block. A more common mechanism is the occurrence of a transient episode of ventricular tachycardia or ventricular fibrillation.

It has often been suggested that the occurrence of ventricular extrasystoles in A.V. block can be explained by the fact that the aetiological conditions which produce A.V. block are common causes of extrasystoles. While this may be true of conditions such as coronary artery disease, diphtheria and digitalis intoxication, we now know that these are not responsible for many cases of A.V. block in which the lesion is confined to the bundle of His or its two main branches. On the other hand, in many cases of A.V. block there is a clear relationship between the incidence of ventricular extrasystoles and the rate of the idioventricular rhythm. The slower the rate, the more frequent are the premature beats. That this relationship is causal is suggested by the observation that increasing the rate of discharge of the dominant pacemaker by intravenous isoprenaline (*see* page 256) will usually abolish the extrasystoles. The same is true when the heart rate is increased by an artificial pacemaker. It would seem reasonable to deduce from these findings that the extrasystoles are due to myocardial ischaemia as a result of a reduction in coronary flow, secondary to a low cardiac output.

Rare instances have been recorded of interpolated ventricular extrasystoles occurring in complete A.V. block. Their occurrence can only be explained by assuming that the dominant ventricular pacemaker is protected by entrance block.

Atrial Extrasystoles

Atrial extrasystoles, in their most characteristic form, can readily be recognized in the electrocardiogram. They are premature in time, and their QRS complexes, which are usually normal in contour, are preceded by P waves, generally of abnormal shape. Since the ectopic stimulus arises in the same part of the heart as the dominant pacemaker, the latter is usually prematurely discharged, so that the timing of the next sinus impulse is altered. In consequence, the post-extrasystolic pause is not compensatory; that is to say, the interval between the last sinus beat before the extrasystole, and first sinus beat following it, measures less than two sinus cycles.

In practice, many variations from this typical pattern occur, and diagnostic difficulties may arise.

Effect of Atrial Extrasystoles on Cardiac Rhythm

The effect of atrial extrasystoles on cardiac rhythm is variable and is influenced by several factors. These include the site in the atria of the ectopic focus, the rate of conduction over the atria of the ectopic stimulus and the time of its occurrence in diastole; that is, its coupling time. The coupling time of atrial extrasystoles is measured from the commencement of the P wave of the preceding sinus beat to the commencement of the P wave of the extrasystole. While this coupling time tends to be constant, slightly wider variations seem to occur with atrial than with ventricular extrasystoles.

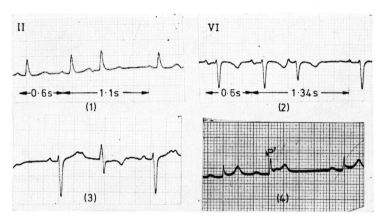

Figure 6.15—Illustrating the four different effects which atrial extrasystoles may produce on cardiac rhythm: (1) shows an atrial extrasystole which is followed by a pause which is less than compensatory, though it is rather more than a normal sinus cycle in length; (2) shows an atrial extrasystole followed by a pause which is rather more than compensatory; (3) the second beat of the record is an atrial extrasystole (with aberrant conduction). Its P–R interval is considerably prolonged so that the ventricular complex is less premature than the atrial; (4) in the ST segment of the second sinus beat, there is a blocked P′ wave. This is followed by a considerable pause in the ventricular rhythm

There are 4 different effects which atrial extrasystoles may produce on the rhythm of the heart.

(1) The atrial extrasystole may discharge the sinus node, so that the pause following it is less than compensatory; it then usually approximates to one sinus cycle in length (*Figure 6.15(1)*).

(2) When the atrial ectopic focus is situated at a distance from the sinus node, and if it discharges late in diastole, its excitation wave may fail to reach the sinus node in time to discharge it prematurely. The post-extra-systolic pause will then be compensatory, just as it usually is following a ventricular extrasystole. In *Figure 6.15 (2)* the post-extrasystolic pause is slightly more than compensatory. This is presumably due to sinus arrhythmia.

(3) When an atrial extrasystole occurs early in diastole, its excitation wave may reach the A.V. junction during its relatively refractory phase, and its P–R interval will thus be prolonged. In consequence, ventricular activation will be less premature than atrial activation (*Figure 6.15(3)*).

(4) Finally an atrial extrasystole may occur so early in diastole that it fails to elicit a ventricular contraction (*Figure 6.15(4)*). Such atrial extrasystoles are termed blocked and since they discharge the sinus node there is a pause in the ventricular rhythm which may give the erroneous clinical impression of partial heart block with 'dropped' beats. The precise site of block cannot be established from the conventional electrocardiogram. Although in the majority this occurs at the A.V. junction, due to the arrival of the excitation wave during its absolute refractory phase, it may also occur within the intraventricular conduction system. This can only be recognized by His bundle electrography (*Figure 6.16*).

Contour of P Waves of Atrial Extrasystoles

The contour of the P waves of atrial extrasystoles is largely determined by their site of origin. If the ectopic focus lies near to the sinus node, the P wave will closely resemble that of a sinus beat. With ectopic foci situated low in the atrial septum, the P waves will have a retrograde contour, being negative in leads II, III and AVF.

P waves originating from other sites in the atria may show contours which differ widely from those of sinus origin. They may be taller or smaller, or widened and notched. Very often they coincide with the T wave of the preceding beat, when they can be seen to deform some part of its contour. Occasionally a hand lens is necessary to identify them.

Contour of QRS Complexes of Atrial Extrasystoles

The QRS complexes of atrial extrasystoles may be identical in contour to those of sinus beats. However, varying degrees of minor aberration are not uncommon. Sometimes aberrant intraventricular conduction of an atrial extrasystole may be so marked that its QRS complex resembles that of a ventricular ectopic beat with a wide QRS and the T wave written in the opposite direction. Differentiation between atrial extrasystoles with aberrant QRST contours and ventricular extrasystoles can occasionally cause diagnostic difficulty. An atrial origin of a bizarre QRST complex is indicated if it is preceded by a premature P wave with a normal (or prolonged) P–R interval. However, the ectopic P wave may be difficult to identify if it is buried in the preceding T wave. In any one lead, aberrant QRST complexes of atrial origin generally show appreciable variations in contour and this may prove helpful in differentiating them from ventricular extrasystoles which are usually constant in shape. The cause of aberrant intraventricular conduction of atrial extrasystoles is usually only their prematurity, for all parts of the conduction system have not fully recovered from the preceding beat. The time available for recovery of the conduction system may conveniently be measured by the R–P interval; that is, by the interval between the commencement of the last QRS complex before the atrial extrasystole and the beginning of the latter. Since the coupling time of atrial extrasystoles may be quite variable, this R–P interval may vary and, in consequence,

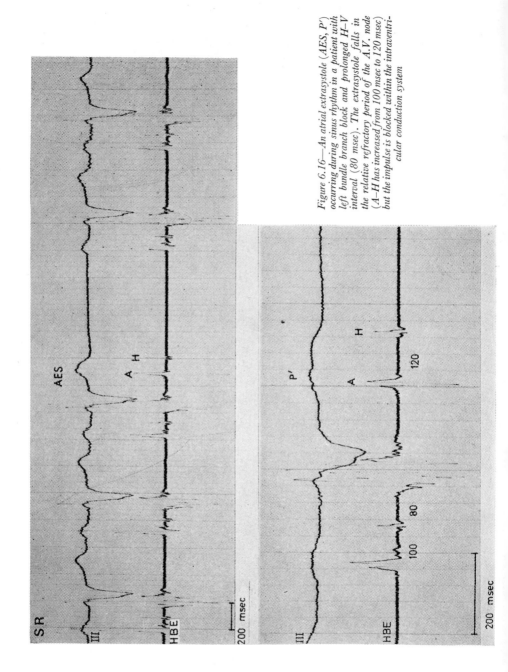

Figure 6.16—An atrial extrasystole (AES, P') occurring during sinus rhythm in a patient with left bundle branch block and prolonged H–V interval (80 msec). The extrasystole falls in the relative refractory period of the A.V. node (A–H has increased from 100 msec to 120 msec) but the impulse is blocked within the intraventricular conduction system

some atrial extrasystoles in a record may show normal intraventricular conduction and others, with slightly shorter coupling times, may have aberrant QRS contours. *Figure 6.17* shows an example of this variation in QRS contour of atrial extrasystoles depending on the coupling time.

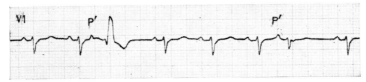

Figure 6.17—Variation of QRS contour of atrial extrasystoles dependent on their coupling time. The QRS complex of the first atrial extrasystole marked P' is very aberrant. The coupling time of the atrial extra-systole measures 0·3 second. The second atrial extrasystole, also marked P', has a coupling time of 0·42 second and its QRS complex is far less aberrant than that of the first

Post-extrasystolic T-wave Changes

Changes in the T wave of the first beat following an atrial extrasystole are occasionally observed. This has the same significance as it does following a ventricular extrasystole, but it is less commonly seen.

Multiple Atrial Extrasystoles

As with ventricular extrasystoles, two or more extrasystoles of atrial origin may occur in succession. Three or more in succession are again arbitrarily defined as a run of atrial tachycardia. Sometimes the first QRST complex of a run of atrial extrasystoles is aberrant, while subsequent ones are not. The

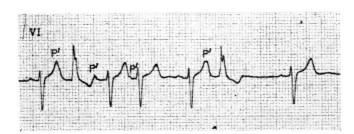

Figure 6.18—A run of three atrial extrasystoles with aberrant contour of the first. Shortening of the re-fractory period by the increased heart rate is suggested by the shortening of successive P–R intervals of the extrasystoles

explanation for this probably lies in the shortening of the refractory period with an increased heart rate. This shortening may take several beats to occur. *Figure 6.18* shows three successive atrial extrasystoles; the first is aberrant in contour but the second and third are not. Shortening of the refractory period is strongly suggested by simultaneous shortening of the P–R interval of the extrasystoles. In this case it is clear that the ectopic impulse coming down the left bundle branch could not have entered the right bundle branch in a retrograde direction and thus render it refractory, as was described on page 31.

Multifocal Atrial Extrasystoles

Figure 6.19 is a record with basic sinus rhythm which is disturbed by frequent atrial extrasystoles. Their multifocal origin is indicated by the variations both in contour and coupling times of the ectopic P waves. Clinically, frequent multifocal atrial extrasystoles result in an irregular ventricular rhythm which may be indistinguishable from atrial fibrillation without an electrocardiogram.

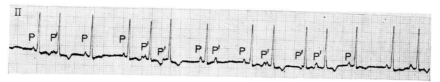

Figure 6.19—Multifocal atrial extrasystoles (lead II). Sinus rhythm is disturbed by frequent atrial extra-systoles, and the P' waves show wide variations both in coupling time and contour

Significance of Atrial Extrasystoles

The occurrence of occasional atrial extrasystoles in an otherwise normal heart is usually an entirely benign finding without any significance. Frequent atrial extrasystoles very commonly herald the onset of atrial fibrillation. This is particularly true when they are multifocal in origin or when they occur in a patient with mitral valve disease.

Distribution of Atrial Extrasystoles

It is unusual for the distribution of atrial extrasystoles to show any clear pattern, although one may follow regularly after every sinus beat, producing one form of bigeminal rhythm, or after every second sinus beat, producing trigeminal rhythm. On rare occasions, a blocked atrial extrasystole may follow

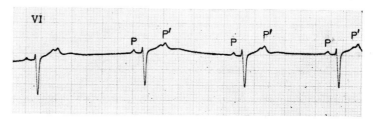

Figure 6.20—Blocked atrial extrasystoles following each sinus beat and simulating 2 : 1 A.V. block (see text)

each sinus beat. If the blocked P wave resembles a sinus P wave in contour, the electrocardiographic appearances may closely simulate 2 : 1 A.V. block, for it is well recognized that in the latter condition the P–P interval which includes a QRS complex is commonly shorter than the P–P interval which does not (*Figure 6.20* shows an example). Differentiation of the two conditions is obviously important since their clinical significance is widely different. The diagnosis can usually be readily established by repeating the electrocardiogram after light exercise (Scherf and Schott, 1953). This will usually transiently abolish atrial extrasystoles, whereas 2 : 1 A.V. block will change either to occasional blocked beats or to a higher degree of block (*see* Chapter 14).

Sometimes the blocked P' wave may not be visible, being hidden in the preceding T wave. The record may then resemble a sinus bradycardia. The differentiation may then be made clinically from inspection of the jugular venous pulse which will show cannon waves following each ventricular contraction due to the ectopic P wave, causing atrial contraction against a closed tricuspid valve.

A.V. Junctional Extrasystoles

A.V. junctional extrasystoles are relatively uncommon. Like A.V. junctional escape rhythms, they used to be divided into upper, middle and lower types, according to whether the P wave precedes, coincides with, or follows the QRS complex. Today however it is probably best to classify as A.V. junctional extrasystoles those with either no visible P wave or those with a retrograde P' wave following the QRS complex; all extrasystoles with a retrograde P' wave preceding the QRS are best regarded as being atrial in origin. There is a third type of A.V. junctional extrasystole which used to be classed as 'main stem' in origin. One of these is illustrated in *Figure 6.21*. The criteria for recognizing these in the electrocardiogram are the occurrence of premature QRS complexes which are identical in contour with those of sinus beats (indicating their origin above the bifurcation of the

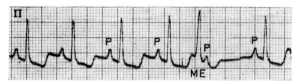

Figure 6.21—The 5th complex of the row is a 'main stem extrasystole' (marked ME) with a blocked sinus P wave falling in its ST segment

bundle of His). The sequence of sinus P waves continues undisturbed and the post-extrasystolic pause is compensatory. Their degree of prematurity varies so that the blocked sinus P wave may precede the QRS (but with a short P–R interval) or more often as in *Figure 6.21* the P wave can be seen in the ST segment of the extrasystole but is clearly of sinus origin. Such ectopic beats are clearly A.V. junctional in origin with retrograde A.V. block.

As with atrial extrasystoles, the pause following an A.V. junctional extrasystole may or may not be compensatory.

The QRS complexes of A.V. junctional extrasystoles are generally normal in duration. They may precisely resemble those of sinus beats or they may, as in A.V. junctional escape beats and rhythms, have a distinctly different contour which is more evident in some leads than others. The mechanism is presumably the same as that already discussed for A.V. junctional escape beats. A wide QRS complex resembling a ventricular extrasystole can presumably occur occasionally but recognition of their A.V. junctional origin would be extremely difficult from the electrocardiogram alone under these conditions.

91

Sinus Extrasystoles

Extrasystoles arising in the sinus node itself are exceedingly rare. It is, however, generally accepted that they occur and they have been produced in experiment on animals by the injection of ouabain into the sinus node. They have to be differentiated from atrial extrasystoles arising close to the sinus node, and strict electrocardiographic criteria are given for their recognition. Sinus extrasystoles are premature in time; their P waves, P–R interval and QRS complexes are identical with those of normal sinus beats in all leads, and the post-extrasystolic pause is never compensatory. In fact, the post-extrasystolic pause is usually a little less than a normal sinus cycle. The explanation given for this slightly shorter post-extrasystolic pause is that, because it is premature, the sinus extrasystole encounters first-degree sino-atrial block and thus its first manifestation in the electrocardiogram, namely its P wave, is a little delayed. By the time the next normal sinus impulse occurs, sino-atrial conduction time is normal and so the post-extrasystolic pause appears shortened. Records fulfilling these strict criteria are rare and even then it is difficult to exclude the possibility of an atrial extrasystole arising close to the sinus node.

One would expect that sinus extrasystoles would arise in a different part of the sinus node from that acting as pacemaker at the time. The direction of spread of the excitation wave over the atria would then be altered and the P waves would have a slightly different contour, as in wandering of the pacemaker within the sinus node (pages 58, 59). It is possible that such extrasystoles of sinus origin are not very rare, but their differentiation from atrial extrasystoles is at present impossible.

Return Extrasystoles or Reciprocal Beats

Return extrasystoles or reciprocal beats are of considerable physiological interest. They are sometimes called echoes. There is convincing evidence, both from animal experiments and from clinical records, that an impulse may traverse the A.V. junction by one pathway and then return in the opposite direction through a different pathway. On completion of its 'return' passage, the same impulse may cause a second contraction of the neighbouring cardiac chambers. This second contraction is called a 'return extrasystole' or a 'reciprocal beat'. The phenomenon is commonly referred to as 'reciprocal rhythm'. Reciprocal beats were first recognized as occurring in that form of A.V. junction rhythm where a retrograde P' wave follows the QRS complex. There is good evidence that the condition necessary for this type of reciprocal beat is unequal depression of conduction in the A.V. junction, so that a longitudinal section will only conduct in an antegrade direction (that is, unidirectional block). An A.V. junctional impulse may then be conducted to the atria in that part of the A.V. node which still conducts in a retrograde direction. The impulse may then enter the section with retrograde block and be conducted back again towards the ventricles. If the sum of the retrograde and antegrade conduction times is sufficiently long, the returning impulse may find the ventricles outside their refractory period and it may then elicit a second ventricular contraction. *Figure 6.22* shows diagrammatically the conditions necessary for this type of reciprocal beat.

In the electrocardiogram, this form of return extrasystole or reciprocal beat is characterized by a retrograde P' wave sandwiched between two QRS complexes. The following electrocardiographic criteria must be satisfied before a diagnosis of this form of return extrasystole can be made. A QRS complex, not preceded by a P wave, must be followed by a P' wave with an R–P interval of at least 0·12 second. A second QRS must follow with an R–R interval between the two ventricular complexes of 0·4 second or less. It is quite common for the contour of the reciprocal beat to be aberrant.

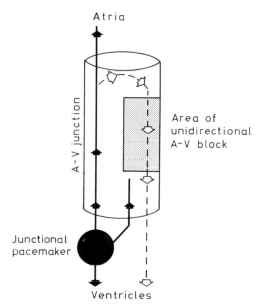

Figure 6.22—Diagram of the conditions believed to be necessary in the A.V. junction for the occurrence of reciprocal beats in A.V. junctional rhythm

Figure 6.23a, b shows 2 examples of reciprocal beats occurring in A.V. junctional rhythm. *Figure 6.23a* shows lower nodal rhythm with progressive lengthening of the R–P' intervals of successive beats, the fifth beat of the strip being a return extrasystole. The P' waves are not easily discernible in the record, but the mechanism is illustrated in the key. On rare occasions the returning impulse which elicits the ventricular reciprocal beat may also return again to the atria, eliciting a second atrial contraction followed by a third ventricular response. *Figure 6.23b* shows two reciprocal beats in succession occurring on two occasions. There is A.V. junctional rhythm with gradual increase of successive R–P' intervals; when the latter exceeds 0·22 second, the P' wave is followed by two successive reciprocal beats with an intervening P' wave. This occurs on two occasions in the record, the third and fourth, the tenth and eleventh beats being, on each occasion, two reciprocal beats in succession.

Return extrasystoles must be differentiated from other conditions in which a P wave is sandwiched between two QRS complexes. This may happen in an irregular sinus bradycardia punctuated by A.V. junctional escape beats

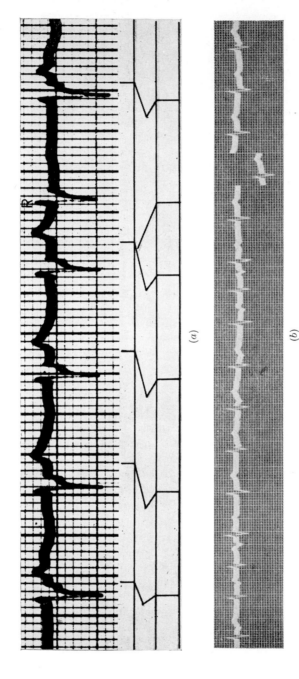

Figure 6.23—(a) A.V. junctional rhythm. The fifth beat is a reciprocal beat (see text). By courtesy of L. Schamroth. (b) Two reciprocal beats occurring in succession. Reproduced from 'Extrasystoles and Allied Arrhythmias' by D. Scherf and A. Schott by courtesy of Heinemann Medical Books

in the presence of retrograde A.V. block. *Figure 6.24* shows an example; two A.V. junctional escape beats are followed by a sinus beat with a prolonged P–R interval of 0·28 second, After two further A.V. junctional escape beats, a second sinus beat occurs.With both sinus beats (marked 1 in the record), a P wave appears sandwiched between two QRS complexes. These cannot be return extrasystoles, since the P waves are upright and of sinus origin. This form of ventricular bigeminy has sometimes been called pseudoreciprocal rhythm. Bradley and Marriott (1958) suggest the more descriptive term 'escape capture bigeminy' for this form of bigeminal rhythm.

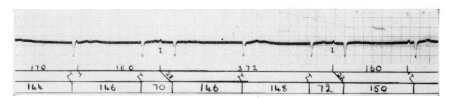

Figure 6.24—Escape capture bigeminy (see text)

Reciprocal Beats following Ventricular Extrasystoles

In the past it was considered that reciprocal beats following ventricular extrasystoles were very rare. However, Kistin (1963) has shown, using oesophageal leads, that in many cases of interpolated ventricular extra-systoles, the QRS complex following the ventricular ectopic beat is in fact a return extrasystole. The oesophageal lead clearly demonstrates a retrograde P' following the ventricular extrasystole, and this is followed in its turn by a supraventricular QRS complex. *Figure 6.25* lead II, shows an example (but without an oesophageal lead). The QRS complexes following the ventricular

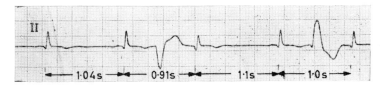

Figure 6.25—Reciprocal beats following ventricular extrasystoles (see text)

extrasystoles are almost certainly reciprocal beats, for although no preceding P' wave is visible, the interval between them and the sinus beat before the ectopic is less than a normal sinus cycle. *Figure 6.26* shows a reciprocal beat terminating a short run of ventricular tachycardia. Although again no preceding P' wave is seen, this complex cannot be sinus in origin for the R–R interval between it and the next sinus beat is 1 second and no sinus cycle approaching this length occurred anywhere else in a very long recording.

Kistin was able to demonstrate in several of his cases that ventricular to atrial conduction times fell into one or other of two different magnitudes. He considered this finding as good evidence for the presence of both 'slow' and 'fast' conduction pathways in the A.V. junction. There is a good deal of physiological evidence from other workers for the presence of at least two different pathways in the A.V. junction, both for atrioventricular and ventriculo-atrial conduction. Since several of Kistin's cases had no evidence of heart disease and were not receiving digitalis or other drugs, he postulated that retrograde followed by antegrade conduction of the ventricular ectopic impulses took place over two different pathways in the A.V. junction, and that there was no necessity to invoke the presence of special conditions to explain the reciprocal beats.

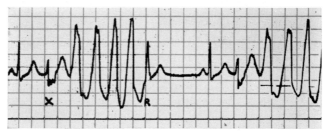

Figure 6.26—A reciprocal beat terminating a run of ventricular tachycardia (see text)

Atrial Reciprocal Beats

The term 'reversed reciprocal rhythm' has been used when two atrial contractions are elicited by the same stimulus. This occasionally occurs in the Wolff–Parkinson–White syndrome, but it has recently been shown by Kistin (1965), again using an oesophageal lead, to be not uncommon following atrial extrasystoles. In two of his cases he found two different magnitudes of A.V. conduction time suggesting again the presence of two different pathways for conduction in the A.V. junction which would provide a mechanism for reciprocal rhythm.

Aetiology of Extrasystoles

The aetiology of benign extrasystoles occurring in an otherwise normal heart is largely unknown. They may persist over years or come and go without any obvious precipitating factor. Certain conditions, such as excess consumption of tobacco, tea or coffee, are thought to precipitate extrasystoles in some subjects. Extrasystoles have also been imputed to reflexes from various parts of the gastro-intestinal tract. Certainly, extrasystoles sometimes seem to be precipitated by meals. The occurrence of extrasystoles is favoured by any of the conditions known to increase the excitability of the heart, such as CO_2 retention. Many drugs may cause extrasystoles, particularly digitalis, quinidine, sympathomimetic amines, amino-oxidase inhibitors and certain anaesthetic agents, particularly cyclopropane or fluothane. Extrasystoles occur in many forms of myocardial disease and the ventricular variety is particularly ominous following recent myocardial infarction.

An important cause of extrasystoles, which is perhaps not generally appreciated, is pregnancy. Both extrasystoles, usually ventricular, or attacks of paroxysmal tachycardia, may appear for the first time during pregnancy and may persist until parturition, when they promptly disappear within an hour. It is important to recognize this for they are usually benign and need not give rise to apprehension in the absence of known heart disease.

The relationship between digitalis and extrasystoles will be discussed in more detail in the chapter on digitalis intoxication.

Mechanism of Origin of Extrasystoles

Despite the frequency of their occurrence, there is still no general agreement about the pathogenesis of extrasystoles. Whatever view is held about their causation, the fixed coupling time of extrasystoles is generally accepted as evidence that they are in some way precipitated by the preceding beat. At present there are two main theories. During the past 20 years, the American literature particularly has been dominated by the so-called 're-entry theory'. Very briefly, this theory postulates, with little supporting evidence, the presence of unidirectional block in a peripheral twig of the conduction system. The normal impulse fails to pass this twig (because of the unidirectional block), so that the muscle it supplies receives its excitation wave from adjacent fibres. The impulse is then said to re-enter the conduction system through the area of unidirectional block, thus setting up a second excitation wave which is responsible for the extrasystole. The adherents to this theory claim that it satisfactorily explains fixed coupling. Moreover, it is said that repeated re-circulation of the excitation wave round the same pathway may explain ectopic tachycardias. Many cogent arguments have been advanced against the re-entry theory, particularly by Scherf and Schott (1953). The only form of extrasystole for which these authors accept a re-entry mechanism are return extrasystoles or reciprocal beats. They have always regarded the common type of extrasystole with fixed coupling as arising from a localized focus in the myocardium; that is, they regard extrasystoles as a manifestation of abnormal impulse formation, rather than as a disturbance of conduction. For a detailed account of their views, the reader is referred to their publications (Scherf and Schott, 1953; 1959). In summary, they regard the stimulus from the ectopic focus to be normally subthreshold, but that it becomes superthreshold when the level of threshold is lowered under certain conditions. Two possible mechanisms responsible for a lowered threshold are considered. The first is the supernormal phase of recovery. A temporary overswing in the recovery curve of excitability following a normal impulse has been demonstrated in some mammalian hearts. Although there is considerable doubt as to whether a supernormal phase of recovery occurs in the normal human heart, its presence in some clinical cases with heart disease seems to be established beyond doubt. However, the duration of the supernormal phase (during which a normally subliminal stimulus might fire off a propagated response) is very short, lasting only a few hundredths of a second. Scherf and Schott do not consider, therefore, that a supernormal phase is an acceptable explanation for all varieties of extrasystoles, though it may possibly account for those with a short coupling following acute myocardial infarction. They propose, as a more satisfactory explanation for a temporary increase in excitability following a conducted beat, the Wedensky effect which was first demonstrated in nerves by Wedensky in 1887. He showed that if, in the sciatic-gastrocnemius preparation of the frog, subliminal faradic stimulation was applied to the nerve, a single induction shock applied more proximally to the nerve would induce tetanus. The Wedensky effect is in fact a temporary period of enhanced excitability

97

following the passage of a normal impulse. Its occurrence has been demonstrated in all excitable tissues, including mammalian Purkinje fibres and, more recently, in the electrically paced human heart, by Castellanos and his colleagues (1966). Moreover, the duration of this phase of increased excitability following a normal impulse lasts as long as 0·2 second.

Nature of Subthreshold Stimulus

The precise nature of the subthreshold stimulus which may produce an extrasystole during the phase of increased excitability following a normal impulse is still uncertain. One suggestion is the occurrence of oscillating after potentials. It has been shown that, under certain conditions, the slow spontaneous diastolic depolarization which takes place in pacemaker fibres may become oscillatory and may form the necessary stimulus for extrasystoles or even sustained ectopic tachycardias. In the present state of our knowledge, much remains uncertain. It is quite possible that there is more than one mechanism responsible for extrasystoles.

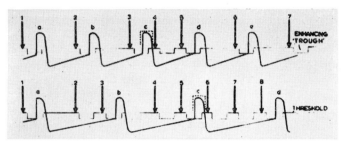

Figure 6.27—Diagram to illustrate Schamroth's theory of the origin of ventricular extrasystoles

Schamroth (1966) has recently proposed an alternative hypothesis to explain the genesis of ventricular extrasystoles. This hypothesis involves the Wedensky effect and explains the distribution of extrasystoles in both manifest and concealed bigeminy and trigeminy. He postulates that an idioventricular pacemaker in some way acquires protection from being discharged by the normal sinus impulse. Its transmembrane potential will therefore continue to undergo spontaneous diastolic depolarization. As this nears threshold, the enhanced excitability following a sinus impulse will cause it to fire a propagated impulse prematurely. Provided the dominant rhythm is substantially regular, this would result in extrasystoles with fixed coupling; the angle which the slope of diastolic depolarization of the pacemaker makes with threshold would determine whether bigeminal or trigeminal rhythm would occur. *Figure 6.27* illustrates this hypothesis diagrammatically. Although this hypothesis is attractive, it lacks any positive proof; moreover, it would certainly not explain the more common variety of ventricular extrasystoles which appear to be scattered at random throughout a record.

Clinical Features of Extrasystoles

The symptoms resulting from extrasystoles vary widely in different subjects. This is partly explicable by the wide variation in individual thresholds of discomfort. Even so, it is occasionally remarkable how an individual having very frequent extrasystoles may be quite unaware of the resulting irregularity of their heart beat. Perhaps one important factor in determining the severity of any symptoms is the presence or absence of ventricular hypertrophy. Patients with large and particularly hypertrophied hearts are probably often aware of their heart beating and will therefore be more immediately conscious of any irregularities. This may also be true of nervous individuals who often seem unduly conscious of their cardiac action, possibly because of more forcible contractions induced by catecholamines.

In general, patients who are aware of their extrasystoles have one or other of two symptoms. Either they complain of 'missed beats' or of 'palpitation'. Patients who complain of their heart 'missing' a beat, fail to feel the extrasystole, since it is usually a less forcible contraction than normal. The first post-extrasystolic beat, on the other hand, is more forcible than normal, partly owing to the greater ventricular filling during the longer diastole, and partly owing to post-extrasystolic potentiation. Patients who are more conscious of this larger beat, tend to complain of palpitation. In either event, the symptoms are more a source of apprehension than disability. In some patients, extrasystoles tend to occur in bouts lasting up to an hour at a time and then disappear. They are often more troublesome in bed at night.

If, during an extrasystole, the right atrium contracts while the tricuspid valve is closed, it results in a cannon wave in the jugular venous pulse. In some patients, this causes a particularly disagreeable sensation located in the neck or even in the head. Nervous individuals may complain of weakness, dizziness or faintness as the result of extrasystoles, but it is doubtful if such symptoms are ever organically determined unless multiple extrasystoles, amounting to runs of ectopic tachycardia, occur. Not rarely, patients are encountered who are found in regular sinus rhythm on clinical examination and in whom no extrasystoles are recorded during a routine electrocardiogram. A diagnosis of extrasystoles will then have to be based on the patient's history. This is not usually difficult if a careful history is taken; a story of 'missed beats' followed by a 'thump' is quite typical. Patients who are more conscious of the forcible post-extrasystolic beat may simply complain of attacks of palpitation. True paroxysmal ectopic tachycardia may be suspected if the attacks are sudden in onset, but this can usually be excluded by the patient's description of the palpitation as being slow and usually irregular.

Relationship of Extrasystoles to Exercise

In the vast majority of cases, extrasystoles are abolished by exercise. Quite light exercise is usually all that is necessary, even getting up and walking round the room. Paradoxically, in some patients, extrasystoles are induced by exertion and disappear with rest. This type is closely related to Gallavardin's 'tachycardie parosystique à centre excitable' (1922) which will be discussed more fully in Chapter 9.

Physical Signs of Extrasystoles

Peripheral Pulse

An extrasystole may or may not produce a palpable pulse at the wrist. Whether it does so depends on many factors, of which the most important is its coupling time. The earlier an extrasystole occurs in diastole, the less time would have been available for ventricular filling and, in consequence, the smaller is its stroke volume. Extrasystoles are by far the commonest cause of a 'dropped' beat at the wrist and can immediately be differentiated from partial heart block by auscultation of the heart.

Extrasystoles occurring later in diastole will usually produce a palpable wave at the wrist, but it is always weaker than that produced by a normal beat. Bigeminal rhythm, sometimes called 'coupled beats', due to an extrasystole following each beat of the dominant rhythm, may be mistaken for pulsus alternans. A correct diagnosis can be made from palpation of the pulse alone, for when there is alternation of strong and weak beats, there is also alternation of cycle lengths. When extrasystoles are the cause, the long cycle follows the weak beat, whereas in pulsus alternans the long cycle follows the stronger beat.

The occurrence of extrasystoles may prove helpful in differentiating between aortic valve stenosis and the hypertrophic variety of sub-aortic stenosis. The first post-extrasystolic beat is usually obviously larger than normal and this is so in aortic valve stenosis. In hypertrophic sub-aortic stenosis, on the other hand, the more forceful post-extrasystolic beat only serves to increase obstruction to left ventricular outflow and the first post-extrasystolic pulse is smaller than normal.

Extrasystoles and the Jugular Venous Pulse

Except in the presence of atrial fibrillation, it is common for an extrasystole to be associated with a cannon wave in the jugular venous pulse due to right atrial contraction occurring when the tricuspid valve is closed. This may be seen irrespective of whether the extrasystole is ventricular, A.V. junctional or atrial in origin. In ventricular extrasystoles, the cannon wave may result either from the atrial contraction of the blocked sinus impulse or from retrograde activation of the atria by the ectopic stimulus. With 'middle' or 'lower' A.V. junctional extrasystoles, there is more or less simultaneous activation of atria and ventricles, so again atrial contraction occurs when the tricuspid valve is closed. Although with atrial extrasystoles, atrial activation precedes ventricular activation, a cannon wave may still occur if the extrasystole has a short coupling time, for then the atria contract before the ventricular systole of the previous beat of the dominant rhythm is over. It may be possible to appreciate this clinically with a finger on one or other carotid artery. The cannon wave may then be seen to coincide with a normal carotid pulse, and the feebler pulse of the extrasystole will be felt to follow. In principle it is possible to recognize blocked atrial extrasystoles by the occurrence of a cannon wave in the neck, coincident with the carotid pulse and followed by a pause.

When the rhythm of the heart is very irregular owing to frequent extrasystoles, coincident cannon waves in the neck immediately exclude atrial fibrillation as the cause, since atrial contractions are absent in the latter arrhythmia.

Auscultatory Findings in Extrasystoles

When extrasystoles fall early in diastole, they may be too feeble to open the pulmonary and aortic valves. Only the first sound of A.V. valve closure will then be heard on auscultation. The nature of this single sound will be apparent since it will coincide with a pause in the peripheral pulse. Extrasystoles occurring later in diastole will normally produce audible first and second heart sounds. When the extrasystoles originate in one or other ventricle, the two ventricles contract asynchronously and both the first and second heart sounds can be heard to be widely split. This finding alone suggests that the extrasystole is ventricular in origin, but it is not diagnostic, for supraventricular extrasystoles with aberrant intraventricular conduction may show the same phenomenon. On the other hand, absence of wide splitting of the heart sounds of an extrasystole may be taken as evidence of its supraventricular origin.

If it can be observed that an extrasystole with widely split first and second sounds is preceded by a venous cannon wave in the neck, a clinical diagnosis of an atrial extrasystole with aberrant intraventricular conduction may at least be suspected at the bedside. It can be an instructive and entertaining clinical exercise to attempt to recognize the site of origin of extrasystoles before the final arbiter, the electrocardiogram, is seen.

Extrasystoles and Murmurs

Cardiac murmurs may be modified by extrasystoles, and analysis of such changes can sometimes be of value in the clinical assessment of a case. For example, the ejection murmur associated with aortic or pulmonary valve stenosis will be perceptibly quieter or even absent during an extrasystole if the lesion is severe. Correspondingly, the murmur of the first post-extra-systolic beat will be louder and associated with a more pronounced thrill. Pan-systolic murmurs of A.V. valve regurgitation are often louder with extrasystoles which are known to accentuate valvular incompetence.

Treatment of Extrasystoles

The treatment of extrasystoles will be discussed in Chapters 12 and 13.

PARASYSTOLE

In addition to escape beats and extrasystoles, there is a third and important variety of ectopic beat called parasystole. Parasystolic beats are most often ventricular, but atrial and nodal parasystole occurs.

Ventricular Parasystole

There is convincing evidence that ventricular parasystole results from an idioventricular pacemaker which is protected from being discharged by impulses of the dominant rhythm by entrance block. The parasystolic focus is thus able to produce regular impulses at its own inherent rate, and these impulses will invade the surrounding myocardium wherever they find it outside its refractory period, producing an ectopic beat. It is important to recognize parasystole, since, in the majority of instances, it is associated with organic heart disease.

Parasystole belongs to the group of arrhythmias called the pararrhythmias. These are defined by Scherf and Schott (1953) as a 'group of arrhythmias in which two (or rarely more) centres concurrently and independently produce impulses which yield contractions of the whole heart or part of the heart, without disturbance of conduction of the normal impulse being responsible for the arrhythmia'.

The commonest situation in which two independent pacemakers control the heart is complete A.V. block, but this is excluded from the pararrhythmias by the above definition. The pararrhythmias fall into two distinct groups, namely parasystole and A.V. dissociation. Both these arrhythmias have in common the presence of two (or more) independent pacemakers in the heart and in this sense are pararrhythmias (two parallel rhythms). They differ, however, in so many other respects that they are not being considered together here. Atrioventricular dissociation, with and without capture beats, is considered on its own in Chapter 10.

There are three electrocardiographic criteria for identifying parasystole. (1) The ectopic beats, being independent of the dominant rhythm, show wide

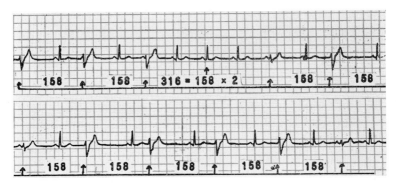

Figure 6.28—Simple ventricular parasystole (see text)

variations in coupling time to the beats preceding them. (2) The interectopic intervals (that is, the time intervals between two successive ectopic beats) always have a simple arithmetical relationship to each other, being all fairly precise multiples of the parasystolic pacemaker rate. (3) From time to time, an impulse of the dominant rhythm may invade part of the ventricles at the same time as an impulse from the parasystolic centre, resulting in a fusion beat which has a contour in the electrocardiogram intermediate between a beat of the dominant rhythm and a parasystolic beat. It is desirable to satisfy all three criteria; that is, variable coupling times, arithmetically related interectopic intervals and occasional fusion beats, before a diagnosis of parasystole is made.

Figure 6.28 shows an example of simple ventricular parasystole. There is basic sinus rhythm which is disturbed by fairly frequent ventricular ectopic beats. Variations in coupling time of the ectopic beats is evident to the naked eye, particularly in the second row. Most interectopic intervals measure 1·58 seconds, but the third interectopic interval (between the third and fourth parasystolic beats) measures 3·16 seconds which is exactly double 1·58 seconds. One parasystolic beat was missed out; the time it was due is indicated on the record by an arrow. Clearly, the parasystolic centre discharged during the refractory period of a sinus beat and its impulse could not,

102

therefore, invade the surrounding myocardium. The fourth parasystolic beat (terminating the longer interectopic interval) is a fusion beat with a contour intermediate between a ventricular ectopic and a sinus beat.

It has already been mentioned that, in order to explain parasystole, it is necessary to assume that the ectopic pacemaker is in some way protected from premature discharge by the impulses of the dominant rhythm. Although the nature of this 'protection' is not yet understood, it is generally referred to as 'entrance block'. Possible mechanisms will be discussed below. The manifest rate of a parasystolic centre is usually slow; when two parasystolic beats occur in succession (without any intervening beats of the dominant rhythm) the interval between them is taken as the 'ectopic cycle length'. *Figure 6.29* shows an example of a rather more complex ventricular parasystole complicating an atrial arrhythmia. The two rows are continuous and, in the

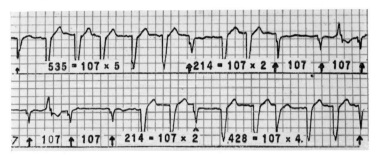

Figure 6.29—Ventricular parasystole complicating an atrial arrhythmia (see text)]

second row, two parasystolic beats occur in succession. The interval between them measures 1·07 seconds which may be taken as the ectopic cycle length. All other interectopic intervals in the record are precise multiples of 1·07 seconds and numerous fusion beats are present.

Figure 6.30 shows an example of ventricular parasystole in atrial fibrillation. When examining records containing extrasystoles, a rough check should always be made that their coupling times remain constant. This can readily be done by eye. If the coupling times appear to vary, a suspicion of parasystole should be raised and the record quickly searched for fusion beats. Finally, the interectopic intervals should be measured to demonstrate any simple arithmetical relationship. This process is simplified if the ectopic cycle length can be readily measured from two successive parasystolic complexes with no intervening beats. While, strictly speaking, all interectopic intervals should be precise multiples of this, minor variations occur. There are at least two reasons for this. The calculated ectopic cycle lengths may show minor variations which rarely exceed 0·05 second, but which may mount up if the manifest interectopic intervals are long. It is also sometimes found that an interectopic interval measures rather less than an exact multiple of the manifest ectopic cycle length. This has been explained on the basis of conduction delay of the second of two successive parasystolic beats. It is suggested that the conduction pathway between the ectopic centre and the surrounding myocardium may still be partially refractory when the second parasystolic beat occurs, so that the manifest cycle length is in fact slightly longer than the true cycle lengths. When several sinus beats intervene, the conduction pathway has fully recovered so that the next parasystolic beat appears without delay and the interectopic interval may then be slightly shorter than a precise multiple of the manifest ectopic cycle length.

Calculations of the interectopic cycle lengths do not always work out as precisely as in *Figures 6.28* and *6.29*. For example, in *Figure 6.30* the calculated interectopic cycle length appeared to range between 159 and 166 hundredths of a second. The question arises as to how much variation in calculated interectopic cycle length can be permitted and still support a diagnosis of parasystole. This difficulty particularly arises when there are very long interectopic intervals. Singer and Winterberg pointed out in 1920 that this difficulty arises when the average in the length of the interectopic intervals

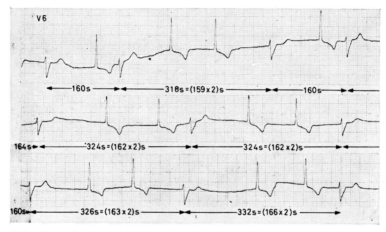

Figure 6.30—Ventricular parasystole occurring in atrial fibrillation. The three rows are continuous. The parasystolic cycle length appears to vary between 1·59 and 1·66 seconds

multiplied by the number of ectopic cycle lengths supposed to be contained in a long interectopic interval attains the length calculated for the ectopic cycle lengths. They express this by a simple formula: $E = x(\pm d)$. In this formula, E is the average cycle length, $\pm d$ the maximum variations from this average, and x the number of ectopic cycle lengths in the interectopic interval. This means that the greatest number (x) of the cycle lengths in a long interectopic interval, which can be used as supporting a parasystolic origin, is that which multiplied by the greatest variations (d) from the average ectopic cycle length does not exceed the cycle length (E) itself (Scherf and Schott, 1953).

In ordinary circumstances the rate of discharge of a parasystolic centre must always be less than that of the dominant rhythm, otherwise the ectopic rhythm would gain control of the whole heart. It would then be indistinguishable from any other variety of ectopic tachycardia.

When records of parasystole are carefully analysed, it is found that from time to time a parasystolic beat fails to appear, although it was due at a time when the surrounding myocardium should have been outside its refractory phase. There are two different reasons why this occurs. First, 'exit block' may develop around the ectopic focus, so that, although it discharges on time, its impulse encounters refractory tissue in its path and is thus prevented from invading the rest of the myocardium which is outside its refractory phase. A second reason is that the activity of the parasystolic mechanism may be intermittent. Intermittent parasystole is not uncommon. For reasons which are not quite clear, the first ectopic beat of a bout of intermittent parasystole

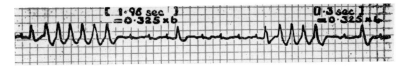

Figure 6.31—Intermittent ventricular parasystole (see text)

always has a fixed coupling to the preceding beat of the dominant rhythm, though of course subsequent ectopics do not. *Figure 6.31* shows a record which illustrates both these mechanisms. It shows two short bouts of ventricular tachycardia with intervening isolated ventricular ectopic beats of the same shape. Both paroxysms of tachycardia commence with an extrasystole which has the same coupling time to the preceding sinus beat. The isolated extrasystoles, however, have obviously different coupling times to the beats which precede them. (This pattern kept repeating itself throughout a long record, of which this is a short extract.) The cycle length of the tachycardia is 0·325 second, and the interval between the end of each paroxysm and the isolated ectopics which follow it is in each case an exact multiple of 0·325 second, clearly indicating that during these intervals the ectopic centre continued to discharge, but its impulses were concealed, owing to exit block. On the other hand, no similar time relationship exists between the isolated ectopic beats and any part of the paroxysms which follow, indicating that the parasystolic mechanism is intermittent. This record may be regarded as showing intermittent parasystolic ventricular tachycardia with exit block. A further example of parasystolic ventricular tachycardia will be given in Chapter 8.

Nature of Entrance Block and Exit Block

The exact nature of the protective block around a parasystolic focus, and of the block which sometimes prevents its impulses becoming manifest, is uncertain. When there is entrance block without exit block, the 'block' is clearly unidirectional and must be physiological rather than anatomical. There is evidence that, at least in some cases, the rate of discharge of the ectopic pacemaker may be much higher than is apparent in the record. If the rate of discharge of the ectopic focus were high, the juxtaposed tissues would be continually maintained in a refractory state, which would act as a barrier to penetration of the focus by impulses of the dominant rhythm. This could well be associated with an exit block with a 2:1, 3:1 or 4:1 conduction ratio which would result in a relatively long manifest ectopic cycle length. In other words, ventricular parasystole could be explained as ventricular tachycardia with exit block. Entrance block need not then be postulated. A number of examples of parasystole have been published (Scherf and

Bornemann, 1961; Schamroth, 1962) in which occasional short runs of ventricular tachycardia occurred revealing the true cycle length of the focus, the manifest ectopic cycle length in other parts of the record being a precise multiple of the much shorter cycle length of the tachycardia.

Effect of Parasystole on the Dominant Cardiac Rhythm

The effect of ventricular parasystole on the dominant rhythm is closely similar to that of ordinary ventricular extrasystoles with fixed coupling. If the dominant rhythm is slow, parasystolic beats may be interpolated. More often the post-ectopic pause is compensatory with no shift of the sinus rhythm. Sometimes the stimulus of a parasystolic beat is conducted in a retrograde direction to the atria and may reach and discharge the sinus node. As with ventricular extrasystoles with retrograde conduction to the atria, the post-ectopic pause may then be shorter than compensatory, fortuitously compensatory or occasionally longer than compensatory, depending on the time of discharge of the sinus node and whether its automaticity is temporarily depressed.

Supraventricular Parasystole

Parasystolic rhythms of atrial or A.V. junctional origin are less common than the ventricular variety. *Figure 6.32* shows an example of A.V. junctional parasystole with aberration.

Atrial parasystole is uncommon but clear-cut cases have been described

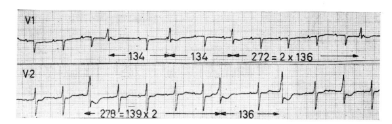

Figure 6.32—A.V. junctional parasystole. The A.V. junctional beats show aberrant conduction

(Schamroth, 1971). The arrhythmia is characterized by P–P' intervals which are very variable (that is, the coupling times of the atrial ectopic beats vary widely) but P'–P' intervals are constant. The variability of the P–P' intervals simply reflect the differences in rate between the sinus rate and that of the ectopic atrial pacemaker. The rate of the parasystolic atrial pacemaker is usually slower than the sinus rate.

Sinus Parasystole

Since the essential feature of parasystole is the simultaneous co-existence of two pacemakers in the heart, one of which is protected by entrance block from being discharged by the other, it is theoretically possible for sinus parasystole to exist where sinus rhythm persists in spite of the presence of a simultaneous rhythm from a lower pacemaker. In the absence of A.V.

dissociation as described in Chapter 10, a convincing example has been described by Schamroth (1971) in which sinus rhythm coincided with an atrial ectopic rhythm which clearly did not discharge the sinus node wherever in the sinus cycle it occurred. This demonstrated that the sinus node was completely protected by entrance block throughout its entire cycle length.

CHAPTER 7

ECTOPIC TACHYCARDIAS—ATRIAL ARRHYTHMIAS

PHYSIOLOGICAL CONSIDERATIONS

Disturbances of normal atrial rhythm may be primary or secondary. 'Secondary' disturbances of atrial rhythm are those in which the atria are activated by ectopic stimuli which have originated outside the atria, either in the A.V. junction or the ventricle. Since the excitation wave reaches the atria in a retrograde direction, the P' waves are inverted in leads II, III and AVF. In primary atrial arrhythmias, the abnormal stimulus originates in one, or more, pacemakers in the atria themselves. They include atrial extrasystoles, atrial tachycardia, with or without A.V. block, atrial flutter, impure flutter and finally atrial fibrillation. Each of these varieties of atrial arrhythmia may occur in paroxysmal or chronic form. This will be discussed in more detail in the clinical section of this chapter.

Until comparatively recently, it was believed that the underlying mechanism of atrial flutter and atrial fibrillation was profoundly different from that of atrial extrasystoles and atrial tachycardia. In 1920 Lewis suggested that atrial flutter and atrial fibrillation were due to an excitation wave which circulated continuously round a ring of muscle surrounding the junctions of the superior and inferior venae cavae with the right atrium. This was known as the 'circus' theory and envisaged the rate of travel of the excitation wave to be such that excitable tissue was always present just ahead. The theory was suggested by the experimental work of Mines (1913), who cut a ring of artial and ventricular muscle from a tortoise's heart and showed that by appropriate electrical stimulation a wave of contraction could be initiated, which would then travel continuously round the ring for periods up to several hours. Lewis attributed both flutter and fibrillation to this primary 'mother wave' circulating round the origins of the two great veins. 'Daughter' waves were said to radiate from this primary wave over the rest of both atria. In flutter, a single circus movement was thought to occur round a fixed unalterable path, while in fibrillation the path followed was thought to be uneven, constantly altering in detail, but in general remaining the same. Lewis produced cogent experimental evidence to support his 'circus' theory; the reader is referred to his original publications for the details. The circus theory became generally accepted and was virtually unopposed for almost 30 years. Since, however, it is a common clinical observation that the same patients might exhibit at different times either atrial extrasystoles, atrial tachycardia, atrial flutter or atrial fibrillation, some physicians were reluctant to accept the view that there was a fundamental difference in their pathogenesis. Towards the end of the 1940s, evidence began to accumulate that the circus theory was incorrect. In 1948, Scherf, Romano and Terranova injected aconitine into the sinus node. This produced atrial tachycardia, and simultaneous stimulation of the vagus often resulted in atrial fibrillation. They found that if the site of aconitine injection was cooled, fibrillation would cease, but it reappeared when cooling was stopped. They considered that a circus movement of excitation was inconsistent with their findings in explaining atrial fibrillation and suggested that atrial flutter and fibrillation were initiated by rapid impulse formation in a single centre. A few years later, Prinzmetal and his colleagues (1952) produced further evidence refuting the circus theory. Very high-speed cinematography of atrial flutter (2,000 frames per second) failed to demonstrate any evidence of a circulating wave of contraction, and this was confirmed by cathode-ray oscillograph recordings of the time of arrival of the excitation wave at different points in the atria. Their general conclusions, like those of Scherf, Romano and Terranova, were that atrial flutter and fibrillation originated from, and were perpetuated by, a single rapidly discharging ectopic focus.

For many years it has been generally accepted that recurrent attacks of supraventricular tachycardia are due to an ectopic pacemaker situated either in the atria or the A.V. junction which has suddenly acquired a rapid rate of spontaneous diastolic depolarization. As will be seen in Chapter 11, very similar attacks of supraventricular tachycardia are a common clinical feature in the Wolff–Parkinson–White syndrome and there is now much evidence that these are due to a circus movement involving two pathways connecting the atria and ventricles. A similar mechanism for attacks of supraventricular tachycardia in the absence of the W.P.W. syndrome was originally suggested by Iliescu and Sebastiani in 1923 and this mechanism was strongly supported by Barker, Wilson and Johnston in 1943. However this view gained little credence presumably because only one pathway was known to connect the atria and ventricles in subjects without the W.P.W. syndrome. However in 1956 Moe and his colleagues produced strong experimental evidence in animals for the presence of a dual A.V. conduction system. They suggested that fibres of the A.V. node could be longitudinally dissociated at least in its upper part, the pathways uniting in the lower node to form a final common pathway. If this were true in the human heart the anatomical basis would exist for a reciprocating tachycardia apart from the Wolff–Parkinson–White syndrome. Indeed the occurrence of reciprocal beats and reciprocal rhythms in clinical traces demand the presence of two A.V. conduction pathways to explain their occurrence (Schamroth and Yoshonis, 1969).

Many authors have recently advanced both clinical and electrophysiological evidence that the underlying mechanism in many cases of supraventricular tachycardia is a reciprocating tachycardia involving two separate pathways in the A.V. node. For example, in a study of six successive cases of supraventricular tachycardia, Bigger and Goldreyer (1970) found, using sophisticated electrophysiological techniques, that a re-entry mechanism for the attacks rather than a rapidly discharging focus was the only acceptable explanation. More recently the same authors have shown, using His bundle electrograms, that the site of re-entry is the A.V. node. The existence of two separate pathways could only become manifest if they had different physiological properties. It is simpler to envisage them as having different refractory periods. A premature supraventricular beat, such as an atrial extrasystole, may find one path in a relative refractory phase and the other still in the absolute refractory phase. The impulse will then be conducted slowly along the relative refractory path and reach the final common pathway at a time when the second pathway has recovered excitability. The excitation wave will then divide into two fronts, one completing the journey to the ventricles down the final common pathway, and the other returning to the atria by the second pathway. Such an event occurring once is termed an 'atrial echo'. Alternatively a circus movement may be started resulting in a reciprocating tachycardia.

One would therefore expect that supraventricular tachycardia should start with an atrial extrasystole falling in the relatively refractory period and having a long P–R interval. In practice this is found to be invariably so, whereas atrial extrasystoles in the same patient falling outside the relative refractory period do not initiate supraventricular tachycardia. Moreover, the

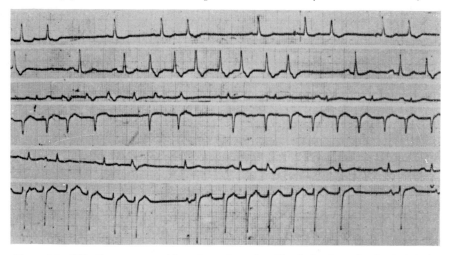

Figure 7.1—This illustrates a repetitive reciprocating tachycardia, the first beat of each episode begins with an atrial extrasystole and a prolonged P–R interval

first few cycles of supraventricular tachycardia are found to alternate in length as one would expect from the reciprocating mechanism but not from a rapidly discharging focus.

Figure 7.1 shows an example of a recurrent reciprocating tachycardia, each bout of which is precipitated by an atrial extrasystole with a long P–R interval. In such a record it is possible confidently to diagnose a reciprocating tachycardia, but not uncommonly in supraventricular tachycardia some degree of A.V. block may occur, as, for example, in the well-known P.A.T. with block due to digitalis intoxication (*see* Chapter 15). The presence of A.V. block of either Wenckebach type or a 2:1 A.V. block must exclude a reciprocating tachycardia for it implies interruption or the reciprocating pathway which would terminate the arrhythmia.

Clinically the atrial arrhythmias appear to fall into five groups; namely, atrial extrasystoles, atrial tachycardia, atrial flutter, impure flutter and atrial fibrillation. These may conveniently be classified according to the atrial rate and this is shown in Table 7.1.

TABLE 7.1

Rhythm	Rate per minute
Atrial extrasystoles	—
Atrial tachycardia	100–250
Atrial flutter	250–350
Impure flutter	350–450
Atrial fibrillation	450–600

Although this classification of the atrial arrhythmias based on the atrial rate is clinically convenient, it is not entirely physiologically satisfactory. The atrial arrhythmias show other differences beside their rate. For example, vagal stimulation (via the carotid sinus) may terminate an atrial tachycardia but in atrial flutter it will only serve to increase the degree of A.V. block without influencing the atrial rate.

Atrial Tachycardia

The majority of cases of paroxysmal tachycardia are due to recurrent episodes of atrial tachycardia. As has already been discussed above, most of these now seem to be due to a re-entry mechanism or reciprocating tachycardia and not, as was previously thought, to a rapidly discharging ectopic focus. With atrial rates between 100 and 180 per minute there is usually 1:1 A.V. conduction. The presence of any degree of A.V. block must imply that this is not a reciprocating tachycardia but is arising from an ectopic focus. The presence of A.V. block depends on many factors in addition to the atrial rate. For example, in children and particularly in infants the A.V. junction may continue to conduct every impulse with the 1:1 ventricular response with rates as high as 300 per minute. In general, however, in adults the maximum rate at which the A.V. junction will conduct with a 1·1 ratio is about 200 per minute. When the atrial rate is higher than this some degree of A.V. block is usually present. Block may also occur at lower rates, particularly in the presence of heart disease or as the result of digitalis medication. The degree of block is variable; it may take the form of 2:1 block with a ventricular rate of half the atrial rate or more irregular bouts of block may occur. Atrial tachycardia with A.V. block is an important manifestation of digitalis intoxication and will be discussed in detail in Chapter 15. On the other hand an apparent identical arrhythmia may occur in undigitalized patients and then digitalis may be the definitive treatment.

Atrial Flutter

Atrial Arrhythmias and Pregnancy

All forms of ectopic atrial rhythms may occur in pregnancy and, as mentioned earlier (page 96), they may be entirely benign and promptly disappear after parturition. However, pregnancy in women with organic heart disease may be associated with atrial extrasystoles, atrial fibrillation and paroxysmal or sustained ectopic rhythms, and it is probable that the majority of cases of post-partum cardiomyopathy with atrial arrhythmias are due to previously unrecognized heart disease. One of the authors has recently reported a family exhibiting a cardiomyopathy principally affecting the atria characterized by ectopic supraventricular arrhythmias progressing to persistent atrial standstill. In one female member two pregnancies were each associated with a variety of atrial arrhythmias 12 years before the cardiomyopathy was clinically recognized. In five of the six women reported with this condition, pregnancy appeared to have been associated with arrhythmias or heart failure which later resolved. Latent cardiac disease should therefore always be considered before arrhythmias associated with pregnancy are considered benign.

With atrial rates between 250 and 350 per minute, atrial flutter is said to be present, and this has distinctive electrocardiographic appearances to be discussed below. The atrial rate is usually perfectly regular, and in the majority of cases there is 2:1 A.V. block with a regular ventricular rate which is exactly half the atrial rate; more complex forms of A.V. block are occasionally seen with regular or irregular Wenckebach periods or sometimes higher degrees of block; that is, 4:1 or greater. With atrial rates up to 350 per minute, co-ordinated atrial contractions will usually be present with regular 'A' waves recordable in atrial pressure traces. With rates above 350 per minute, co-ordinated mechanical contractions of the atria disappear and pressure records show no 'A' waves but simply 'V' waves. Coincident with the disappearance of effective mechanical atrial contraction, the ventricular rhythm always becomes completely irregular. The physiology of these two characteristics of very rapid atrial rates, that is, disappearance of mechanical atrial contraction and a totally irregular ventricular response, merit further discussion.

Physiology of Atrial Fibrillation

Burn (1960) and his colleagues at Oxford devised a simple technique for producing atrial fibrillation in the experimental animal and their work has shed considerable light on the physiology of this arrhythmia. They found that rapid electrical stimulation of the exposed atrium (800 per minute) would not of itself induce any lasting effect on the electrocardiogram. As soon as stimulation was stopped, normal rhythm returned. If, however, the specimen was perfused with a solution of acetylcholine and then rapidly stimulated electrically, atrial fibrillation developed which persisted after stimulation was stopped for as long as the infusion of acetylcholine continued. As soon as the infusion was stopped, fibrillation changed to flutter and normal rhythm reappeared within a minute. It has been shown by means of intracellular recordings that the effect of acetylcholine on atrial muscle fibres is to shorten the duration of the action potential by increasing the rate of repolarization. In other words, acetylcholine shortens the refractory period of atrial fibres so that they become excitable again much more quickly.

Infusion of acetylcholine alone is insufficient by itself to induce atrial fibrillation. Its only obvious effect on the cardiogram is to slow the rate of discharge of the pacemaker of the preparation. A short period of rapid electrical stimulation will immediately induce atrial fibrillation during acetylcholine infusion, so that, in the experimental preparation, both factors are required.

There is ample experimental evidence that rapid stimulation of the atria slows atrial conduction velocity but does so unevenly in different parts of the atria. Burn and his colleagues explain (experimental) atrial fibrillation as being due to two factors: a short refractory period, and uneven rates of conduction from a rapid source of stimulation. To quote Burn's words—'if the rate of conduction varied along different paths, an impulse proceeding to a distant point A (in the atria) might arrive sooner than it would arrive at a distant point B, even though B was adjacent to A. Thus, A would contract before B. When B contracted a little later, excitation from B would spread to A'. This could not happen if the refractory period of A was normal; since, however, the refractory period of A is very short (owing to acetylcholine), A is again responsive when the stimulus reaches B. As long as the refractory period remains short, A and B will continue to excite each other alternately without the necessity for a further stimulus. Once fibrillation starts, individual parts of the atria contract out of phase with each other, but with a short refractory period they will continue to stimulate each other indefinitely. Since the different areas of the atria are contracting out of phase with each other, co-ordinated contraction is lost and there is no mechanical effect.

It is of interest that Mackenzie (1908), who first differentiated atrial fibrillation from other forms of irregular pulse, first called it atrial paralysis. He used simultaneous recordings of the arterial and jugular venous pulses and found that, in atrial fibrillation, evidence of atrial contraction disappeared from the venous pulse tracing.

Bennett and Pentecost (1970) have shown in patients with acute myocardial infarction that atrial extrasystoles will precipitate atrial fibrillation if they fall in the vulnerable period of the atria while those falling later in the cardiac cycle than this do not do so.

Ventricular Response in Atrial Fibrillation

Atrial fibrillation is characterized clinically by an irregularly irregular ventricular rhythm, the length of successive ventricular cycles showing a completely haphazard pattern. This complete irregularity is difficult to explain. Presumably the A.V. junction is bombarded by a rapid series of atrial impulses which it cannot possibly conduct. One would expect that the A.V. junction would conduct at its maximum rate in a substantially regular fashion. Almost certainly the explanation lies in concealed conduction. If the stimuli reaching the A.V. junction vary in strength, some will be conducted decrementally, failing to reach the ventricle, but will leave refractory tissue in their wake. Decremental conduction of an impulse in the A.V. junction, so that it fails to reach the ventricles, will not be recorded on the electrocardiogram but may be deduced from unexpected delay of a subsequent impulse.

As Langendorf, Pick and Katz (1965) have pointed out, if atrial fibrillation in a digitalized patient changes to atrial flutter, the ventricular rate may become appreciably faster. They suggest that this is owing to the absence of repeated concealed conduction of atrial impulses, which occurs in fibrillation and which limits the number of completely conducted impulses which the A.V. junction can pass. It is certainly a common experience in practice that it is much more difficult to slow the ventricular rate in atrial flutter with digitalis than it is in atrial fibrillation, and this is probably owing to absence of frequent abortive and concealed conduction in the former arrhythmia.

There is, of course, no direct evidence that atrial fibrillation in the human heart is the result of the same two factors which are responsible for it in the experimental animal; that is, rapid stimulation and a short refractory period initiating a self perpetuating mechanism. Atrial fibrillation is often heralded by frequent atrial extrasystoles indicating the presence of a potential fast ectopic pacemaker, and it is not uncommon to record a rapid sequence of atrial ectopic beats changing into atrial fibrillation (*Figure 7.2*). It is well known that stretching potential ectopic pacemakers increases the slope of

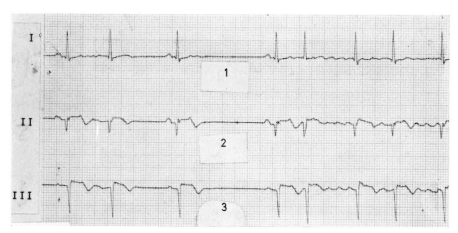

Figure 7.2—Development of atrial fibrillation in a patient with sinus rhythm and frequent atrial extra-systoles

diastolic depolarization and hence their inherent rate. This may well be a contributory factor to the high incidence of atrial fibrillation in mitral valve disease which is associated with distension of the left atrium. Patients, particularly with mitral valve disease, are commonly found with frequent atrial extrasystoles for several weeks or months as a prelude to atrial fibrillation. This seems particularly to be so when the atrial ectopics are multifocal in origin, and some authorities believe that human atrial fibrillation is due to rapid, asynchronous discharge of several ectopic pacemakers simultaneously.

In his study of the human sino-atrial node, Hudson (1960) found evidence that disease of the primary pacemaker itself was invariably present post-mortem in hearts which had manifested atrial fibrillation in life. There is other evidence, to be discussed in Chapter 12, that disease of the sinus node itself may be an important contributory factor preventing restoration of sinus rhythm by modern techniques or leading to early relapse after successful reversion.

Variation in Ventricular Rate in Chronic Atrial Arrhythmias

In chronic established atrial arrhythmias, such as atrial fibrillation, atrial tachycardia with block and even in atrial flutter, the ventricular rate can still increase in response to exercise or emotion. Since the atrial rate is fixed and largely or wholly uninfluenced by nervous control, it is at first sight difficult to see how this is achieved. It is known that the duration of both the relative and absolute refractory periods of the A.V. junction are influenced by autonomic nervous tone. A decrease in vagal or an increase in sympathetic tone, in response to exercise, would shorten the refractory period of the A.V. junction and permit more impulses to be transmitted to the ventricle. *Figure 7.3a* shows the electrocardiogram of a patient with an atrial tachycardia of 220 per minute and varying A.V. block. At rest the ventricular rate is 86 per minute. *Figure 7.3b* recorded after exercise shows a fixed 2:1 A.V. conduction ratio with a ventricular rate of 110 per minute. *Figure 7.3c,*

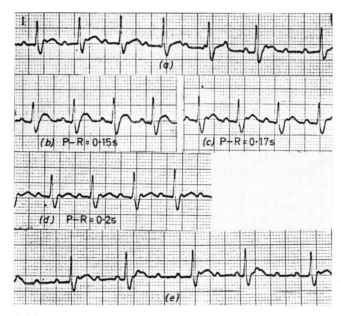

Figure 7.3—Atrial tachycardia with A.V. block. Changes in the P–R interval of the conducted beats following exercise are well shown

d and *e* were recorded at intervals of approximately one minute during recovery from exercise. Although at first a 2:1 A.V. conduction ratio is maintained, the P–R interval of the conducted atrial impulse shows progressive lengthening until, in *Figure 7.3e*, the original higher degree of A.V. block returns and the ventricular rate falls again to 86 per minute. Clearly, the mechanism of the changed ventricular rate is alteration in the refractory period of the A.V. junction in response to exercise. It is well known that with normal sinus rhythm the refractory period of the heart shortens as the rate increases. In atrial arrhythmias (with A.V. block) the converse mechanism operates. A shortened refractory period results in an increased ventricular rate. The variation of the ventricular rate is very restricted in atrial tachycardia but is much more flexible in atrial fibrillation, particularly in digitalized patients, when the ventricular rate in response to exercise may increase from a resting value in the low seventies per minute to over 150 per minute.

The Electrocardiogram in Atrial Arrhythmias

The electrocardiographic appearances of atrial extrasystoles has already been discussed. In simple atrial tachycardia without A.V. block, the electrocardiogram is characterized by a rapid succession of QRS complexes which are usually normal in duration and resemble more or less precisely those of normal sinus beats. Each QRS complex is preceded by a P wave which is usually of abnormal contour. With rapid rates, the P waves may be difficult

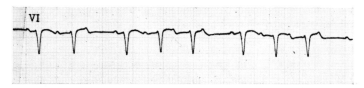

Figure 7.4—Atrial tachycardia with a Wenckebach type of A.V. conduction anomaly

to identify, often being buried in the preceding T waves. In children, very rapid atrial rates may still be conducted in a 1:1 ratio to the ventricles, with normal QRS complexes. In adults, when the atrial rate exceeds about 180 per minute, some degree of A.V. block develops; sometimes A.V. block appears at slower atrial rates, particularly in the presence of heart disease or with digitalis medication. A diagnosis of atrial tachycardia may be made

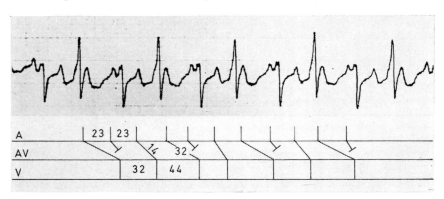

Figure 7.5—Atrial flutter with Wenckebach conduction and a 3:2 conduction ratio with alternating ventricular aberration. For further explanation see text

when QRS complexes of normal duration are preceded by P waves of abnormal contour with an atrial rate of 100 per minute or more.

Atrial tachycardias are usually precisely regular, but irregularities in the ventricular rhythm may result from varying degrees of A.V. block. *Figure 7.4* shows a regular atrial tachycardia with a rate of 150 per minute. The ventricular rhythm is irregular owing to a Wenckebach type of A.V. conduction.

An instructive example of atrial flutter recorded from an undigitalized patient with mitral valve disease is illustrated in *Figure 7.5*. The atrial rate is 300 per minute and there is a Wenckebach type of A.V. conduction with

116

a 3:2 ratio. Alternate QRS complexes are different in contour due to aberration. The key below the record shows the conduction sequence. The P–R interval of the first beat of each Wenckebach period is 0·14 second and the QRS complex is aberrant. The second atrial impulse of each period is conducted with a P–R interval of 0·32 second and the QRS complex of this beat is normal. The third atrial impulse is blocked and just precedes the second conducted QRS. This mechanism results in a bigeminal ventricular rhythm with alternating ventricular aberration. As was described on page 40, Damato and colleagues (1969) have shown that the P–R interval is divisible into two parts. The first atrial impulse of each Wenckebach period in *Figure 7.5* is conducted with a normal P–R interval and therefore presumably a normal P–H interval. Since the H–Q interval is not altered, the impulse arrives at the division of the bundle of His before the right bundle branch has recovered. The second atrial impulse of each period is conducted with a prolonged P–R interval of 0·32 second which is presumably mainly due to prolongation of the P–H interval. This delay permits full recovery of the right bundle branch so that when the impulse reaches the division of the bundle of His, it is normally conducted.

Atrial Tachycardia with Exit Block

It has already been pointed out that exit block may develop round ventricular ectopic pacemakers. Phibbs (1963) reported a case of atrial tachycardia showing exit block. *Figure 7.6a, b* shows two examples of apparent irregularity of an atrial pacemaker due to this cause.

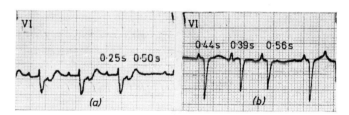

Figure 7.6—Atrial tachycardia with exit block: (a) shows a sudden doubling of the atrial cycle length due to 2:1 exit block; (b) shows a Wenckebach type of exit block with characteristic progressive shortening of successive cycles

Difficulties in the Electrocardiographic Diagnosis of Atrial Tachycardia

There are three main sources of difficulty in the electrocardiographic diagnosis of atrial tachycardia. (1) The P waves may be difficult to identify when they are buried in the preceding T waves. (2) In atrial tachycardia with 2:1 A.V. block, the blocked atrial impulse may again be hidden in the T wave and, since the ventricular rate may be relatively slow, the condition may be mistaken for sinus rhythm. (3) A third source of difficulty occurs when the QRS complexes are aberrant in contour, suggesting a ventricular origin of the tachycardia.

Difficulty in Identifying the P Wave

Figure 7.7 is an example of this problem. It shows a strip of lead II with QRS complexes of normal duration occurring at a rate of 240 per minute. No P waves can be clearly identified in this or any other lead. While, almost

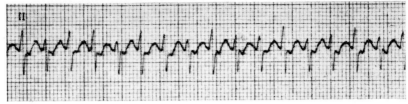

Figure 7.7—*Supraventricular ectopic tachycardia with no P waves clearly visible*

certainly, this is an atrial tachycardia, the possibility that it is A.V. junctional in origin, with retrograde P waves coinciding with and hidden in the QRS complexes, cannot be excluded with certainty. For this reason, some authorities prefer to use the non-committal term 'supraventricular tachycardia' for this type of record in which the QRS complexes are normal, but in which no P waves can be clearly identified.

Atrial Tachycardia with 2:1 A.V. Block

Since the P waves in atrial tachycardia are generally small, in the presence of 2:1 A.V. block, the blocked atrial impulse may be invisible in the QRST complexes. *Figure 7.8* shows an example which could readily be mistaken for sinus rhythm. A correct diagnosis may be suggested if the visible P waves

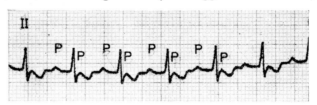

Figure 7.8—*Atrial tachycardia (rate 240 per minute) 2:1 A.V. block. The blocked P waves could readily be missed and the rhythm might be mistaken for sinus tachycardia*

are noticed to be abnormal, or by the complete regularity of the ventricular complexes which would be unusual in normal sinus rhythm. If suspected, the diagnosis may be confirmed by carotid sinus stimulation. This may transiently increase the degree of A.V. block and reveal the true atrial rate. Clinical inspection of the jugular venous pulse may be of diagnostic help, but in difficult cases the use of an eosophageal or a right atrial lead will clearly reveal atrial activity and enable a firm diagnosis to be established.

Atrial Tachycardia with Aberrant QRS Complexes

Sometimes in atrial tachycardia, the QRS complexes are widened to 0·12 second or more in duration. Such records require to be differentiated from ventricular tachycardia. A widened QRS in atrial tachycardia may result from two causes; the patient may already have bundle branch block, and, if this is known, no difficulty in diagnosis should arise. A second possibility which is more likely to cause difficulty is an aberrant QRS contour due to the rapid heart rate. If an orthograde P wave can be seen to precede each QRS complex, the diagnosis of atrial tachycardia with aberrant ventricular conduction can be made with confidence. More often, no definite P waves can be identified and the differentiation from ventricular tachycardia can then be very difficult. This problem will be discussed more fully in Chapter 8.

Electrocardiogram in Atrial Flutter

When the atrial rate recorded by the electrocardiogram lies between 250 and 350 per minute, atrial flutter is said to be present. Although this is a purely arbitrary definition, it is useful, for both the clinical picture and the electrocardiogram are distinctive. The characteristic feature of the electrocardiogram is that the atrial rate is so fast that the P waves merge into each other, producing a 'saw-tooth' or 'picket fence' appearance. In consequence, the baseline is in continual movement and no isoelectric intervals occur. It is customary to refer to the individual undulations of the baseline in flutter as F waves. These F waves usually remain regular, both in size and rhythm. The typical appearance of the baseline is usually most obvious in leads II and III but less obvious in the praecordial leads. However, as Grant (1957) has pointed out, if the direction of the P vectors during part of the P cycle is mainly at right angles to either the frontal or horizontal plane, the limb or praecordial leads may fail to record this part of the P force and isoelectric intervals may occur. Correspondingly, when a fast atrial rate develops in patients with mitral valve disease and a large left atrium, the broad P waves, characteristic of this condition, will fuse together at slower atrial rates than usual. It is sometimes stated that the presence or absence of isoelectric intervals between P waves is the important criterion for differentiating between atrial tachycardia and atrial flutter. This statement implies that there is some subtle difference between the two arrhythmias, other than rate, and there is no evidence to support this view. In the present state of our knowledge it would seem simplest to define and identify the different atrial arrhythmias purely on a basis of the atrial rate as has been done in Table 7.1.

In my experience, the atrial rate in flutter is almost always exactly 300 per minute, and usually there is 2:1 A.V. block with a regular ventricular rate of 150 per minute. The superimposition of the QRST complexes may tend to obscure the continuous undulations of the baseline. The electrocardiographic diagnosis may then be clarified by right carotid sinus stimulation which transiently increases the degree of A.V. block and reveals the typical flutter waves (*Figure 7.9*). The atrial rate may occasionally be less than 300 per minute and occasionally it is faster; the A.V. conduction ratio is still usually 2:1, with rates as high as 350 per minute.

Variations of A.V. Conduction Ratio in Flutter

Although a 2:1 A.V. conduction ratio is the commonest finding in atrial flutter, it is by no means invariable. 1:1 A.V. conduction is occasionally

119

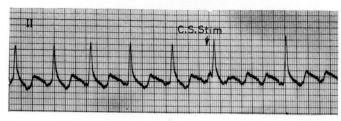

Figure 7.9—Atrial flutter with 2:1 A.V. block. Carotid sinus stimulation (C.S. Stim) increases the degree of A.V. block and reveals the characteristic flutter waves (time markings $\frac{1}{10}$ second)

seen with atrial rates of 250 per minute or more (*Figure 7.10*). Higher degrees of A.V. block with a fixed conduction ratio may occur; that is, 4:1 block (*Figure 7.11*). In these cases the ventricular rate usually doubles on exertion.

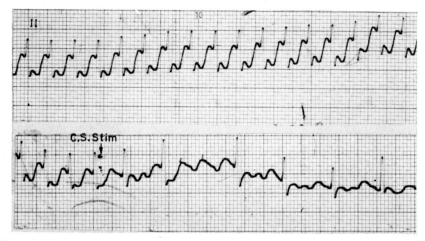

Figure 7.10—Atrial flutter with 1:1 A.V. conduction. Atrial rate 250 per minute. Carotid sinus stimulation increases the degree of A.V. block and reveals the diagnosis

In other patients, different types of A.V. block may be seen. A Wenckebach type of conduction is fairly common. This may result in an apparently varying conduction ratio; for example 2:1 A.V. conduction may seem to

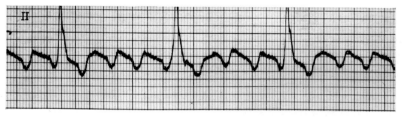

Figure 7.11—Atrial flutter with 4:1 A.V. block in an undigitalized patient (time markings $\frac{1}{10}$ second)

alternate with 4:1, causing a bigeminal ventricular rhythm (*Figure 7.12*). Atrial flutter may co-exist with complete heart block when the ventricular rate will be slow with no evidence of a conduction ratio. Careful inspection

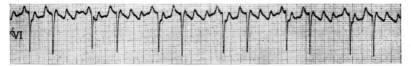

Figure 7.12—Atrial flutter with an A.V. conduction ratio apparently alternating between 2:1 and 4:1. In fact the apparent bigeminal ventricular rhythm is due to a Wenckebach type of conduction anomaly. The first FR interval of each pair is always shorter than the second FR interval. For an unknown reason, if the F waves in flutter are numbered consecutively, only the odd ones or the even ones are conducted except in, of course, 1:1 conduction

will be necessary to differentiate this from examples of 4:1 block. The last part of the record illustrated in *Figure 7.13* shows atrial flutter with a slow ventricular rate. Complete heart block was confirmed in the first part of the rhythm strip when the atria were controlled by the sinus node.

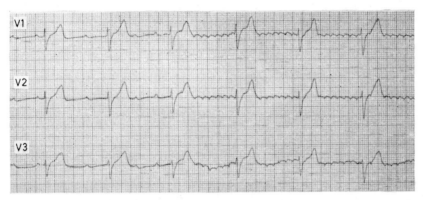

Figure 7.13—Complete heart block, initially with the atria controlled by the sinus node. Atrial flutter develops during the recording

'Impure Flutter'

When the atrial rate exceeds 350 per minute, it is common to use the term 'impure flutter' or sometimes 'flutter fibrillation'. There is no clear dividing line between 'impure flutter' and atrial fibrillation. Once the atrial rate exceeds 350 per minute, the features characteristic of atrial fibrillation usually appear, that is, co-ordinated contraction of the atria disappears and the ventricular response becomes irregularly irregular. The condition tends to be unstable and usually progresses to frank atrial fibrillation.

Electrocardiogram in Atrial Fibrillation

Since the fundamental characteristic of atrial fibrillation is loss of mechanical contraction of the atria, it would seem at first sight to be illogical to speak of the atrial rate. However, in the electrocardiogram, atrial fibrillation is recognized by continual rapid undulations of the baseline, usually designated as 'f' waves, the rate of which can be measured, and it is a matter of experience that when the rate of the f waves exceeds 350 per minute, mechanical contraction of the atria no longer occurs.

121

There are three electrocardiographic criteria for the diagnosis of atrial fibrillation: (1) the absence of P waves, (2) the presence of rapid undulations of the baseline (f waves) at rates of 350–600 per minute and (3) an irregularly irregular ventricular rhythm.

In the majority of patients with atrial fibrillation, particularly of recent onset, the electrocardiogram fulfils all three criteria and the diagnosis is simple. However, diagnostic difficulties may be encountered. It should be emphasized that the only diagnostic electrocardiographic evidence of atrial fibrillation is the presence of fibrillatory f waves disturbing the baseline. These may be evident in all leads, though most commonly they are best seen in the praecordial leads V1 and V2. Both the frequency and amplitude of these fibrillatory waves show almost continuous variation, in contrast to the F waves of flutter which are usually quite regular in time and uniform in size. The f waves of fibrillation must be differentiated from artefacts caused by muscle tremor or A.C. interference, which may obscure the presence of P waves. The distinction is seldom difficult, the undulations of muscle tremor being slower than those of fibrillation, and those of a.c. interference being faster (that is, 10 per large square at 25 mm per second paper speed). Difficulties are more likely to arise if fibrillatory waves are small or indiscernible. A diagnosis of atrial fibrillation must then be based on other criteria, for example, absence of P waves and an irregularly irregular ventricular rhythm. In cases of doubt, the use of special leads may reveal atrial activity. Lian, Cassimatis and Hebert (1952) introduced a bipolar lead, which they termed S_5, for delineating atrial activity more clearly. The negative electrode is placed over the manubrium sterni and the positive electrode in the fifth left intercostal space at the left sternal edge. An oesophageal or right atrial lead may similarly be of value in demonstrating fibrillatory waves when these cannot be clearly identified in conventional leads

Significance of Fibrillatory Wave Size

The amplitude of the fibrillation waves in lead V1 appears to have some diagnostic importance and to be related to the contour of the P wave of the same patient when in sinus rhythm. Morris and colleagues (1964) reported that the contour of the P wave in lead V1 was significantly altered in the presence of left atrial (and left ventricular) hypertrophy. A normal sinus P wave in V1 is a small positive deflection, aeproximately 1 mm in amplitude and 0·04 second in duration. In the presence of left atrial hypertrophy, the terminal P forces point posteriorly and the P wave becomes biphasic, the initial positive deflection being followed by a terminal negative deflection. A terminal negative deflection 0·04 second in duration and 1 mm in amplitude (corresponding to one small square of electrocardiograph paper) was found to correlate well with the presence of left atrial hypertrophy, and sometimes of left ventricular hypertrophy (*Figure 7.14a*). Later, Morris, Peter and McIntosh (1966) found a close correlation between the contour of the P wave in sinus rhythm and the fibrillatory wave size of the same patient when in atrial fibrillation. Fibrillatory wave size is classified as fine or coarse. Fine fibrillation waves measure less than 1 mm in lead V1, whereas coarse waves measure more than 1 mm. Patients with coarse fibrillation waves in lead V1 are almost always found to have diphasic P waves in V1 when in sinus rhythm, with a marked terminal negative 'dip'. When, therefore, coarse fibrillation waves measuring more than 1 mm in amplitude are observed in V1, there is a high probability that left atrial hypertrophy is present (*Figure 7.14b*). In

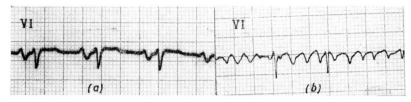

Figure 7.14—Shows lead V1 in the same patient with mitral stenosis: (a) in sinus rhythm; (b) after the development of atrial fibrillation (see text)

long-standing atrial fibrillation, there is a general tendency for fibrillatory wave size to diminish, probably reflecting progressive atrial disease with a reduction in atrial muscle mass. It is common experience that patients with very fine fibrillation waves are often much more difficult to revert to sinus rhythm than those with coarse fibrillation waves.

Ventricular Rate and Rhythm in Atrial Fibrillation

In untreated atrial fibrillation, the ventricular rate is generally between 150 and 170 per minute. Faster ventricular rates up to 190 per minute are occasionally seen, particularly in thyrotoxicosis and in the Wolff–Parkinson–White syndrome complicated by atrial fibrillation. On the other hand, the resting ventricular rate is occasionally normal in untreated patients. This is invariably true in so-called 'lone' atrial fibrillation. In patients with heart disease, a normal resting ventricular rate suggests the presence of first-degree A.V. block and this may be confirmed when the patient is reverted to sinus rhythm by finding a prolonged P–R interval. It has already been stressed that, in atrial fibrillation, the ventricular rhythm is characterized by being completely irregular. It should be emphasized that a regular ventricular rhythm never occurs in uncomplicated atrial fibrillation. Regularity of the ventricular rhythm implies the presence of A.V. dissociation with the ventricles controlled by a pacemaker situated below the atria, most often in the A.V. junction. This may occur in complete A.V. block when the ventricular rate is slow. Atrial fibrillation with A.V. dissociation, the ventricles being controlled by junctional pacemaker, may also occur in digitalis intoxication (page 275). The ventricular rate may then be relatively fast.

Aetiology of Atrial Arrhythmias

Any of the atrial arrhythmias so far described may occur in otherwise perfectly normal hearts, including both atrial flutter and atrial fibrillation. Episodes of atrial tachycardia are probably the commonest form of paroxysmal arrhythmia (page 144), and the majority of these patients have normal hearts. Atrial fibrillation and atrial flutter occurring in otherwise normal hearts will be further discussed later. Probably the commonest cause of atrial arrhythmia is rheumatic heart disease, particularly when the mitral valve is involved. Isolated aortic valve disease, whether of rheumatic or other aetiology, is much less commonly associated with atrial arrhythmia. Hypertensive and chronic ischaemic heart disease are frequent causes, and atrial arrhythmias, usually transient, are common in acute myocardial infarction. Thyrotoxicosis is often associated with atrial fibrillation, particularly in patients over the age of 45 years. In elderly subjects atrial fibrillation is occasionally the only clinical manifestation of thyrotoxicosis. Chronic atrial arrhythmias are very unusual in congenital heart disease. Atrial septal defect is the commonest congenital lesion in which atrial fibrillation occurs, but rarely before the age of 40 years. It is sometimes an ominous complication in Ebstein's anomaly of the tricuspid valve since atrial transport function is lost. The cardiomyopathies are occasionally associated with atrial fibrillation, particularly the alcoholic variety. Transient atrial fibrillation is not uncommon following pulmonary embolism, although it is rare in chronic cor pulmonale; less common causes are bronchial carcinoma with secondary invasion of the atria, and even thoracotomy may precipitate atrial fibrillation. An important cause of atrial arrhythmias is digitalis intoxication and this will be more fully discussed in Chapter 15.

From time to time, patients are encountered with atrial fibrillation, in whom no obvious cause for the arrhythmia can be found. These cases cannot be regarded as 'lone atrial fibrillation' (discussed later) since they present with cardiac symptoms and show radiological evidence of cardiac enlargement. There is nothing to suggest underlying ischaemic heart disease and at present they must be termed idiopathic.

Clinical Features of Atrial Arrhythmias

It is generally recognized that atrial fibrillation and atrial flutter occur in both paroxysmal and chronic forms. Atrial tachycardia, on the other hand, seems to be regarded as only occurring in paroxysms. In consequence, in medical literature, it is often referred to as paroxysmal atrial tachycardia or, more shortly, as P.A.T. Since so-called 'paroxysmal' atrial tachycardia may last for as long as ten years, this would seem to be a misuse of the term paroxysm. It is true that when, in any discipline, words are used as technical terms, they often acquire a special connotation, largely unrelated to their meaning in common use. The word paroxysm as generally employed in medicine implies an event of sudden onset and short duration. Such a meaning is consistent with the literal translation of paroxysm from Greek. There are other paroxysmal medical conditions in which a different term is employed when an attack is unusually prolonged. For example, when a paroxysm of bronchial asthma has lasted for several days, the patient is said to be in status asthmaticus. It has already been mentioned that, by a purely arbitrary definition, three or more extrasystoles in succession constitute a paroxysm of tachycardia. This definition fixes the lower limit to the duration of a paroxysm. It seems desirable from the practical point of view to fix some upper limit to the duration of a paroxysm, after which some other term should be employed. It is suggested that a convenient upper limit would be 24 hours, after which any ectopic tachycardia should be regarded as 'sustained'. Admittedly, such a definition is entirely arbitrary, but the use of the term 'sustained' tachycardia is useful in practice.

Symptomatology of Atrial Arrhythmias

The symptoms of atrial extrasystoles have already been dealt with in Chapter 6, and those of paroxysmal tachycardia as defined above will be reviewed in Chapter 9. The symptoms of 'sustained' atrial tachycardia vary widely according to the duration of the attack, the ventricular rate and the severity of any associated heart disease.

In healthy individuals there is evidence that the cardiac output continues to rise with heart rates up to 190 per minute. Patients with normal hearts will tolerate a sustained atrial tachycardia with ventricular rates as high as 180 per minute for up to a week or more, without developing heart failure or indeed any symptoms apart from the discomfort of palpitation. In the presence of heart disease, however, cardiac output begins to fall at much lower heart rates. Patients with mitral stenosis are particularly intolerant of tachycardia, and acute pulmonary oedema may rapidly complicate an episode of atrial tachycardia.

Atrial Tachycardia in Infants and Children

Atrial tachycardia may occur in infants and young children, either in paroxysmal or sustained form. Very fast heart rates may occur without QRS widening, and when the arrhythmia lasts for more than 24 hours, heart failure may develop. Nadas and colleagues (1952) reviewed 41 cases. In 24 patients no aetiological cause could be identified, but 5 of these had the Wolff–Parkinson–White syndrome. Most of the remaining patients had some form of congenital heart lesion. They divided their cases into two groups; namely, male infants below the age of four months, in whom no cause could be found, and older children of either sex, some with obvious heart disease and some without. The development of heart failure appeared to be determined by a rate in excess of 180 per minute, which lasted for more than 24 hours.

Symptoms

When heart failure develops, the infants are extremely ill. They are pale and cyanosed with tachypnoea, vomiting and sweating. The heart is usually enlarged and there is hepatomegaly and pulmonary congestion. The

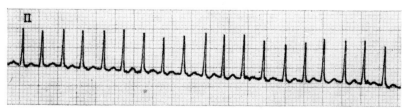

Figure 7.15—Supraventricular tachycardia in a child (lead II). Heart rate 280 per minute. Normal intraventricular conduction

diagnosis is often overlooked. *Figure 7.15* shows an extract from lead II of an infant aged three months who became moribund after the attack had lasted three days. The heart rate is 280 per minute. After full digitalization, the tachycardia reverted to sinus rhythm, and complete recovery ensued. No evidence of underlying heart disease was subsequently found. Treatment of this condition is discussed on page 211.

Clinical Picture in Atrial Flutter

Atrial flutter presents a distinctive clinical picture which makes a bedside diagnosis relatively easy in the majority of cases. The diagnosis is immediately suggested by finding a precisely regular apex rate of 150 per minute. With the patient propped up at 45 degrees, careful inspection of the neck will reveal 'flutter' waves in the jugular venous pulse at a rate of 300 per minute. Right carotid sinus stimulation will nearly always slow the ventricular rate abruptly by producing 4:1 or even higher degrees of A.V. block, with a prompt return to 150 per minute when stimulation is stopped. Carotid sinus stimulation in atrial tachycardia may promptly restore sinus rhythm; occasionally it may transiently slow the rate without increasing A.V. block.

Atrial Fibrillation

The clinical picture of atrial fibrillation is too well known to require detailed description here; there are, however, a number of features which merit discussion. Atrial fibrillation may occur in paroxysmal or chronic form. Paroxysmal fibrillation may never become chronic and constitutes one variety of paroxysmal tachycardia to be described in Chapter 9. Some patients who progress to chronic atrial fibrillation begin with paroxysmal attacks and this is particularly characteristic of thyrotoxicosis.

Even when the ventricular rate is satisfactorily controlled by digitalis, cardiac function is always impaired in atrial fibrillation owing to the loss of atrial systole. The extent to which this matters is determined by the presence and severity of any associated heart disease. In 'lone' atrial fibrillation, to be discussed later, disability is virtually absent. One of the main hazards of atrial fibrillation is clot formation in the left atrial appendage due to stasis; this may be responsible for disastrous systemic emboli, even in patients with no heart disease.

Atrial Fibrillation in Ischaemic Heart Disease

Atrial fibrillation may complicate acute myocardial infarction. It is usually transient and reverts spontaneously to sinus rhythm after a few days. Persistent atrial fibrillation occurs quite commonly in elderly patients with chronic ischaemic heart disease, and these patients are often free of anginal pain and may have painless myocardial infarcts. It is very unusual to see atrial fibrillation in cor pulmonale and its occurrence is at least suggestive of associated coronary artery disease.

Atrial Fibrillation in Rheumatic Heart Disease

Rheumatic heart disease is the commonest cause of chronic atrial fibrillation. It is particularly associated with mitral or tricuspid valve disease, but is very unusual if the lesion is confined to the aortic valve.

Once atrial fibrillation has become established in either mitral or tricuspid valve disease, or both, even when the ventricular rate is adequately controlled by digitalis, the patient's disability is almost always increased by at least one clinical grade. It is common to see patients with mitral stenosis and relatively little disability, while in sinus rhythm, deteriorate abruptly when atrial fibrillation develops and then require mitral valvotomy, despite adequate digitalization.

In mitral valve disease, systemic emboli rarely occur in sinus rhythm but are a constant risk to patients with atrial fibrillation. There is good evidence that systemic emboli are commoner in patients with radiological evidence of a large left atrial appendage. Following mitral valvotomy, with amputation of the left atrial appendage, the danger of systemic emboli is very substantially reduced, even if atrial fibrillation persists. There is probably a good case for recommending prophylactic amputation of a large left atrial appendage, even in relatively asymptomatic patients with mitral valve disease and atrial fibrillation, as the best insurance against systemic embolus.

In mitral valve disease, the onset of atrial fibrillation may be rapidly followed by clot formation in the left atrial appendage, with systemic embolization within 2–3 days. The late Paul Wood used to teach that the onset of atrial fibrillation in a patient with mitral valve disease should be regarded as a grave medical emergency demanding immediate treatment with intravenous digitalis and heparin.

'Lone' Atrial Fibrillation

It has been recognized for many years that chronic atrial fibrillation may be encountered in patients with no other evidence of heart disease. The incidence has been put as high as 6 per cent of patients with this arrhythmia. Evans and Swann (1954) proposed the term 'lone atrial fibrillation' for this condition, and they described the clinical picture and diagnostic criteria.

Since lone atrial fibrillation is asymptomatic, it is usually an accidental finding during routine medical examination. The vast majority, if not all, of the patients are males, and apart from the arrhythmia, there are no other abnormal findings. The only complaint the patient may have is palpitation on strenuous exertion. The resting ventricular rate is 90 per minute or less, and the heart sounds are normal. There is no radiological evidence of cardiac enlargement (or of selective left atrial enlargement). Before making a diagnosis of lone atrial fibrillation, care must be taken to exclude minimal mitral stenosis, and auscultation should be carried out in the left lateral position after exercise. Occasional cases have been recorded, who fulfilled the criteria for lone atrial fibrillation but suffered a systemic embolus. For this reason, some authorities consider that an attempt should be made to revert these patients to sinus rhythm. It is a curious finding that lone atrial fibrillation proves extremely resistant to both drug therapy and electric shock.

Lone atrial fibrillation is a chronic arrhythmia, and Evans and Swann considered it was different from paroxysmal atrial fibrillation which also occurs in otherwise normal hearts. Clinically the main differences are that in the paroxysmal variety the ventricular rate is fast and that women are affected as often as men.

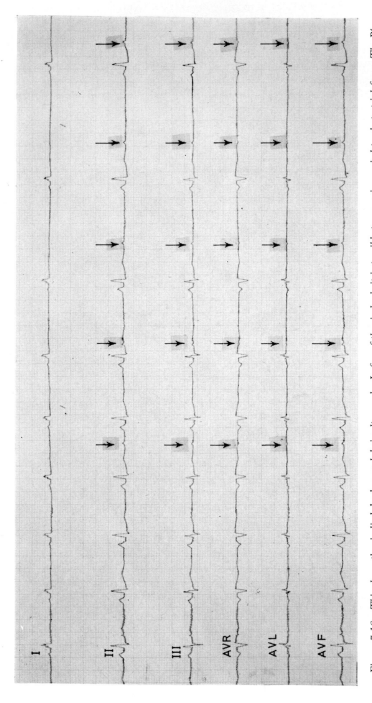

Figure 7.16—This shows the six limb leads recorded simultaneously. In five of the six leads it is possible to recognize an independent atrial focus. The P' waves of each are marked by an arrow. None of these ectopic P' waves are conducted to the ventricles and they do not disturb the normal sinus rhythm

Atrial Dissociation

Dissociated contraction of the two atria has repeatedly been observed in the exposed heart of the experimental animal. From time to time electrocardiographic records from human patients are seen which exhibit apparent atrial waves which are independent of the conducted sinus P waves. The accessory atrial waves are usually slower than sinus P waves and are never conducted to the ventricles. Numerous examples of such tracings have now been published and have been interpreted as implying dissociation of the two atria or at least of part of one atrium from the remaining atrial musculature. The French have termed the condition 'la double commande auriculaire'.

The right atrium usually remains in sinus rhythm while the left atrium (or part of it) is the seat of the independent ectopic focus. Sometimes the left atrium exhibits atrial fibrillation or flutter or an atrial tachycardia. Most often the independent atrial rhythm is slow. *Figure 7.16* shows an example, Such a situation necessarily implies that an area of protective block must exist between the two atria since otherwise the impulses of one centre would necessarily reach and discharge the other and the fast centre would then control both atria whereas the accessory atrial centre does not disturb the normal sinus rhythm.

When such records are published, critics are quick to point out that the accessory P waves could in fact be artefacts from some external source of interference such as a dial telephone, an electric saw or buzzer, or from hiccoughs. However, very convincing cases have been published, for example, by Dimond and Hayes (1958) and Dietz and colleagues (1957).

'Malignant' Atrial Arrhythmia

Dewhurst (1957) introduced the term 'malignant atrial arrhythmia' for a condition with a fairly well defined clinical picture, electrocardiographic changes and progressive course. The patients are over the age of 45 years

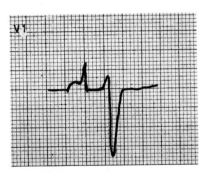

Figure 7.17—Left atrial rhythm

and present with attacks of palpitation and dyspnoea on effort. The distinctive features claimed for the condition are the great variability of the arrhythmia, its resistance to treatment, absence of any demonstrable cause and the tendency to progressive left ventricular enlargement. The arrhythmia tends to be paroxysmal with protean manifestations, the cardiograph showing more or less abrupt variations between sinus rhythm, atrial extra-systoles, atrial tachycardia, flutter and fibrillation. Left ventricular enlargement is characteristic and appears relatively late in the disease; that is, it appears to be a sequel to the arrhythmia and not a cause of it. The prognosis appears to be serious, but it is questionable whether it justifies the term 'malignant'.

It has recently been recognized that quite rarely the dominant pacemaker of the heart is not the sinus node but an ectopic focus in the left atrium which discharges at a relatively slow rate. The clinical significance of this is not clear but it does not seem to be related to any drugs or to follow myocardial infarction. Left atrial rhythm may be diagnosed when the P waves are inverted in all the limb leads and when the P waves in lead V1 show the 'dome and dart' configuration. The P wave is then notched with a rounded low voltage initial component which is followed by a tall peaked component (*Figure 7.17*).

CHAPTER 8

ECTOPIC TACHYCARDIAS—A.V. JUNCTIONAL AND VENTRICULAR TACHYCARDIAS

In Chapter 7 (page 124) it was suggested that the term 'paroxysmal', when used in relation to ectopic tachycardias, should have a more restricted meaning, and that when such a rhythm had persisted for more than 24 hours, it should be termed 'sustained'. Paroxysmal tachycardia is a well defined clinical entity occurring usually in otherwise normal hearts, and it will be discussed in detail in Chapter 9. In the present chapter the cardiographic appearances and electrocardiographic diagnosis of ectopic tachycardias originating in the A.V. junction and the ventricles will be described, and the clinical features of these arrhythmias, when they occur in sustained form, will be discussed.

A.V. JUNCTIONAL TACHYCARDIAS

The normal A.V. junction has a dual function. It transmits the excitation wave from the atria to the ventricles after an appropriate delay, the purpose of which has already been discussed. It is also the main subsidiary pacemaker of the heart and takes over control for one or more beats, when, for any reason, the sinus node fails to produce an impulse. The rates of such 'escape' A.V. junctional rhythms usually lie between 40 and 60 per minute. Although in the past it was considered that pacemaking cells were present in the A.V. node itself, recent electrophysiological studies suggest that pacemaking cells are only present in the so-called 'H–N' portion of the node immediately adjacent to the bundle of His. In fact it seems likely that the pacemaking cells for most of the rhythms which used to be called 'nodal' lie in the bundle of His itself. Sometimes the inherent rate of discharge of an A.V. junctional pacemaker becomes, for some reason, temporarily enhanced, and, if its rate exceeds that of the sinus pacemaker, it will assume control of the heart. When it does so in paroxysmal form, the rate may lie between 150 and 220 per minute. Pick and Dominguez (1957) have described what they term a non-paroxysmal form of nodal tachycardia. They use the term 'non-paroxysmal' in the sense that the onset is not sudden, nor the offset abrupt; they point out that this variety of nodal tachycardia differs from the paroxysmal variety in having a substantially slower rate (between 70 and 130 per minute), and that, whereas the paroxysmal form occurs most often in otherwise normal hearts, the non-paroxysmal form is generally a manifestation of organic disease or digitalis intoxication. In practice, it almost always results in A.V. dissociation and detailed discussion of this will be deferred until Chapter 10.

Electrocardiogram in A.V. Junctional Tachycardia

A.V. junctional tachycardia may be diagnosed with confidence in the electrocardiogram under two conditions. (1) When the QRS complexes are normal in duration (though they may differ in contour from sinus beats as in junctional escape rhythms) and a retrograde P′ wave is visible in the ST segments. *Figure 8.1* shows an example. (2) When the QRS complexes are normal in duration and regular in rhythm, but A.V. dissociation is present. This most commonly occurs in non-paroxysmal A.V. junctional tachycardia and will be discussed in Chapter 10.

When no evidence of atrial activity is visible in the electrocardiogram and the QRS complexes are normal in duration, it is usually impossible to differentiate A.V. junctional from atrial tachycardia. It is then generally simplest to use the non-committal term 'supraventricular tachycardia'.

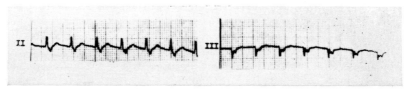

Figure 8.1—Junctional tachycardia. In leads II and III, a retrograde P′ wave can be seen in the ST segments of the QRS complexes

As in atrial tachycardia, the QRS complexes in A.V. junctional tachycardia may be aberrant. If they are 0·12 second or more in duration, the differentiation from ventricular tachycardia may be difficult or impossible from the electrocardiogram. This problem will be further discussed later under ventricular tachycardia.

A.V. Junctional Tachycardia with Block

Both paroxysmal and non-paroxysmal junctional tachycardia may be associated with either antegrade or retrograde block. The block may take the form of a fixed conduction ratio; that is, with antegrade block, the ventricular rate may be relatively slow, with twice the number of retrograde P′ waves being visible. More often, the block is retrograde, P′ waves only appearing after every second or third QRS complex, indicating 2:1 or 3:1 retrograde block. Occasionally, a Wenckebach type of conduction anomaly may be present in either a retrograde or antegrade direction. Pick, Langendorf and Katz (1961) have described at least six varieties of block complicating junctional tachycardias of both paroxysmal and non-paroxysmal varieties, and have drawn attention to the frequency of digitalis intoxication as a cause. The subject will be reviewed more fully in Chapter 15.

Clinical Features of A.V. Junctional Tachycardias

Since in A.V. junctional tachycardia, the atria and ventricles contract virtually simultaneously, cannon waves in the jugular venous pulse with each heart beat are a characteristic clinical feature. While this has sometimes been stated as diagnostic of junctional tachycardia, it is certainly not. In atrial tachycardia with a rapid rate, the atria may contract before the tricuspid valve has opened and produce a cannon wave. Ventricular tachycardia with retrograde conduction to the atria will similarly result in jugular venous cannon waves.

A sustained form of A.V. junctional tachycardia may follow the trauma of open heart surgery. Dreifus, Bartolucci and Likoff (1960) described 57 cases of A.V. junctional tachycardia: 40 per cent were due to digitalis excess and a further 30 per cent followed cardiac surgery. They found surgically induced A.V. junctional tachycardia to last from 1 to 5 days, after which it reverted to the preoperative rhythm. They considered it was always wiser to continue digitalis, for if this were stopped a rapid atrial mechanism always ensued.

VENTRICULAR TACHYCARDIA

Ventricular tachycardia is a disorder of cardiac rhythm which must always be regarded with apprehension. Although it is known that it may occur in otherwise normal hearts, it is much more commonly associated with serious organic heart disease, and even attacks occurring in the absence of heart disease have proved fatal. Ventricular tachycardia may occur in paroxysmal or sustained form in the sense already defined.

Aetiology of Ventricular Tachycardia

In a study of 131 episodes of ventricular tachycardia in 107 subjects, Armbrust and Levine (1950) found the following types of underlying heart disease.

(1) Coronary artery disease, 79 (74 per cent) (In 44 of these cases the episode of ventricular tachycardia occurred during the acute stage of myocardial infarction.)
(2) Rheumatic heart disease, 9 (8 per cent)
(3) No evidence of heart disease, 13 (12 per cent)
(4) Wolff–Parkinson–White syndrome, 5 (4·7 per cent) (Today these cases would almost certainly be classified not as ventricular tachycardia but as atrial fibrillation with preferential conduction over the bypass, *see* page 179.)
(5) Congenital heart disease, 1 (0·9 per cent)

They did not consider that digitalis intoxication was a frequent or important cause, although this is probably not true today (*see* Chapter 15).

Thus, it seems that by far the commonest cause of ventricular tachycardia is ischaemic heart disease. Over half the attacks occur during the acute stage of myocardial infarction. Herman, Park and Hejtmanciak (1959), reporting on 84 episodes of ventricular tachycardia in 60 patients, give closely similar figures. They consider that ventricular tachycardia in the Wolff–Parkinson–White syndrome should be treated separately as 'pseudo-ventricular tachycardia'. They considered that digitalis intoxication was a precipitating factor in 10 per cent of their patients, and certainly the rise in incidence of toxic digitalis rhythms, since the introduction and widespread use of oral diuretics has increased the frequency of digitalis as a causal factor (*see* Chapter 15).

A common cause of transient and usually benign ventricular tachycardia today is cardiac catheterization and cardiac surgery. When the catheter tip lies in the right or left ventricle during catheterization, ventricular ectopic beats or short runs of ventricular tachycardia are often induced. They usually revert spontaneously when the catheter is re-positioned, but they are always a source of anxiety to the operator. Occasionally such arrhythmias persist, even after withdrawal of the catheter.

Electrocardiogram in Ventricular Tachycardia

The electrocardiogram in ventricular tachycardia is usually characterized by QRS complexes which are widened to 0·12 second or more, and they are generally notched. As in ventricular extrasystoles, the T waves are written in the opposite direction with no intervening S–T segment. In some cases there is retrograde conduction of the ectopic stimulus to the atria, with either a 1:1 conduction ratio or, perhaps, 2:1 or 3:1 retrograde block. In other cases there is A.V. dissociation, the atria remaining under control of the sinus node. Independent P waves at a slower rate may then be discernible in the record. Often no evidence of atrial activity can be identified in ordinary leads and an oesophageal lead may be necessary. The ventricular rate is usually fast, between 140 and 180 per minute, but slower rates (between 100 and 140 per minute) are sometimes encountered, and occasionally much faster rates (up to 280 per minute) are seen. In many cases the ventricular rhythm is slightly irregular; when counted over successive periods of a minute, the rate may vary by 7 per minute, and contiguous cycles may differ by as much as 0·13 second in length. (In atrial and A.V. junctional tachycardias, cycle lengths rarely vary by more than 0·01 second.) While generally successive QRS complexes are identical in contour, variations in contour may occur, including bi-directional ventricular tachycardia, in which alternate complexes are written in opposite directions. Bi-directional ventricular tachycardia is always suggestive of digitalis intoxication, but is not diagnostic, for it has occasionally been reported in undigitalized patients. In occasional cases a ventricular 'capture' by a sinus impulse may transiently interrupt the tachycardia, or a fusion beat (partial 'capture') may occur. *Figure 8.2* illustrates some of these features.

Electrocardiographic Diagnosis

The diagnosis of ventricular tachycardia from the electrocardiogram often presents considerable difficulty. The main problem is the difficulty in differentiating between an ectopic ventricular tachycardia and a supraventricular arrhythmia with intraventricular conduction disturbance. The latter may be due to the presence of bundle branch block or to aberrant intraventricular conduction, as a result of the rapid rate. It used to be considered that an electrocardiographic diagnosis of ventricular tachycardia could be made with confidence if three criteria were fulfilled; namely, wide QRS complexes (0·12 second or more in duration), slight irregularity in rate and the demonstration of P waves at a slower, independent rate. Unfortunately all three of these criteria may prove misleading. The demonstration of independent P waves of sinus origin, either by conventional or oesophageal leads, is often quoted as diagnostic of a ventricular origin of the tachycardia. This, however, is not so, for the tachycardia may be A.V. junctional in origin with retrograde A.V. block and aberrant ventricular conduction. Slight irregularity of contiguous QRS cycle lengths up to 0·03 second is strongly suggestive of ventricular tachycardia, but again is not absolutely diagnostic, for a similar irregularity is occasionally seen in supraventricular tachycardias, as a result of conduction disturbances (Schott, 1955). Conversely, ventricular tachycardias can often be perfectly regular, particularly in the sustained variety. If a P wave is clearly seen to precede

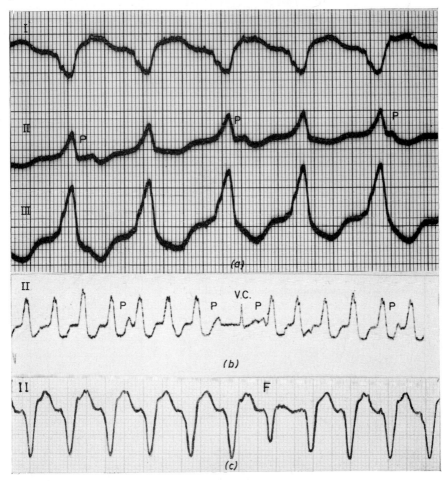

Figure 8.2—(a) Leads I, II and III recorded simultaneously on a multichannel machine. There is apparently ventricular tachycardia, and independent sinus P waves at a slower rate can be seen in lead II (line markings $\frac{1}{10}$ second). (b) There is apparently a ventricular tachycardia; independent sinus P waves are visible (marked P) and in the middle of the strip there is a ventricular capture (V.C.) by the sinus impulse. The P–R interval of the capture is considerably prolonged, presumably due to concealed retrograde conduction of the ectopic ventricular impulse. (c) Ventricular tachycardia with a partial sinus capture producing a fusion beat marked F

each QRS complex, a supraventricular origin of the tachycardia with aberrant intraventricular conduction is virtually certain, provided that the atrial wave is not retrograde in contour. In 80 per cent of supraventricular tachycardias with aberrant intraventricular conduction, the QRS complexes show the pattern of right bundle branch block. When, therefore, the QRS complexes show a left bundle branch block pattern, a diagnosis of ventricular tachycardia is much more probable. If the QRS complexes show the pattern of right bundle branch block and have a triphasic RSR pattern in lead VI, aberrant conduction of a supraventricular tachycardia is very probable (*see* page 74). The occurrence of occasional ventricular captures by the sinus impulse, or the occurrence of fusion beats, strongly favours a ventricular origin for the tachycardia. Thus, the electrocardiographic diagnosis of ventricular tachycardia, although apparently easy, may present considerable problems, and the electrocardiogram should always be considered in conjunction with the clinical findings. *Figure 8.3* illustrates some of the difficulties.

Clinical Features of Ventricular Tachycardia

The clinical picture of ventricular tachycardia is frequently striking. Since the normal peristaltic action of ventricular systole is often lost, a ventricular tachycardia tends to be an inefficient rhythm. This is occasionally strikingly illustrated when a patient in heart failure with a relative slow ventricular tachycardia (say 120 per minute) is reverted to sinus rhythm with a rate of, say, 110 per minute and immediately comes out of heart failure. In addition, since ventricular tachycardia is most commonly associated with serious organic heart disease, the patients are often very ill. A sense of oppression in the chest, often amounting to anginal pain, may be present, and cardiogenic shock is common. The site of the ectopic focus within the ventricle may also determine the clinical severity of the arrhythmia, since contraction will commence in the area of early activation. If this lies in the infundibular region, the effective ejection volume will be severely reduced, whereas stimulation in the inflow region may preserve an adequate stroke volume. Certainly in some patients, particularly those with normal hearts, the attack may be virtually symptomless.

On clinical examination, the jugular venous pulse should be carefully inspected. Gallavardin (1920) first drew attention to the typical findings which occur when the sinus node retains control of the atria. The pulsation of the right atrium may be seen in the neck at a much slower rate than that of the ventricles, and occasional cannon waves occur when the atrial contraction coincides with ventricular systole. Such findings may be particularly helpful when P waves cannot be identified in the electrocardiogram. On auscultation of the heart, changing intensity of the first heart sound is heard in 50 per cent of cases (Armbrust and Levine, 1950). This sign is very obvious when present and, as in complete A.V. block, it depends upon the variation in the time of contraction of the atria and ventricles. It is not, therefore, present when there is 1:1 retrograde conduction to the atria and it has the same significance as occasional cannon waves in the jugular venous pulse. A second auscultatory sign of ventricular tachycardia is the presence of multiple low-frequency sounds, up to 4 or 6 per cycle, which may be heard in many cases at the apex or left sternal edge. These were described by Harvey (1959). He attributed them to wide splitting of the first and second heart sounds, together with gallop sounds. Although similar sounds may also be heard in atrial flutter or atrial tachycardia with

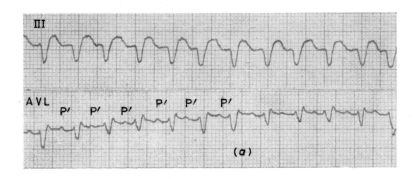

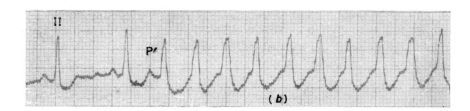

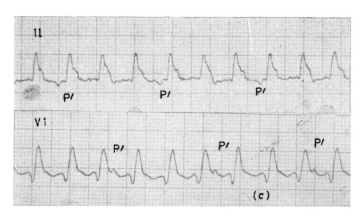

Figure 8.3—The tracings (a), (b) and (c) illustrate some of the difficulties in the diagnosis of ventricular tachycardia: (a) All leads except AVL suggested a ventricular tachycardia. Lead III is illustrative. However, in lead AVL, a distinct P′ wave can be seen preceding each QRS complex, indicating that it is an atrial tachycardia with aberrant ventricular conduction. (b) The strip commences with two sinus beats followed by a run of wide QRS complexes resembling a ventricular tachycardia. However, the first ectopic beat is preceded by a P′ wave indicating an atrial origin of the tachycardia. All subsequent P′ waves are buried in the wide QRS complexes. (c) Leads II and V1 show an ectopic tachycardia with widened QRS complexes suggesting a ventricular origin. Every third QRS complex is followed by (or preceded by) an atrial wave which is inverted in lead II and positive in lead V1. This may be a ventricular tachycardia with 3:1 retrograde block. Alternatively, it could be an A.V. junctional tachycardia with aberrant conduction and 3:1 retrograde block

block, these latter arrhythmias may be influenced by carotid sinus stimulation, which ventricular tachycardia is not. A further occasional auscultatory sign in ventricular tachycardia was pointed out by Armbrust and Levine. In 3 out of their 107 cases, only one heart sound could be heard. This may lead to the presence of a rapid tachycardia being overlooked. They instance one case in which the single heart sound alternated in intensity, so that it was difficult at the bedside to tell whether it was two heart sounds with a rate of 115 per minute or a single heart sound with a rate of 230 per minute. This difficulty was accentuated by inability to feel the pulse or record a blood pressure.

While at times it is impossible to be sure of the presence of ventricular tachycardia, even by combining the clinical and electrocardiographic findings, immediate clarification of the diagnosis is now less important than in the past, since the treatment of both supraventricular and ventricular varieties is the same; namely, synchronized d.c. shock (provided that digitalis as a cause of the arrhythmia has been excluded). Once sinus rhythm has been restored, a correct retrospective diagnosis is sometimes possible, and this may be important in considering prognosis.

T-wave Changes following Ventricular Tachycardia

Following prolonged attacks of ventricular tachycardia, long lasting abnormal T waves may occur in the electrocardiogram. It is important to appreciate this, for they may occur in otherwise normal hearts and arouse the suspicion that the attack was due to myocardial infarction. Inverted T waves may be present for as long as 54 days following an attack, without necessarily implying the presence of myocardial disease. (Similar, though less marked, T-wave changes may follow attacks of supraventricular tachycardia.)

Possible Re-entry Mechanism in Ventricular Tachycardia

Recently Wellens and his colleagues have shown (1972) in five patients subject to recurrent ventricular tachycardia that they could initiate and terminate episodes of tachycardia at will by electrical stimulation of the right ventricle. They considered that their results could best be explained by a re-entry mechanism, the circus re-entry pathways involved being composed of (1) the bundle branches, (2) Purkinje fibres with or without adjacent ventricular myocardium, (3) infarcted or fibrotic ventricular tissue, and (4) combinations of (1), (2), and (3).

Classification of Ventricular Tachycardia

Ventricular tachycardia may be classified on either electrocardiographic or clinical grounds.

Electrocardiographic Classification of Ventricular Tachycardia

Ventricular tachycardia may be classified on electrocardiographic grounds into four main types.

(1) Extrasystolic ventricular tachycardia
(2) Parasystolic ventricular tachycardia

(3) Idioventricular tachycardia (Schamroth, 1966)
(4) Repetitive paroxysmal ventricular tachycardia

Extrasystolic Ventricular Tachycardia

This is the commonest type and may be regarded as a succession of ventricular extrasystoles. Each paroxysm commences with a premature beat, and the duration of the attack varies from seconds up to hours, days or even weeks. The heart rate is usually between 140 and 180 per minute.

Parasystolic Ventricular Tachycardia

This is a much less common variety which may only be recognizable if it manifests exit block, allowing intervening sinus beats to appear between paroxysms. It will then be found that the first beat of each paroxysm has a variable coupling time to the preceding sinus beat, but the interval between paroxysms is always a precise multiple of the cycle length of the tachycardia. Since the parasystolic focus is protected by entrance block from being discharged by the sinus impulse, these cases may prove refractory to treatment by direct current shock. The cycle length of the tachycardia is often longer than in extrasystolic ventricular tachycardia, corresponding to rates of 75 to 120 per minute.

Intermittent parasystolic ventricular tachycardia is occasionally encountered. This again can only be recognized if exit block occurs, permitting one or more conducted beats to intervene. Like intermittent parasystole (*see* page 105), the first beat of any bout of intermittent parasystolic tachycardia always has a fixed coupling time to the initiating sinus beat. An example of this arrhythmia was shown in *Figure 6.29*.

Idioventricular Tachycardia

Schamroth (1966) described idioventricular tachycardia as a specific variety. It is closely analogous to so-called shifting pacemaker between the sinus and A.V. nodes. It is postulated that an idioventricular focus acquires an inherent discharge rate just above the sinus rate. In this sense, therefore, it is a tachycardia rather than an escape rhythm, but the rate is relatively slow. Ventricular 'captures' by the sinus impulse are frequent and these discharge the idioventricular focus, which is not protected by entrance

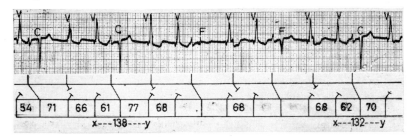

Figure 8.4—There are numerous ventricular ectopic beats marked V, and several sinus captures marked C, and fusion beats marked F. The ectopic ventricular cycle length measures usually 0·68 second, but the first two consecutive ventricular beats have a cycle length of 0·66 second. When a sinus capture intervenes between two ventricular ectopic beats, the interval between the latter (marked x and y on the record) does not precisely equal two ventricular ectopic cycle lengths, suggesting that the capture beat has discharged the ventricular pacemaker. By courtesy of L. Schamroth

block, and so cause a shift in the timing of the ventricular rhythm (*Figure 8.4* shows an example).

Another variety of a relatively slow ventricular rhythm is often seen following acute myocardial infarction. This has been termed by Marriott 'accelerated idioventricular rhythm'. This variety will be more fully described in Chapter 16.

Repetitive Paroxysmal Ventricular Tachycardia

This is a distinctive variety of paroxysmal ventricular tachycardia characterized by short individual paroxysms separated by only a few sinus beats. It will be considered in greater detail in Chapter 9.

Clinical Classification of Ventricular Tachycardia

From personal observations and a survey of reported cases, Froment, Gallavardin and Cohen (1953) have suggested a clinical classification which divides ventricular tachycardia into the following four groups.

(1) Terminal pre-fibrillatory ventricular tachycardia.

(2) Ventricular extrasystoles with paroxysms of tachycardia usually affecting healthy hearts.

(3) Ventricular tachycardia due to a septal lesion (either infarction or, rarely, a syphilitic lesion).

(4) Prolonged attacks of ventricular tachycardia occurring in young subjects with otherwise normal hearts.

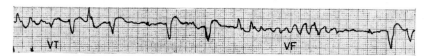

Figure 8.5—The record shows runs of ventricular tachycardia (marked VT) and a short run of ventricular fibrillation (marked VF) lasting just over 2 seconds

(1) *Pre-fibrillatory ventricular tachycardia* was first described by Gallavardin in 1920. It is always associated with advanced myocardial disease and is generally a terminal or pre-terminal event. The electrocardiogram usually shows a polymorphic ventricular tachycardia (that is, one with frequent changes in QRS contour or frank alternation). Digitalis toxicity is an important contributory factor. Such paroxysms have an ominous prognosis and commonly precede terminal ventricular fibrillation. *Figure 8.5* shows an example with a short paroxysm of ventricular fibrillation.

(2) *Ventricular extrasystoles with short paroxysms of ventricular tachycardia* appear to be identical with repetitive paroxysmal ventricular tachycardia. This will be further discussed in Chapter 9.

(3) *Ventricular tachycardia due to a septal lesion* is the common variety seen in ischaemic heart disease. In over 50 per cent of the cases, the arrhythmia follows a recent infarct involving the septum. It is most common in elderly subjects and may be the first evidence that infarction has occurred. On the other hand, the onset may occur at any time during the first month following infarction. Its occurrence is always serious; attacks tend to be prolonged unless treated promptly and often lead to the rapid onset of cardiac failure or cardiogenic shock. Recurrence of the tachycardia after

successful reversion is common. In the remaining patients with ischaemic heart disease who develop ventricular tachycardia, a microscopic lesion, without frank infarction, but involving the septum, is presumably responsible. If such attacks are prolonged they may be associated with fever, leucocytosis and cardiac failure, and frank infarction can only be excluded by the electrocardiogram after reversion to sinus rhythm has been achieved.

In exceptional cases, ventricular tachycardia may be caused by a syphilitic lesion involving the septum. Several such cases have been published and, while individual attacks respond promptly to treatment, they tend to keep recurring until anti-syphilitic treatment has been given. In unexplained recurrent ventricular tachycardia, the possibility of a syphilitic origin should always be borne in mind.

(4) *Prolonged attacks of ventricular tachycardia* may occur in younger subjects with otherwise normal hearts. Such attacks may last from an hour or so, up to several days. In the more prolonged episodes, evidence of congestive heart failure may occur. Sometimes such attacks may keep recurring frequently and produce considerable invalidism.

This form of ventricular tachycardia is relatively uncommon; it differs from repetitive paroxysmal ventricular tachycardia in that between attacks the electrocardiogram reveals no extrasystoles. It is clearly not of the pre-fibrillatory variety, for there is no associated evidence of heart disease and the prognosis is generally good. Although most authors regard the condition as benign, it is questionable whether 'benign' is an appropriate term, since many reported cases have had disabling symptoms, sometimes with frank heart failure during prolonged attacks, and others without serious symptoms have died suddenly. The condition is relatively rare; one of us has seen three examples in the past ten years, and although all have fully recovered and now have apparently normal hearts, each has had several episodes requiring hospital admission.

Ventricular tachycardia is also a late complication of myocardial infarction complicated by ventricular aneurysm formation. This arrhythmia is often refractory to drug treatment and the negative inotrophic effect of large doses of most suppressive agents only serves further to compromise ventricular function. It is of some practical importance to appreciate that resection of the aneurysm may abolish the arrhythmia. In 1969 the first patient was reported in whom this was the sole indication for surgery (Hunt, Sloman and Westlake, 1969), and the same year, Magidson (1969) reported three patients who had a successful aneurysmectomy for refractory life-threatening arrhythmias.

Ventricular Flutter

The term ventricular flutter is sometimes used for very fast ectopic ventricular rhythms that do not fulfil the electrocardiographic criteria for ventricular fibrillation (*vide infra*). The cardiogram shows large, very rapid, continuous fluctuations of voltage with no separate QRS complexes or T waves. The resulting waves on the record remain constant in amplitude and size, analogous to the F waves of atrial flutter. *Figure 8.6* shows a typical record from a patient during a Stokes–Adams attack. Such a rapid ventricular rate, although probably associated with a more or less co-ordinated

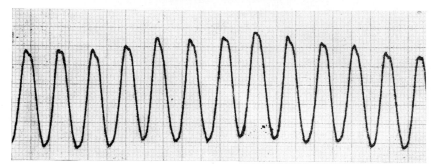

Figure 8.6—Ventricular flutter. There is no distinction between QRS complexes and T waves in the record

ventricular contraction, would not produce an effective cardiac output, and consciousness is quickly lost. Ventricular flutter may precede ventricular fibrillation; it is a fairly frequent cause of Stokes–Adams attacks in patients with complete heart block. It also occurs during open heart surgery, particularly during rewarming from profound hypothermia.

Ventricular Fibrillation

In ventricular fibrillation, co-ordinated mechanical contraction of the ventricles ceases, just as does mechanical contraction of the atria in atrial fibrillation. In ventricular fibrillation, cardiac output necessarily ceases immediately, and it is almost certainly the commonest cause of cardiac arrest. In ischaemic heart disease, it is not infrequently responsible for sudden death occurring in previously apparently healthy individuals.

The Electrocardiogram of Ventricular Fibrillation

Figure 8.7 shows the typical cardiographic appearances of ventricular fibrillation. In contrast to ventricular flutter, successive waves are inconstant both in amplitude and in time.

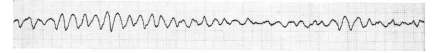

Figure 8.7—Ventricular fibrillation. This is characterized by amorphous fluctuations in voltage varying both in amplitude and frequency

Physiological Considerations

Burn (1960) and his colleagues have shown that the physiological conditions for producing experimental ventricular fibrillation are not quite the same as for atrial fibrillation. They stimulated the left ventricle electrically at rates between 12 and 25 per second. This would almost always induce ventricular fibrillation, but when stimulation stopped, reversion to sinus rhythm occurred within about one minute. In contradistinction to the atria, addition of acetylcholine to the perfusing fluid did not maintain ventricular fibrillation. The difference appears to be due to the fact that acetylcholine does not shorten the refractory period of the ventricles as it does that of the atria. Four different factors were found which would perpetuate ventricular fibrillation induced by rapid electrical stimulation. These were hypoxia (that is, by halving the saturation of O_2 in the perfusing fluid), removal of glucose from the perfusing fluid, metabolic inhibitors like dinitrophenol and, perhaps surprisingly, high concentrations of calcium. In each case there was evidence that the ventricular refractory period was shortened, and Burn postulates that ventricular fibrillation tends to be self perpetuating because fibres are contracting out of phase with each other, but recovering in time to be re-excited by their neighbours. Further discussion of the pathogenesis of ventricular fibrillation in acute myocardial infarction will be found in Chapter 16, page 288.

Aetiology of Ventricular Fibrillation

The commonest cause of ventricular fibrillation is ischaemic heart disease, and it is responsible for many deaths from acute myocardial infarction. Other causes include digitalis intoxication, particularly following intravenous administration of the drug, and quinidine toxicity. It is also caused by electric shock and lightning stroke. The combination of chloroform anaesthesia and the parenteral administration of adrenaline has been known to cause ventricular fibrillation since the work of Levy (1915). In artificial hypothermia, ventricular fibrillation almost always ensues when the body temperature falls below about 28°C. Spontaneous reversion to sinus rhythm is not uncommon on re-warming. Sudden deaths following the intravascular injection of radio-opaque media are sometimes due to ventricular fibrillation. This is apparently an idiosyncrasy, for I have seen ventricular fibrillation follow the injection of only 10 ml into the ascending aorta.

Although, unless promptly treated, ventricular fibrillation is usually a terminal event, it can also occur in paroxysmal form reverting spontaneously to sinus rhythm. A typical example of paroxysmal ventricular fibrillation is quinidine syncope (page 188). Paroxysmal ventricular fibrillation may also occur in complete heart block and be responsible for Stokes–Adams attacks.

Paroxysmal Ventricular Fibrillation in Children

In 1957 Jervell and Lange-Neilson described a family in which four out of the five children were affected by congenital deafness whose electrocardiograms showed a prolonged Q–T interval and who were subject to recurrent syncopal attacks. Many similar families have since been described in which often a syncopal attack proved fatal. Ward (1964) was the first to appreciate that the syncopal attacks were due to ventricular fibrillation. The attacks were often precipitated by exertion or emotion. Similar families have since been described in which the affected children were not deaf. A case of particular interest was described by Wellens and colleagues (1972) in which attacks of ventricular fibrillation were provoked on arousal from sleep by auditory stimuli. The most effective treatment so far advanced is propranolol with diphenylhydantoin. On this combination Wellens' patient appeared to be cured.

The clinical picture and management of ventricular fibrillation will be discussed in detail in Chapter 16.

CHAPTER 9

ECTOPIC TACHYCARDIAS—PAROXYSMAL TACHYCARDIA

A classical account of attacks of rapid heart action, together with pulse tracings, was first given by Cotton in 1867. The condition was given its name by Bouveret in 1889 in his paper entitled 'De la tachycardie essentielle parosystique'. The name paroxysmal tachycardia type Bouveret still persists in the French literature.

Paroxysmal tachycardia may be defined as attacks of rapid heart action of abrupt onset due to an ectopic focus situated either in the atria, the A.V. junction or the ventricles. Since paroxysmal attacks of atrial flutter or fibrillation have a closely similar clinical picture, they are included in the syndrome. The duration of attacks may vary from a few seconds up to several days or even weeks. However, reasons have already been given why an attack which has lasted for more than 24 hours should be termed a sustained ectopic tachycardia. It is, however, unusual for attacks to last for more than 2–3 hours, and a duration of 2–3 minutes is common. Though in individual patients there may be variability in the length of attacks, they often show a tendency to have a more or less uniform pattern.

Aetiology

In approximately 60 per cent of patients with paroxysmal tachycardia, there is no other evidence of heart disease, and the cause in these cases is at present unknown. The remaining patients have organic heart disease of widely varying type. Thyrotoxicosis is an important cause of paroxysmal tachycardia, often atrial fibrillation, and may be overlooked. Other organic conditions commonly associated with paroxysmal tachycardia include rheumatic, syphilitic, ischaemic and congenital heart disease and the cardiomyopathies. An important cause, particularly in children, is the Wolff–Parkinson–White syndrome. Approximately 80 per cent of patients with this type of cardiographic anomaly exhibit attacks of paroxysmal tachycardia.

An unusual but clear-cut cause of paroxysmal tachycardia is pregnancy. It was mentioned in Chapter 6 that extrasystoles may develop in pregnancy, disappearing with parturition. The same is true of paroxysmal tachycardia, usually of atrial origin, which may appear for the first time in the middle trimester and attacks may continue with increasing severity until parturition, but always disappear within an hour or so of delivery. There is a tendency for recurrence of attacks with subsequent pregnancies, although no attacks occur in the non-pregnant state.

Electrocardiogram in Paroxysmal Tachycardia

When an electrocardiogram has been recorded during an attack, it usually enables the nature of the abnormal rhythm to be determined. If the QRS complexes are normal in duration, the tachycardia is supraventricular in origin. There is usually no difficulty in recognizing the presence of atrial flutter or atrial fibrillation. The usual difficulty in differentiating between atrial and A.V. junctional tachycardia, when no P waves are discernible, is common, and a non-committal diagnosis of supraventricular tachycardia may only be possible. When the QRS complexes are widened to 0·12 second or more, difficulty may arise in deciding whether the tachycardia is ventricular in origin or supraventricular with pre-existing bundle branch block or aberrant intraventricular conduction due to the rapid rate. This difficulty has already been discussed in the preceding chapter.

The heart rate in attacks of paroxysmal tachycardia usually lies between 160 and 200 per min. A rate of 150 per minute is always suggestive of atrial flutter. Slower rates between 110 and 150 per minute are occasionally seen. In children with paroxysmal atrial tachycardia, extremely rapid rates up to 300 per minute or more (with 1:1 A.V. conduction and normal QRS complexes) may occur.

When the change from sinus rhythm to paroxysmal tachycardia is recorded in the electrocardiogram, the first beat of the paroxysm is seen to be premature, and if the end of the paroxysm is recorded, it is usually, but not always, followed by a pause.

Between attacks, in the majority of cases, the electrocardiogram is normal. It is generally stated that when isolated extrasystoles are seen in the cardiogram between attacks, they are of the same origin as the tachycardia. This, in general, is true but it cannot be accepted as an invariable rule. In the first place, it is quite common for no extrasystoles to be recorded between attacks. In the second place, an isolated extrasystole between attacks may have a wide aberrant QRS and be mistaken for a ventricular ectopic, when it is actually supraventricular in origin. In such cases, if the commencement of a paroxysm is recorded, the QRS complex of the first one or two beats may be aberrant, while subsequent ones are normal in duration as the refractory period of the conduction system shortens with the increased rate. An example of this was shown in *Figure 6.18* (page 89).

Davis and Ross (1963) noted that between attacks of paroxysmal tachycardia, due either to paroxysmal atrial fibrillation or supraventricular tachycardia, the P waves were often abnormal. The incidence of this change was 21 per cent in 200 cases. The abnormal P waves are best seen in lead II; they are increased in duration from 0·12 to 0·16 second and are frequently notched, resembling a P mitrale. The precise cause of this change could not be determined but appears to reflect an abnormality in the left atrial component of the P wave.

When the electrocardiogram reveals bundle branch block between attacks, it may serve to clear up any doubt about their possible ventricular origin.

Transient S–T-segment and T-wave changes may follow attacks, especially if they are prolonged for several hours, but such changes rarely last as long as after a sustained attack of ventricular tachycardia.

Clinical Features of Paroxysmal Tachycardia

A diagnosis of paroxysmal tachycardia very commonly has to be made entirely from the patient's history. Very often there are no abnormal findings on clinical, radiological or electrocardiographic examination, and even if there are, they have usually no relevance as to whether the patient's complaint of palpitation is due to attacks of an abnormal rhythm. On the other hand, the diagnosis is quite simple if the patient is asked certain questions. When the complaint is of attacks of palpitation, it is first necessary to establish that the patient understands the meaning of the word. Occasionally patients confuse palpitation with a sense of distressed breathing or even with pain. When it is clear that the patient gets attacks in which he is conscious of a rapid heart action (often described as fluttering), it is first necessary to enquire if the attacks start abruptly or come on gradually. For a diagnosis of paroxysmal tachycardia, it is necessary to establish that the attacks come on abruptly; one moment all is normal, the next instant the attack has started; there is no preliminary build up of rate. An attempt should be made to estimate the heart rate in an attack. The patient should be asked to indicate the rate by tapping his own chest or the desk with a hand. If the rate indicated is slow (below 100 per minute), a diagnosis of a paroxysmal arrhythmia is very unlikely. If the diagnosis is correct, patients are generally surprisingly accurate in demonstrating rates up to 180 per minute; with rates above this they usually manage to indicate that it is extremely fast. It is always useful to enquire if the rhythm during an attack is regular or irregular. If the answer is irregular, the rhythm may well be paroxysmal atrial fibrillation, but flutter or atrial tachycardia with some irregular type of A.V. conduction anomaly cannot be excluded. A final question which should always be put is an enquiry as to the date, time and duration of the last attack. When the patient is able to give precise dates, times and duration of attacks, the diagnosis of paroxysmal tachycardia is certain. If the palpitation is of nervous origin, a common reply is 'I have it now', or the answer may be otherwise vague and unconvincing. A history of an abrupt termination of the attack is not necessarily always obtainable. Cessation of the tachycardia is often followed by transient sinus tachycardia which gives the patient the impression that the attack has died away gradually. Moreover, following reversion to sinus rhythm there may be a period with fairly frequent extrasystoles which can also convey to the patient the impression that the attack did not terminate suddenly. Many patients, however, are aware of the moment when reversion to sinus rhythm occurs. A confident diagnosis of paroxysmal tachycardia may always be made from a history of attacks of rapid palpitation, of abrupt onset, and where the patient can give precise dates, times and durations of recent episodes.

Frequency and Duration of Attacks

This is very variable, both from patient to patient, and in the same patient at different times. Attacks may be very infrequent, occurring once in two months or at even longer intervals. At the other extreme, patients are occasionally encountered who seem to have almost continuous paroxysmal tachycardia. Whenever they are seen, a fast abnormal rhythm is present, but they cannot be classified as sustained ectopic tachycardias, for it is clear from their histories that brief spells of normal rhythm occur many times in 24 hours. Although uncommon, such cases appear to form a distinct clinical entity. In much the commonest type of history, the patient experiences attacks two or three times a week, each attack lasting from a few minutes up to an hour, but with no very consistent pattern.

Associated Symptoms

The nature and severity of associated symptoms during attacks of tachycardia are determined by several factors, including the heart rate, the duration, the presence of organic heart disease and probably the integrity of the cerebral arterial supply. Most patients, including those without heart disease, are alarmed or even terrified by the attacks. In the absence of heart disease and with rates up to 180 per minute, the discomfort of the rapid palpitation, combined with apprehension as to the outcome, is generally the only symptom present. Some patients with cannon waves in the jugular venous pulse complain of a disagreeable throbbing sensation in the neck. Patients with organic heart disease may experience dyspnoea and orthopnoea during attacks. This is particularly true in mitral stenosis, for these patients are particularly intolerant of a rapid heart rate, and pulmonary oedema is an occasional urgent complication. In subjects with ischaemic heart disease or aortic stenosis, attacks may induce typical anginal pain. If such a patient is seen after the attack is over, the history of anginal pain which lasted for an hour or so may suggest a diagnosis of myocardial infarction, and this may appear to be substantiated by S–T segment and T-wave changes in the cardiograph following the arrhythmia. A history of coincident rapid palpitation and the transient nature of the ST T changes will usually make the diagnosis clear.

Cerebral symptoms are quite common, particularly in patients with organic heart disease or in elderly patients with cerebral vascular disease. Symptoms include various visual disturbances, particularly transient monocular visual loss, true vertigo and syncope. Occasionally patients develop frank hemiplegia during attacks, particularly those with rheumatic heart disease (Hutchinson and Stock, 1960). A woman aged 21 years was seen recently who described attacks occurring at weekly intervals, which all followed the same pattern. She first noticed the abrupt onset of rapid palpitation which was followed within seconds by true vertigo and then loss of consciousness. The duration of the attacks was about five minutes. There was no clinical, radiological or electrocardiographic evidence of heart disease. There were no abnormal signs in the central nervous system, but the symptoms suggested acute brain-stem ischaemia and were presumably triggered off by a fall in cardiac output or blood pressure, or both. The focal nature of the symptoms suggests that they may have been determined by the presence of a congenital anomaly of the vertebro-basilar arterial system.

Polyuria in Paroxysmal Tachycardia

Although it has been known for some time that attacks of paroxysmal tachycardia are sometimes associated with polyuria, a systematic study of the phenomenon was first undertaken by the late Dr Paul Wood and reported in a communication to the British Cardiac Society in 1961. His data were published posthumously in 1963. In summary, his findings were that polyuria might occur in any form of rapid paroxysmal arrhythmia. It

147

is most frequent in patients whose attacks last at least half an hour, with heart rates over 120 per minute. He found a total incidence of 50 per cent with polyuria in such patients. It seemed to occur rather more frequently in paroxysmal atrial flutter and fibrillation than in atrial tachycardia and was commoner in patients with otherwise normal hearts.

Posture is related to the amount of diuresis, which is more profuse and starts earlier in nocturnal attacks than when the patient is up and about. Although patients may fail to mention polyuria unless directly questioned, in some subjects the diuresis is a major symptom of an attack. For example, one of Wood's patients, whose attacks were nocturnal, was in conflict whether to get up to pass water and lose consciousness, or to stay where she was and risk the consequences.

The diuresis usually commences in about 20–30 minutes after the onset of the attack, and urine is passed about every half hour for one and a half hours up to 8 hours. At its peak, the volume of urine passed per hour is about 10 times greater than normal.

Nature of Diuresis

The volume of urine passed is considerable in quantity, pale in colour, of low specific gravity and electrolyte content. It is, in fact, a water diuresis, with the features of diabetes insipidus. Even so, large quantities of sodium chloride, and rather less of potassium, are lost during the diuresis. The pathogenesis may be inhibition of secretion of anti-diuretic hormone from the posterior pituitary. An alternative explanation may lie in the volume receptors of the left atrium, which are believed to play an important part in the control of blood volume. It has been shown that a large diuresis can be induced in a dog by distending a balloon in the left atrium. It is known that the left atrial pressure rises in paroxysmal tachycardia and it is an attractive hypothesis that left atrial distension is responsible for the diuresis. Against this view is the finding that patients with mitral stenosis do not have a diuresis during paroxysmal tachycardia, despite a very sharp rise in left atrial pressure. This objection is not necessarily insuperable, however, for in mitral stenosis, tachycardia may be associated with a sharp fall in cardiac output and in renal blood flow.

Although the diuresis of paroxysmal tachycardia is mainly of water, the excretion of Na in one of Wood's cases rose from an average normal of 4·1 m. equiv. per hour to 49·0 m. equiv. per hour, one and a half hours after the onset of an attack. This represents a considerable sodium loss and may explain a curious feature sometimes seen in children with paroxysmal tachycardia. The parents of a child aged 3 years with this condition, reported that during attacks the child flooded her cot with urine. They had also noted that the child had a craving for salt, so that all salt in the house had to be hidden; otherwise the child would be found eating it by the handful.

Ghose, Joekes and Kyriacov (1965) have recently suggested that the polyuria of paroxysmal tachycardia may simply be of emotional origin due to the associated anxiety and apprehension engendered by the attack. Such an explanation seems scarcely convincing for children, who are usually emotionally unconcerned.

Precipitating Factors in Attacks

In the majority of patients with paroxysmal tachycardia, no obvious precipitating factor for individual attacks can be elicited. The condition behaves in a capricious manner, attacks occurring without warning at any time of the night or day. Occasionally, in women, attacks are related to the menstrual cycle, occurring only in the pre-menstrual week or during menstruation. There is one important group of cases in which attacks are provoked by exertion or emotion. Gallavardin first separated this group, to which he applied the term 'tachycardie parosystique à centre excitable' (Gallavardin, 1922). This is an important group which can readily be overlooked if an accurate history is not taken. Patients with this condition may or may not have associated heart disease. Those with normal hearts may

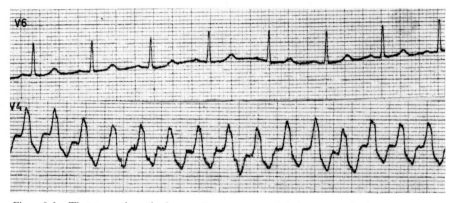

Figure 9.1—The top row shows the electrocardiogram at rest and the bottom row after light exercise. After light exercise there is an ectopic tachycardia with a rate of 190 per minute. Although the QRS complexes are wide, there is nothing in the record to indicate whether the tachycardia is ventricular or supraventricular in origin

only experience the discomfort of rapid palpitation induced by exertion. In taking the history, it is essential to establish that the onset of the palpitation is abrupt during exercise and not gradual. The attacks usually terminate abruptly with rest. In patients with organic heart disease, dyspnoea or cardiac pain may accompany the palpitation and may be severe enough to overshadow it, so that the tachycardia may not be mentioned. Similar attacks of tachycardia may result from emotional causes or may sometimes occur without evident reason. The condition should always be considered when the patient's symptoms in response to exercise are greater than would be anticipated from the clinical findings. The diagnosis can generally be readily confirmed by direct enquiry into the sudden onset of palpitation accompanying the symptoms produced by exertion or, more convincingly, by exercising the patient and recording an electrocardiogram. Symptoms in this variety of paroxysmal tachycardia can be very disabling, and it is clearly important not to miss the condition, since the response to antiarrhythmic drugs can be dramatic. *Figure 9.1* shows an example of an electrocardiogram before and after effort in a patient with mild aortic regurgitation, whose symptoms on exertion were disproportionate to the clinical findings.

Paroxysmal Tachycardia in Infancy and Childhood

Paroxysmal supraventricular tachycardias are not uncommon in infants and young children; the features of sustained attacks were described in Chapter 7. A characteristic feature in this age group is the ability of the atria to contract at rates well over 200 per minute without fibrillating and of the A.V. junction to conduct the rapid stimuli to the ventricles in a 1:1 ratio. In 10 per cent of children the attacks are virtually symptomless and may be accidentally noted during routine physical examination. In the record shown in *Figure 9.2*, an attack of supraventricular tachycardia developed with a ventricular rate of 260 per minute which occurred during a

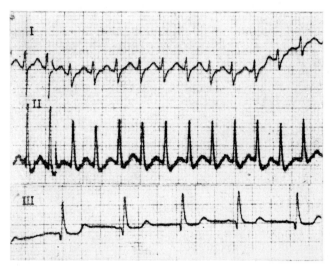

Figure 9.2—Leads I and II, recorded simultaneously, show a short burst of supraventricular tachycardia which had spontaneously subsided by the time lead III was recorded (see text)

routine cardiographic recording. The child, a boy aged 4 years, referred to his heart as his 'fire engine'; he remarked that his 'fire engine was at it again'. The attacks seldom lasted as long as a minute. When an attack becomes a sustained tachycardia lasting more than 24 hours, heart failure may develop (page 125).

Treatment of Paroxysmal Tachycardia

This will be considered in Chapter 12.

Repetitive Paroxysmal Tachycardia

Although relatively uncommon, it is important to be aware of this condition since, in general, its outlook is benign, despite a bizarre and often ominous-looking electrocardiogram. Gallavardin was the first to describe it and to insist on its distinction from ordinary paroxysmal tachycardia (type Bouveret). He called it first 'extrasystolie à paroxysmes tachycardiques' and later used the term 'tachycardie en salves'. Parkinson and Papp (1947) described a series of 40 patients and re-named the condition repetitive paroxysmal tachycardia. These authors stressed the continuous nature of the arrhythmia, so that it was rare to record an electrocardiogram free from ectopic beats, in contrast to ordinary paroxysmal tachycardia where the difficulty is often to obtain a record of an attack. The electrocardiogram shows repetitive short paroxysms of either supraventricular or ventricular tachycardia separated by only a few sinus beats. The number of ectopic beats in each 'paroxysm' varies from one to about twenty. The atrial variety is generally said to be the most common, though in my personal series of 33 cases, 21 were of the ventricular variety. There is rarely any evidence of organic heart disease, although the heart may show generalized enlargement radiologically, which reverts to normal when the arrhythmia is controlled or ceases. Occasionally, patients with frank organic heart disease, usually ischaemic, have electrocardiograms showing repetitive runs of tachycardia, generally ventricular. Such cases are not examples of the condition under consideration here. The distinction is not easy from the electrocardiogram alone, but clinically the difference is usually clear, the patients with organic heart disease being obviously seriously ill. Occasionally, patients with sustained ventricular tachycardia, when treated with quinidine, are converted into a rhythm which cardiographically resembles repetitive paroxysmal ventricular tachycardia. Obviously, this condition is essentially different, but it may provide a link between the two arrhythmias.

Aetiology

The cause of the condition is entirely unknown. It appears to be a functional derangement of the specialized tissues of the heart, with a tendency to spontaneous recovery after the passage of time. In most reported series, the sex ratio shows a 2:1 preponderance in males.

Clinical Features

The arrhythmia is commonest in children and young adults, but no age appears exempt. Symptoms are remarkably few, the commonest complaint being one of palpitation, with perhaps mild dyspnoea on effort. Syncopal episodes have occasionally been reported in the ventricular form, but I have never encountered this. Once established, the arrhythmia tends to persist over months or years but seems almost always to disappear eventually. Clinically, at first, the impression may be given of atrial fibrillation. The diagnosis can only be established by the electrocardiogram which also differentiates between the supraventricular and ventricular varieties.

Although the clinical course of most patients with repetitive paroxysmal tachycardia is uneventful, occasional cases have been reported who died suddenly, and some, with ventricular variety, have developed prolonged episodes of sustained ventricular tachycardia with heart failure. Even in these, the eventual prognosis is generally good, as, for instance, the oft-quoted patient of Gallavardin's who, after long years of chronic invalidism, eventually recovered completely and was actively following a career as a midwife at the age of 61 years.

As in ordinary paroxysmal tachycardia, an occasional case is seen in which the arrhythmia is provoked only by emotion or exertion. Illustrative electrocardiograms of the arrhythmia are shown in *Figures 9.3, 9.4* and *9.5.*

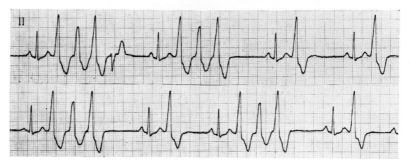

Figure 9.3—The two rows are continuous. There is a repetitive paroxysmal ventricular tachycardia in a man aged 45 years. The patient had no symptoms and was not conscious of palpitation. He was referred because of the irregular heart action which had been noted on a routine examination

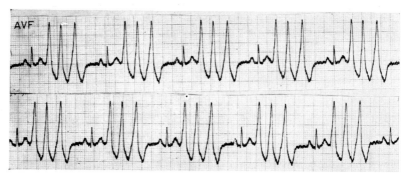

Figure 9.4—The two rows are continuous. This is another example of a benign repetitive paroxysmal ventricular tachycardia. The patient, a woman aged 22 years, was again symptomless and the arrhythmia was an incidental finding

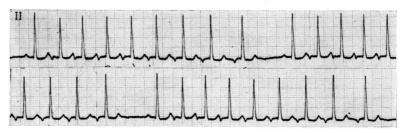

Figure 9.5—This shows a repetitive atrial tachycardia which was an incidental finding in an otherwise symptomless patient, a man aged 25 years

Treatment

Most cases of repetitive paroxysmal tachycardia prove resistant to anti-arrhythmic drugs. Some cases respond to quinidine, but usually the effect is only temporary and the arrhythmia recurs despite continued treatment. One case of the ventricular variety, which was only induced by effort, has been completely controlled by propranolol in a dose of 40 mg t.d.s.

CHAPTER 10

ATRIOVENTRICULAR DISSOCIATION (NOT DUE TO ANTEGRADE BLOCK)

Atrioventricular dissociation belongs to the group of pararrhythmias, which include parasystole, and which were defined on page 101. It is an arrhythmia of considerable physiological and clinical interest. Its interest is probably out of all proportion to its importance, for symptoms are trivial or absent (apart from those due to the underlying cause), and all authorities agree that it has little prognostic significance.

In its commonest form, a faster A.V. junctional pacemaker controls the ventricles and coincides with a slower sino-atrial rhythm controlling the atria. As the timing of the two rhythms shift, sinus impulses will periodically reach the A.V. junction outside its refractory period and will then be conducted to, and 'capture', the ventricles.

Terminology

Unfortunately, in published descriptions of this arrhythmia, terminology has become very confused, mainly owing to the use of the term 'interference' in two completely different senses by different authors. This term is generally understood to mean that when the sinus impulse captures the ventricles, it 'interferes' with the A.V. junctional rhythm and the ventricular capture is called an 'interference beat'. Authors using the word in this sense speak of 'A.V. dissociation with interference'. Other authors, on the other hand, have used the term 'interference' quite differently. When in A.V. dissociation, the timing of the sino-atrial and A.V. junctional impulses is such that the oncoming sinus impulse encounters the junctional impulse travelling in a retrograde direction towards the atria, they mutually extinguish each other, and this 'physiological' block is termed 'interference'. In consequence, these authors refer to this arrhythmia as 'interference dissociation', implying that the independence of the two rhythms is maintained by 'interference'. As Marriott (1957) has pointed out, this discrepancy in the use of the term 'interference' is particularly unfortunate because the two interpretations conflict, for the 'interference beats' of the first school are the only beats in which 'interference', as interpreted by the second school, plays no part. After careful consideration, it seems best to avoid the term 'interference' altogether and it will not be used in this book. Unfortunately, this still leaves a rather unsatisfactory semantic difficulty, for it is necessary to restrict the term A.V. dissociation, arbitrarily, to those cases in which complete antegrade A.V. block is not the cause, although the atria and ventricles necessarily beat independently in the latter condition.

Physiology

Atrioventricular dissociation may be defined as an arrhythmia in which, for one or more beats, the atria and ventricles are controlled by different pacemakers in the absence of antegrade block. In most instances this occurs when, for any reason, the rate of discharge of an A.V. junctional pacemaker exceeds that of the sino-atrial node. Much less commonly, the faster pacemaker may be situated in the ventricles. The precipitating mechanism may be a slowing in the rate of discharge of the sinus node below that of the inherent rate of the lower pacemaker, which then 'escapes'. Alternatively, there may be acceleration in the rate of the lower pacemaker so that it exceeds that of the sinus rate. Whichever mechanism operates, the essential condition is that the rate of the lower pacemaker exceeds that of the atrial pacemaker. Since it is a fundamental rule in cardiac physiology that normally the pacemaker with the faster rate of discharge controls the

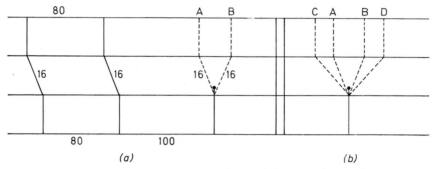

Figure 10.1—Diagram to illustrate the zone of potential dissociation (see text for discussion)

whole heart, a further factor must be present if dissociation is to persist. As in parasystole, the slower pacemaker must be protected from being discharged by the impulses of the faster pacemaker. In A.V. dissociation, the slower atrial pacemaker is protected from discharge by the presence of retrograde block in the A.V. junction above the ventricular pacemaker. This prevents the faster A.V. junctional impulses from reaching the atria and discharging the sinus node. Since antegrade conduction is usually unimpaired, the gradual shift in the timing of atrial and ventricular activation will permit, sooner or later, a sinus impulse to reach the A.V. junction outside its absolute refractory period, and it will be conducted to, and 'capture', the ventricles. Thus, A.V. dissociation is never complete if a long enough record is taken. The physiological principles involved in A.V. dissociation may be illustrated most simply by considering an A.V. junctional escape beat due to a pause in the sinus rhythm. *Figure 10.1a* shows the time relationship diagrammatically employing the conventional key. The first two beats show a sinus cycle of 0·8 second (rate 75 per minute) with a P–R interval of 0·16 second. There is then a sudden pause in the sinus rhythm. An A.V. junctional escape interval of 1·0 second is assumed. The point A is marked 0·16 second before this. If the sinus node discharged after this point, its impulse would fail to reach the A.V. junctional pacemaker before it discharged, and dissociation would occur. If retrograde conduction time were the same as antegrade conduction time, and the sinus pause persisted, the A.V. junctional impulse would control the whole heart and would capture the atria, reaching and discharging the sinus node at the point marked B. On the other hand, if the sinus node discharges at any time between the points A and B, it would control the atria but not the ventricles. The time interval between A and B has been termed the 'zone of potential dissociation' and is equal to the sum of the conduction times between the two centres (that is, the sino-atrial and atrioventricular nodes). This zone of potential dissociation will clearly be lengthened if either antegrade or retrograde conduction times are prolonged. This is illustrated in *Figure 10.1b*. With equal prolongation of conduction time in both directions, the zone of potential dissociation would be from point C to point D. In practice, it is usually

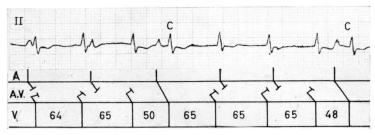

Figure 10.2—Simple A.V. dissociation with two capture beats

only retrograde conduction time which is prolonged, so the zone is between point A and point D. If the sinus node discharges anywhere between these two points, A.V. dissociation would result. If the discharge rate of the two centres were to remain the same, dissociation would continue indefinitely. However, when, as is more usual, the rates are different, a gradual shift in the timing of the two centres results, and when a sinus impulse falls outside the zone of potential dissociation, it will be conducted to and will capture the ventricles. A capture beat can normally be recognized because it is premature in time, disturbing the otherwise orderly sequence of A.V. junctional beats. In its passage through the A.V. junction, the sinus impulse necessarily discharges the immature impulse forming in the A.V. junctional pacemaker. As would be expected, the interval between the conducted (capture) beat and the next junctional beat is equal to the usual interval between two junctional beats, for a new impulse starts forming in the junctional pacemaker immediately following its discharge.

Electrocardiogram

The most common form of A.V. dissociation is due to non-paroxysmal A.V. junctional tachycardia, the A.V. junctional rate being somewhat faster than the sinus rate. *Figure 10.2* shows an example. Atrioventricular dissociation is immediately apparent from the characteristic wandering of successive P waves through the QRS complexes (indicating that the atrial rate is slower than the ventricular). When the P wave has emerged beyond the QRS complex, the sinus impulse finds the A.V. junction non-refractory and it is conducted to and captures the ventricles. The capture beat is premature and the interval between it and the next junctional beat corresponds to the A.V. junctional cycle length.

While capture beats are normally recognizable by their prematurity, sometimes their QRS complexes are different in contour from those of A.V. junctional beats. This difference in contour was discussed on page 63.

155

Figure 10.3 shows an example of A.V. dissociation in which captures can immediately be recognized by their different contour. The mechanism of the arrhythmia is best seen in the short strip of lead I where the P waves are more readily discernible. Atrioventricular dissociation is apparent from the regular ventricular rate (cycle length 58) while successive P waves wander through the QRS complexes. The last P wave of the strip is conducted, and the QRS complex is slightly different from the A.V. junctional ones and is premature. The difference in contour between nodal and conducted beats is most evident in lead III where sinus beats have a mainly positive deflection

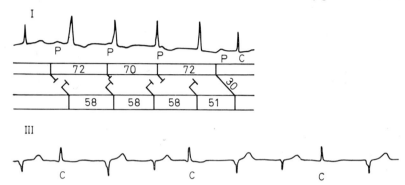

Figure 10.3—A.V. dissociation with capture beats. The sinus and junctional beats have different contours, most evident in lead III (see text)

and junctional beats a mainly negative one. (In this case in lead III the P waves are not visible.)

If the rates of the two pacemakers in A.V. dissociation remain constant, two successive capture beats should not occur. The first capturing sinus impulse necessarily discharges the faster junctional pacemaker, the next impulse of which will be due before the next sinus impulse could arrive. However, two consecutive (rarely three) capture beats may occur, and this phenomenon has been studied by Schamroth (1966). He described two possible mechanisms. First, if concealed retrograde conduction of the junctional impulses occurs, this will render the A.V. node above the junctional pacemaker partially refractory to a capturing sinus impulse which, in consequence, will be delayed in reaching and discharging the junctional pacemaker. The next sinus impulse will find the upper part of the A.V. junction in a non-refractory phase and will therefore reach the junctional pacemaker before it has discharged, and a second capture beat results. An alternative mechanism is the depression of the junctional pacemaker following its premature discharge, so that its next impulse is unduly delayed, enabling a second sinus impulse to effect another capture. Whichever mechanism operates, the P–R interval of the first capture beat is always appreciably longer than the second. An example of the two successive captures is shown in *Figure 10.4*.

Duration of Cycle Following Capture Beat

If the conduction time through the A.V. junction of a capture beat is normal, and the junctional pacemaker immediately commences to generate a fresh impulse following its discharge, the cycle length following a capture beat will equal a 'normal' junctional cycle. Sometimes, however, it is shorter and in other instances it is longer. Shortening of the first ventricular cycle following a capture may be due to prolongation of the conduction time (P–R interval) of the capture beat. This will necessarily shorten the next ventricular cycle. Lengthening of this cycle, on the other hand, is sometimes seen. It has already been mentioned that premature discharge of any pacemaker may result in temporary depression of its activity. When the junctional pacemaker is discharged by a capture beat, such transient depression may

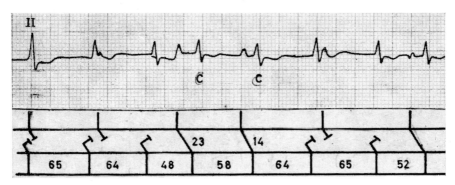

Figure 10.4—A.V. dissociation with two consecutive capture beats, marked C (see text)

delay the appearance of the next junctional beat and the first post-capture ventricular cycle is prolonged. According to Scherf and Schott (1953), occasionally following a captured beat, the next ventricular cycle length is far longer than can be accounted for by transient depression of the junctional pacemaker. They attribute this to concealed conduction of the next sinus impulse which, although it becomes blocked before reaching the ventricles, effects a partial capture and again discharges the junctional pacemaker. Such long cycles are usually terminated by a second capture beat.

Rate of Lower Pacemaker

In most cases of A.V. dissociation, the lower pacemaker (usually A.V. junctional) is only slightly faster than the atrial pacemaker. The usual mechanism is non-paroxysmal 'nodal' tachycardia (Pick and Dominguez, 1957). Miller and Sharrett (1957) termed these 'homogenetic rhythms', in contrast to those in which the lower centre was very much faster than the upper centre. They termed these 'heterogenetic rhythms'. A good example is ventricular tachycardia without retrograde conduction. An independent slower atrial rhythm is maintained and, at least in this sense, many cases of ventricular tachycardia may manifest A.V. dissociation. A similar situation may be present in A.V. junctional tachycardia with a fast rate.

Atrioventricular Dissociation in Atrial Arrhythmias

In atrial arrhythmias, whether atrial tachycardia, fibrillation or flutter, A.V. dissociation may occur. This is usually a manifestation of digitalis intoxication and will be discussed in detail in Chapter 15. *Figure 10.5* shows an example due to digitalis intoxication. There is atrial tachycardia with A.V. dissociation and bigeminy due to ventricular extrasystoles. The third beat of the dominant rhythm is a ventricular capture.

Atrial Captures

In the majority of cases of A.V. dissociation, disturbance of one rhythm by the other takes the form of ventricular captures by a sinus impulse. This is because of the presence of retrograde block in the A.V. junction,

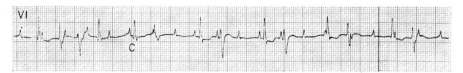

Figure 10.5—Extract from lead VI from a patient with digitalis intoxication. The atrial rate is 142/min. and there is A.V. dissociation with a capture beat marked C recognized because of its prematurity. Most of the junctional beats are followed by ventricular extrasystoles with a fixed coupling time of ·046 second

with preservation of normal antegrade conduction. Cases have been described, however, in which both ventricular and atrial captures occur. (An atrial capture is recognized by the occurrence of a retrograde P′ wave following a junctional QRS, the P′ wave being premature in the atrial rhythm.) It is difficult to explain the occurrence of both ventricular and atrial captures in the same case unless the retrograde block is assumed to be intermittent. An atrial capture may discharge the sinus node and be followed by a period in which the A.V. junction controls the whole heart.

Fusion Beats in Atrioventricular Dissociation

In A.V. dissociation between an atrial and an idioventricular pacemaker, a fusion beat may occur when the ventricles are invaded simultaneously by impulses from both pacemakers. More rarely, fusion may occur between

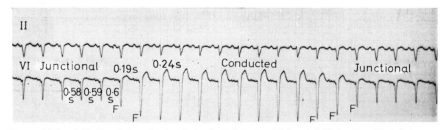

Figure 10.6—A.V. dissociation showing fusion beats between atrial and A.V. junctional impulses as one rhythm merges into and out of the other (see text)

an atrial and a junctional impulse if the latter are using a different pathway in the A.V. junction. *Figure 10.6* shows an example of this phenomenon. The record is an extract from a 20 minute recording of a patient with a complex arrhythmia due to digitalis intoxication. Leads II and VI were recorded simultaneously with a twin channel machine. QRS complexes with two distinct contours are seen, the difference being much more evident in lead VI. Most of the QRS complexes have S waves only 12 mm in depth, but in the middle of the strip, the QRS complexes have S waves which are 30 mm in depth. The deep QRS complexes are preceded by P waves with a fixed P–R interval of 0·24 second, whereas the shallow ones have no constant relation to P waves. Clearly, therefore, the deep QRS complexes are conducted beats and the shallow ones are junctional beats with A.V. dissociation. The strip commences with A.V. dissociation, the ventricles being controlled by the junctional pacemaker. In the middle of the strip there is a run of conducted beats with a P–R interval of 0·24 second, and then junctional rhythm with A.V. dissociation recurs. As one rhythm merges into the other, QRS complexes of intermediate contour occur. These intermediate QRS complexes have all the characteristics of fusion beats resulting from simultaneous invasion of the ventricles by atrial and junctional impulses using different pathways in the A.V. junction. The rhythm change is initiated by slight slowing of the junctional pacemaker, its cycle lengthening from 0·58 to 0·6 second, while the atrial rate remains constant. This results in gradual separation of the P wave and QRS complexes, and when the P–R interval reaches 0·19 second, the first fusion beat occurs. Following a second fusion beat, there is a run of eight consecutive complete ventricular captures by the atrial pacemaker, slight acceleration of the junctional pacemaker results in two more fusion beats and then the A.V. junction resumes full control of the ventricles. A striking feature throughout the whole of this record was that the atrial and A.V. junctional rates remained virtually identical.

Atrioventricular Dissociation with Upper Pacemaker Faster than Lower

Occasionally, in A.V. dissociation, the actual sinus rate is faster than the A.V. junctional rate. There are several sets of conditions in which this apparent anomaly may occur. In patients with incomplete A.V. block, the site of which is above the A.V. junctional pacemaker, the rate of the *conductible* impulses which reach the region of the pacemaker may be slower than the A.V. junctional rate. This may happen in 2:1 A.V. block if the sinus rate slows for any reason. The electrocardiogram may then be indistinguishable from complete A.V. block unless capture beats occur. Obviously, for a conducted beat to occur, the refractory period of the A.V. junction (expressed as the shortest R–P interval allowing conduction), plus the A.V. conduction time, must be shorter than the A.V. junctional cycle length. An example of this type of A.V. dissociation is shown in *Figure 10.7*.

Figure 10.8 shows an unusual example of A.V. dissociation with a faster sinus rate than the A.V. junctional rate. In this record there is a striking difference between the contour of the QRS complexes of the sinus and junctional beats. It may, therefore, be presumed that the junctional impulses are using an accessory pathway in the A.V. junction. The sinus cycle length is 0·84 second (72 per minute) and the junctional cycle length is 0·88 second (68 per minute). Each spell of junctional rhythm is initiated by a ventricular extrasystole. This prevents the descent of the next sinus beat. The junctional pacemaker is thus transiently enabled to assume control of the ventricles until the faster sinus impulse overtakes it and regains control of the whole heart.

Accrochage in Atrioventricular Dissociation

The atrial and ventricular rates are sometimes almost identical. Where this happens, it is common for the atria and ventricles to beat simultaneously

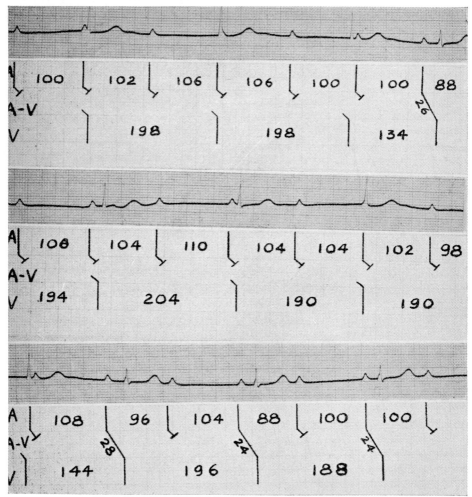

Figure 10.7—A.V. dissociation occurring during 2:1 A.V. block. Reproduced from 'Atrioventricular Dissociation with and without Interference,' by A. Schott by courtesy of Grune and Stratton

and the condition is sometimes called A.V. synchrony. It is rare for such synchronization to persist for very long, but it happens with sufficient frequency to suggest that there may be some underlying mechanism responsible. For example, it is not uncommon to see records of A.V. dissociation in which the initially slower P wave gets closer and closer to successive QRS complexes, but instead of going through them, the sinus rate accelerates as soon as the two complexes (P and QRS) coincide and a period of synchronization results. These findings suggest that when there are two independent pacemakers in the heart at the same time, the rate of one may influence the rate of the other. There is experimental support for such a concept. Segers (1946) reported that if two excised strips of cardiac muscle which were beating spontaneously were placed in contact or were joined by a drop of Ringer's solution, they would begin to beat synchronously, provided

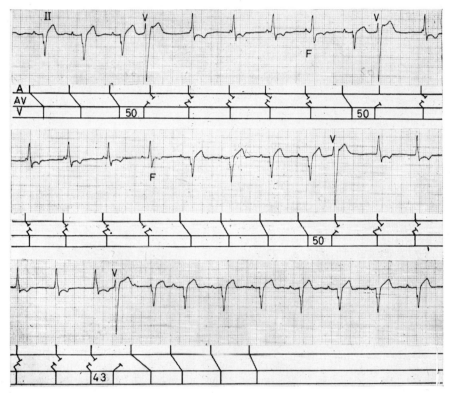

Figure 10.8—Unusual case of A.V. dissociation in which the sinus rate is faster than the junctional rate (for full description see text). The three rows are continuous, and towards the end of the first and at the beginning of the second row, there are beats strongly suggestive of fusion beats between atrial and junctional impulses

their original rates were within 25 per cent of each other. The synchronized rate was usually that of the faster beating strip, the slower beating strip accelerating. He also noted synchronization to occur in a 2:1 ratio, especially when a strip of atrial muscle was placed in contact with a ventricular strip. It has long been observed that, in complete A.V. block, the atrial and ventricular rates are not always completely independent. In 1947, Segers, Lequime and Denolin described a case of complete A.V. block in which the atrial rate was consistently double that of the ventricles, although the time relations of the P waves to the QRS complexes showed constant minor variations. They considered that this approximate synchronization resulted from the same mechanism as that which Segers had observed in the isolated strips of cardiac muscle. When simultaneous beating of cardiac fragments or chambers (in the intact heart) was short-lived, lasting for only a few beats, Segers used the term 'accrochage' (which literally means a hooking together), whereas when it lasted for long periods, he used the term synchronization. Used in this sense, therefore, accrochage is merely a brief

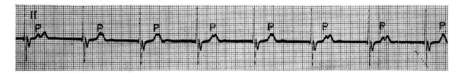

Figure 10.9—A.V. dissociation with accrochage. This has sometimes been referred to as iso-rhythmic dissociation

spell of synchronization. However, it would seem better to use the term 'accrochage' for all forms of synchronization of two otherwise independent pacemakers, in order to imply some active process rather than a fortuitous coincidence. *Figure 10.9* shows an example of A.V. dissociation with accrochage. The QRS complexes show a fixed cycle length of 1·2 seconds. An upright P wave is seen lying in the ST segment of each QRS complex. Since this is lead II, it cannot be a retrograde P' wave, which excludes a diagnosis of junctional rhythm.

The underlying mechanism responsible for accrochage is not yet understood. There is experimental and clinical evidence for both a mechanical and an electrical mechanism.

Termination of Atrioventricular Dissociation

Atrioventricular dissociation is generally a transient arrhythmia, although occasional cases are seen who are always found to show it, whenever they are reviewed. When dissociation is between the sino-atrial and atrioventricular pacemakers, normal sinus rhythm will follow either slowing of the

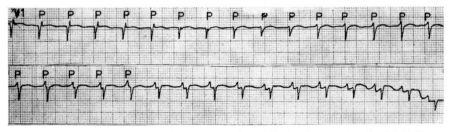

Figure 10.10—A.V. dissociation with transient accrochage following d.c. reversion of atrial fibrillation (for further discussion see text)

lower pacemaker or acceleration of the sinus rate. *Figure 10.10* illustrates the termination of A.V. dissociation by acceleration of the sinus rate. This record was obtained from a patient following reversion of atrial fibrillation by direct current shock. After a shock of 50 watt-seconds, the ventricular rhythm, which had previously been completely irregular, was found to be quite regular, but no P waves were visible. The rate was 120 per minute. After about two minutes a diagnosis of A.V. junctional tachycardia was made, but before a further shock could be given to terminate this, the cardiogram illustrated in *Figure 10.10* was recorded. This reveals that A.V. dissociation with accrochage was present; the record shows acceleration of the sinus rate which gradually brings the P wave back from its position at the end of QRS complex to preceding it, and finally gaining control with discharge of the junctional pacemaker. The sinus rate gradually slowed down to 80 per minute over the next five minutes without recurrence of arrhythmia.

Diagnosis of Atrioventricular Dissociation

When the lower pacemaker is faster than the atrial pacemaker, the diagnosis is usually quite easy. Successive P waves are seen to get closer to the QRS complexes and then to wander through them. Once a P wave has reached the ST segment, it is usually followed by a premature QRS complex, indicating a ventricular capture. In more complex forms of A.V. dissociation, it can be very helpful if the conducted and A.V. junctional QRS complexes differ in contour. This may enable the origin of a QRS complex to be recognized at a glance, without the necessity for measurement. At one time it was thought that a diagnostic feature of A.V. dissociation was that the atrial pacemaker was slower than the ventricular pacemaker, thus distinguishing the arrhythmia from complete A.V. block. Exceptions to this, however, occur and have been discussed above.

Aetiology of Atrioventricular Dissociation

Occasional cases of A.V. dissociation are seen in otherwise normal hearts. This is, however, extremely rare but has been recorded in subjects with coronary sinus rhythm. There are three conditions in which A.V. dissociation is particularly liable to occur; namely, digitalis intoxication, active rheumatic carditis and recent diaphragmatic myocardial infarction. All three conditions are known to involve the A.V. junction and to produce impaired conduction, especially retrograde conduction, and at the same time to enhance the rhythmicity of the A.V. junctional pacemakers. An identical situation may follow the trauma of open heart surgery.

Clinical Features of Atrioventricular Dissociation

In the common type of A.V. dissociation in which the ventricular rate is only slightly faster than the atrial rate, no symptoms may be present or the patient may complain of palpitation due to the capture beats. Clinically, without an electrocardiogram, the arrhythmia is indistinguishable from extrasystoles. It has no particular prognostic significance of itself, though it may give early warning of serious digitalis intoxication (*see* Chapter 15).

CHAPTER 11

THE WOLFF–PARKINSON–WHITE SYNDROME

Wolff, Parkinson and White (1930) described a group of 11 cases under the title 'Bundle branch block with short P–R interval in healthy young people prone to paroxysmal tachycardia'. This was the first time that an abnormal electrocardiogram associated with a tendency to attacks of tachycardia had been recognized as a definite clinical syndrome, although similar isolated cases had been published previously, the first by Wilson in 1915. The syndrome is important for several reasons. First, the electrocardiogram may simulate that of serious organic heart disease when none is present and, secondly, studies of the recurrent arrhythmias which are commonly associated with this syndrome have shed a good deal of light on the mechanisms of arrhythmias in general. Although the syndrome is relatively uncommon, numerous theories have been advanced to explain the underlying mechanism and these will be discussed in some detail below.

There is some evidence that the syndrome is hereditary and at least seven families have been described in the literature where the mode of transmission appeared to be that of an autosomal dominant trait.

Terminology

Ten years after the original publication, the term 'Wolff–Parkinson–White Syndrome' (or W.P.W. syndrome) was introduced by Öehnell in 1940. He later called it the pre-excitation syndrome (Öehnell, 1944). In 1945 Rosenbaum and colleagues re-named the condition 'anomalous atrioventricular conduction'. Although these three terms are used interchangeably in the literature, the eponymous title 'Wolff–Parkinson–White Syndrome' seems preferable on historical grounds. Moreover, pre-excitation of the ventricles is absent in that variety of the condition in which there is a short P–R interval, a normal QRS and recurrent attacks of supraventricular tachycardia.

Electrocardiographic Criteria

In the classical electrocardiogram of the Wolff–Parkinson–White syndrome, the P waves are usually normal. The P–R interval measures less than 0·12 second in 85 per cent of the cases and is often less than 0·1 second. The QRS complexes are widened to more than 0·1 second but in the majority of cases the P–J interval (measured from the onset of the P wave to the end of the QRS complex) remains normal. In many leads, the first part of the widened QRS complex is slurred and this slurring is referred to as the delta wave. In consequence of the delta wave, Q waves are usually absent in leads I, AVL and left praecordial leads. In some cases the direction of the delta wave is such that Q waves or QS complexes may be seen in leads II, III and AVF which may mimic diaphragmatic myocardial infarction

(*Figure 11.1*). Secondary changes in the ST segments and T waves are commonly present, the T waves pointing in the opposite direction from the delta wave.

Types of Wolff–Parkinson–White Syndrome

Rosenbaum and colleagues (1945) divided the Wolff–Parkinson–White syndrome into two types, according to the direction of the delta wave. In

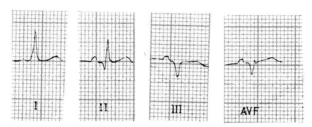

Figure 11.1—Traces showing the Wolff–Parkinson–White syndrome with a short P–R interval most evident in lead I and the delta wave has produced Q waves in leads II, III and AVF, mimicking diaphragmatic myocardial infarction

Type A, the delta force is directed anteriorly, inferiorly and to the right, producing mainly positive deflections in the right praecordial leads (*Figure 11.2*). In Type B the delta forces are directed posteriorly and to the left,

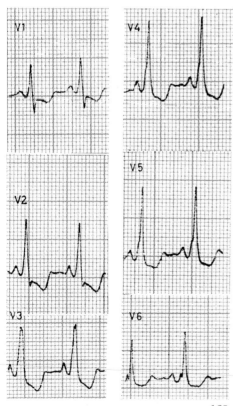

Figure 11.2—Praecordial leads from a patient with Wolff–Parkinson–White Type A. The P–R interval is short and the QRS complex is widened. In the right praecordial leads the dominant deflection of the QRS is positive. However, the P–R interval is short and the QRS complex is widened. This pattern should not be confused with right ventricular hypertrophy or right bundle branch block

producing slurred downward deflections in the right praecordial leads (*Figure 11.3*). According to Grant, Tomlinson and van Buren (1958), the delta forces may also have a direction intermediate between these two.

Variations of Anomalous Atrio-ventricular Conduction in the Wolff–Parkinson–White Syndrome

There are three variations of atrio-ventricular conduction in the W.P.W. electrocardiographic pattern. The first was called by Öhnell the 'concertina effect'. In these electrocardiograms there are variations in the length of the

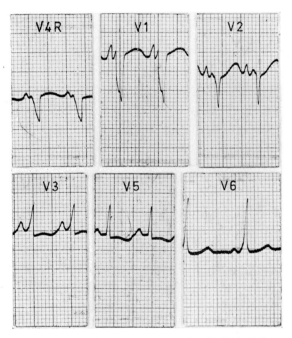

Figure 11.3—Praecordial leads in Wolff–Parkinson–White Type B. In the right praecordial leads there is a downward slurred QRS complex. (Reproduced by courtesy of Dr. A Hudson.)

P–R interval, the longer P–R intervals being associated with a reduction in height and duration of the delta waves and a consequent narrowing of the QRS complex, although the P–J interval remains constant (*Figure 11.4*). This variation has been attributed to differences in the amount of ventricular myocardium which undergoes pre-excitation. The second variant has been called the 'Lown–Ganong–Levine Syndrome'. In this syndrome, the P–R interval is short, measuring 0·12 second or less, but the QRS complexes are normal and no delta wave is present. These patients however are similarly prone to attacks of ectopic tachycardia (*Figure 11.5*). In the third variation, which is rare, the P–R interval is normal or even prolonged, but delta waves are present with widened QRS complexes.

The pre-excitation pattern may be found every time an electrocardiogram is done. On the other hand, in some subjects it may be quite transitory,

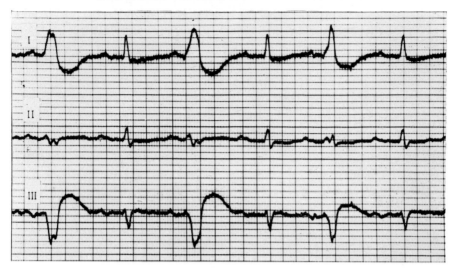

Figure 11.4—This shows the three standard leads recorded simultaneously. The Wolff–Parkinson–White pattern is present in alternate beats. It shows moreover the 'concertina effect'. In the fifth beat of the record the P–R interval is a little longer and the QRS complex a little narrower than the other beats with pre-excitation. The P–J interval remains constant throughout. (Time markings 1/10 second.)

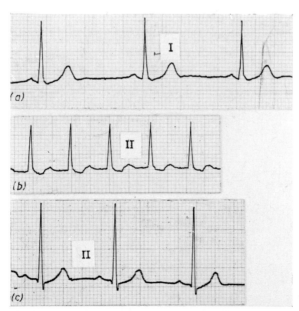

Figure 11.5—Illustrating the Lown-Ganong-Levine syndrome occurring in one of a pair of identical twins. All three records are of lead II. (a) Shows a short P–R interval (0·11 second) and a normal QRS complex. This child was subject to attacks of paroxysmal tachycardia. (b) Shows a record during such an attack with a rate of 144/min. (c) Shows lead II from the identical twin who had no attacks of paroxysmal tachycardia. The P–R interval in (c) is normal, measuring 0·17 second. (Reproduced by courtesy of Dr. Robinson and Dr. R. Gibson.)

being present for only a few beats, or appearing and disappearing in successive electrocardiograms (*Figure 11.6*). Many children presenting with the syndrome and attacks of ectopic tachycardia have been recorded in whom the electrocardiogram has later reverted to normal with disappearance of the paroxysms of arrhythmia.

Electrocardiographic Diagnosis

The electrocardiographic diagnosis is usually easy and is based on the presence of a short P–R interval with a deformed and widened QRS complex. The first part of the QRS complex or delta wave represents pre-excitation

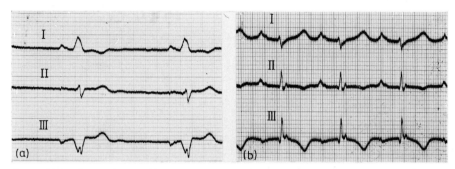

Figure 11.6—Showing leads I, II and III recorded simultaneously on 2 successive days from a girl aged 14 years with Ebstein's anomaly of the tricuspid valve. (a) Shows the Wolff–Parkinson–White pattern with a short P–R interval and wide QRS complex. (b) Recorded the following day, shows a normal P–R interval and the pattern of incomplete right bundle branch block. (Time markings 1/10 second.)

of part of the ventricular musculature and this is fused with the last part of the QRS which represents normal excitation of the remainder of the ventricular musculature via the normal conduction pathways. Occasionally the Wolff–Parkinson–White pattern may only be present in alternate beats (*Figure 11.4*).

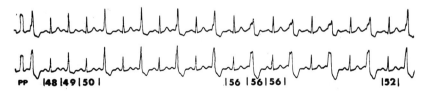

PP |48 |49 |50 | |56 |56 |56| |52|

Figure 11.7—Showing leads I and II recorded simultaneously from a patient having a ventricular extrasystole with a fixed coupling time of 0·48 second occurring after every beat. Wolff–Parkinson–White syndrome in alternate beats is mimicked. For fuller explanation, see text. (Reproduced by courtesy of Dr. R. Gold.)

It may then be difficult to differentiate from a ventricular extrasystole with a long coupling time which fuses with the QRS complex of the next sinus beat. This difficulty is illustrated in *Figure 11.7*. In this record, each sinus beat is followed by a ventricular extrasystole with a long but fixed coupling time. When the P–P interval is short, the extrasystole is fused with the next sinus beat and closely mimics the pattern of W.P.W. in alternate beats. However, when the P–P interval lengthens, the ventricular extrasystole is seen to commence simultaneously with the P wave and to be responsible for the whole QRS complex. This record could readily be mistaken for the Wolff–Parkinson–White syndrome occurring in alternate beats and showing the so-called 'concertina effect'.

Type A Wolff–Parkinson–White with tall positive deflections in all praecordial leads can sometimes be mistaken for right ventricular hypertrophy or right bundle branch block (*Figure 11.2*). The diagnosis, however, should be clear from the presence of the short P–R interval and the slurred QRS complex produced by the delta wave. Similarly, when the delta wave

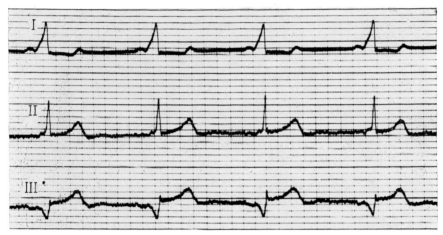

Figure 11.8—Three standard leads recorded simultaneously from a patient with the W.P.W. syndrome. The complexes superficially resemble left bundle branch block

is directed leftwards, the pattern of left bundle branch may be simulated (*Figure 11.8*).

It has already been mentioned that the Wolff-Parkinson–White syndrome can mimic myocardial infarction. This is because the delta wave may deform the first part of the QRS and produce apparent Q waves. This usually happens when the delta force is directed leftwards and superiorly, producing Q waves in II, III and AVF, simulating diaphragmatic infarction (*see Figure 11.1*); much less commonly the delta force is directed rightwards and inferiorly, producing Q waves in leads I and AVL, suggesting anterolateral myocardial infarction. On the other hand, some cases have been reported in the literature where the delta wave of pre-excitation has apparently supplanted and obscured the Q waves of infarction. Thus, the Wolff–Parkinson–White deformity of the QRS complex may either simulate infarction or may mask it.

Effect of Certain Procedures and Drugs

In some patients, the W.P.W. pattern in the electrocardiogram is abolished by exercise. On the other hand, in others, it may appear on exercise although it was absent at rest. The Valsalva manoeuvre can occasionally transiently restore normal conduction and so also may carotid sinus stimulation.

Several drugs have been claimed to abolish the pre-excitation pattern; the best known is quinidine but it is not always effective.

Incidence of Wolff–Parkinson–White Syndrome

The incidence of the Wolff–Parkinson–White electrocardiographic anomaly (as distinct from the W.P.W. clinical syndrome with recurrent attacks of ectopic tachycardia) has been variously reported as between 0·1 and 3·1 per thousand otherwise healthy subjects. About 70 per cent of the patients with the W.P.W. anomaly are men but this preponderance is probably biased by large surveys of armed forces personnel who have been mainly men. (For example, Averill and colleagues (1960) found an incidence of 0·16 per thousand among 67,375 normal men in the United States Air Force.) One difficulty in estimating the incidence is that the electrocardiographic anomaly may be intermittent and not necessarily present when the electrocardiogram is recorded.

Aetiology of the W.P.W. Syndrome

Seventy per cent of adults presenting with the Wolff–Parkinson–White syndrome show no other evidence of heart disease, whereas in children referred for cardiac investigation, the figure varies from 32 to 58 per cent. The W.P.W. syndrome in otherwise normal subjects has several times been shown to be familial and to be transmitted as an autosomal dominant trait. In a genetic study, Warner and McKussick (1958) did not confirm this but McKussick (1966) lists W.P.W. as being transmitted as an autosomal dominant trait. If the condition is familial, this would certainly explain its widely varying incidence in different reported series. (For example, Swiderski, Lees and Nadas (1962) found estimations of the incidence of the syndrome in unselected children in different series to vary from no case in 3,400 electrocardiograms to 17 cases in 5,500 electrocardiograms.)

On the other hand, the W.P.W. syndrome can appear for the first time in association with acquired organic heart disease. It has been noted to appear for the first time in acute rheumatic carditis, thyrotoxicosis and myocardial infarction. It also occurs in congenital heart disease, including atrial and ventricular septal defect, coarctation of the aorta, corrected transposition of the great vessels, tricuspid atresia and in Ebstein's anomaly of the tricuspid valve. Schiebler and colleagues (1959) found the W.P.W. syndrome in 6 of 23 patients with Ebstein's disease. They suggest that the finding of the W.P.W. electrocardiographic pattern in a cyanosed child with ischaemic lung fields strongly suggests a diagnosis of Ebstein's anomaly. Several families have been described in which the Wolff–Parkinson–White syndrome was associated with familial cardiomyopathy.

Mechanism of the Wolff–Parkinson–White Syndrome

In 1932, Holtzmann and Scherf suggested two possible mechanisms for the Wolff–Parkinson–White syndrome; either that there was an irritable centre high in the ventricular septum which was triggered off by the mechanical (or electrical) contraction of the atria producing pre-excitation of part of the ventricular musculature, or that there was an accessory muscular pathway connecting the atria and ventricles; they suggested that the bundle of Kent might act as the bypass down which the sinus impulse could pass rapidly without delay to produce pre-excitation of part of the ventricle, later fusing with the normal impulse coming down through the A.V. junction. By 1944, Öhnell was able to cite 40 different mechanisms which had been put forward to explain the anomalous E.C.G. pattern. The concept of an irritable focus high in the ventricular septum being 'triggered' by the mechanical jarring of atrial systole seems to be untenable in view of the fact that the Wolff–Parkinson–White pattern persists in the presence of atrial fibrillation when mechanical contraction of the atria is absent. Today there are three main theories put forward to explain the production of the syndrome.

(1) Accelerated conduction through part of the A.V. node (Prinzmetal and colleagues, 1952).

(2) The presence of a rapidly conducting accessory pathway, bypassing the normal A.V. junction and being either the bundle of Kent or actually lying in the A.V. junction but bypassing the A.V. node.

(3) Recently Sherf and James (1969) have suggested that the pre-excitation syndrome could be explained as a functional disorder of normal, synchronized sino-ventricular conduction.

Accelerated Conduction

Prinzmetal and colleagues (1952) pointed out that since the main function of the A.V. node was to delay conduction of the impulse to the ventricles, damage or disease of part of the A.V. node might result in accelerated conduction through that part rather than slowing or block. In consequence, the site of the ventricles supplied by that portion of the node would be activated prematurely, resulting in pre-excitation. They claimed support for this hypothesis by producing in animals experimental damage to the A.V. node resulting in a W.P.W. pattern. They suggested that acquired Wolff–Parkinson–White syndrome was due to focal disease in the A.V. node.

Pick and Katz (1955) rejected this theory on the grounds that the published tracings could better be explained as A.V. junctional rhythms with A.V. dissociation. Moreover, Grant Tomlinson and van Buren (1958) in studies on ventricular activation in the pre-excitation syndrome denied that accelerated A.V. conduction could explain the pattern. It also seems clear that accelerated conduction in part of the A.V. node could not explain the frequency of supraventricular arrhythmias encountered in the W.P.W. syndrome. It seems probable that accelerated conduction in part of the A.V. node is an unacceptable explanation for the mechanism of the syndrome.

Accessory Conduction Pathways Bypassing the A.V. Node

There is a good deal of evidence to support the view that pre-excitation can best be explained by the presence of an anomalous anatomical muscular pathway which bypasses the A.V. junction. Type B pre-excitation (with mainly negative deflections in the right praecordial leads) can be accounted for by the presence of a bundle of Kent connecting the right atrium to the right ventricle in the right atrio-ventricular groove. Two recent observations strongly support this view. Durrer and Roos (1967) studied the order of epicardial excitation of the ventricle at operation in a patient with an atrial septal defect of the secundum type and an electrocardiogram which showed the Wolff–Parkinson–White syndrome. They demonstrated very early excitation occurring 10 milliseconds after the end of the P wave at the right lateral border of the right ventricle near the atrio-ventricular sulcus. They concluded that in this case pre-excitation was by a muscular bypass between the right atrial musculature and the closely adjacent right ventricle. They found that the right ventricle was activated predominantly by the bypass whereas the left ventricle was activated normally by the A.V. junction. Even more convincing was the case described by Cobb and colleagues (1968) who had the Wolff–Parkinson–White syndrome and was in congestive heart failure from almost continuous supraventricular tachycardia. By careful electrocardiographic techniques they demonstrated both before and at operation that pre-excitation was occurring at the right lateral border of the right ventricle. Surgical division of the right atrio-ventricular sulcus immediately abolished the Wolff–Parkinson–White pattern in the electrocardiogram and the patient was cured of his attacks of supraventricular tachycardia.

Not all cases of Type B Wolff–Parkinson–White syndrome are explained by the presence of a bundle of Kent. Lev and colleagues (1966) fully described a case with the Type B Wolff–Parkinson–White electrocardiographic anomaly which terminated in complete A.V. block. Detailed histological studies post-mortem failed to demonstrate a bundle of Kent in either atrioventricular groove, but revealed a tract in the A.V. junction which bypassed the A.V. node and joined the bundle of His direct. This tract explained the short P–R interval, and copious Mahaim fibres passing from the bundle to the posterior portion of the muscular septum accounted for the delta wave. In Type A Wolff–Parkinson–White there is pre-excitation of the left ventricle so that the delta force is directed anteriorly, inferiorly and to the right. This is probably most commonly due to the presence of the bundle of Kent connecting the left atrium to the left ventricle and the presence of such bundles has been described.

Sherf and James Theory

Sherf and James (1969) have recently suggested that Wolff–Parkinson–White conduction may be due to a disturbance of the normal synchronized sino-ventricular conduction. They point out that there are two phenomena which are difficult to explain by the presence of an anomalous A.V. bypass. One is the frequency of extrasystoles in patients with Wolff–Parkinson–White; they were found in 23·4 per cent of patients with W.P.W. compared with 1·4 per cent in normal subjects. Moreover, in contrast to the extrasystoles of normal subjects which were mostly ventricular, in patients with W.P.W. there were twice as many supraventricular extrasystoles. The other phenomenon is the occasional occurrence of first-degree heart block with pre-excitation (Pick and Katz, 1955). They postulate that the pre-excitation pattern is due to an ectopic centre in the posterior internodal tract whose impulses bypass most of the A.V. junction. An alternative explanation would be a functional disorder in the sinus node so that exciting impulses were preferentially conducted down the posterior internodal tract. Marriott (1969) comments that for the moment 'Scherf and James hypotheses, though they compel us to re-examine our conventional concepts of conduction, must be regarded as tentative and sub judice; their acceptance must await the verdict of further ingenious anatomic and electrophysio-logical studies'.

It is of some interest that Brashear and Edmands (1972) were able to pro-duce a reversible Wolff–Parkinson–White type of conduction disturbance in dogs by artificially elevating their cerebrospinal fluid pressure. This was associated with significant changes in heart rate and blood pressure and indicated that anomalous conduction may result from neurohumoral factors and need not be dependent on abnormal anatomical pathways.

Value of His Bundle Electrography

The basic abnormalities in the classical Wolff–Parkinson–White syndrome were described earlier (page 54). The shortened P–R interval is caused by a reduction in H–V time due to premature activation along the anomalous pathway, and the QRS complexes represent fusion between the two activa-tion fronts (*Figure 11.9*). Atrial pacing at increasing rates allows a greater contribution from the abnormal pathway, with further reduction in the H–V interval (*Figure 11.10*). The response to atrial pacing may vary from patient to patient since the conduction properties of the bypass are unrelated to those of the normal A.V. pathway. Thus first-, second- and third-degree block have been demonstrated in both pathways during atrial pacing in varying combinations. The resulting QRS complexes may be normal, repre-sent pre-excitation fusion or total pre-excitation (Roelandt and colleagues, 1973).

It is important to determine the functional characteristics of the dual con-ducting mechanism in this way since those patients who are vulnerable to life-threatening arrhythmias may be identified. If the refractory period of the accessory pathway is shorter than that of the A.V. node, an appropriately timed atrial extrasystole will establish re-entry with antegrade conduction along the bypass. If there is no appreciable delay in conduction along this route, the ventricles will lose their protection and may be stimulated in their vulnerable phase. Under such circumstances, rapid atrial arrhythmias such as atrial fibrillation may be extremely dangerous and certainly many reported fatalities have occurred in patients with anomalous A.V. conduction.

Anatomical Considerations

At present the weight of evidence is very convincing that the Wolff–Parkinson–White syndrome is due to the presence of one or more functioning anatomical pathways which bypass the normal A.V. junction. In 1967 Ferrer pointed out that the three main variants of A.V. conduction in the Wolff–Parkinson–White syndrome could be explained on an anatomical basis. These three variations are (1) a short P–R interval with a wide QRS and a delta wave, (2) a short P–R interval and a normal QRS com-plex (the Lown–Ganong–Levine syndrome) and (3) a normal or even prolonged P–R interval with a wide QRS and delta wave. There are three bypass tracts which are known to exist. The first is a bundle of Kent which may be present either in the right or left atrio-ventricular sulcus. The second is the bypass tract of James (that is, the posterior internodal tract), which connects the atrium to the lower part of the A.V. *node*, and third are the Mahaim fibres which connect the A.V. *node* direct to the interventricular

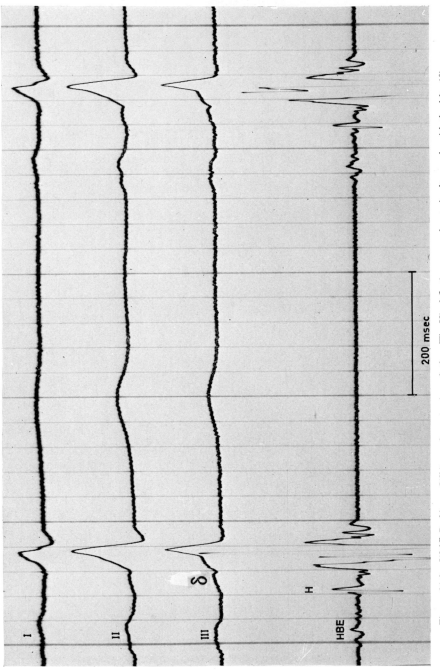

Figure 11.9—Wolff–Parkinson–White syndrome in sinus rhythm. The His deflection occurs almost simultaneously with the delta (δ) wave

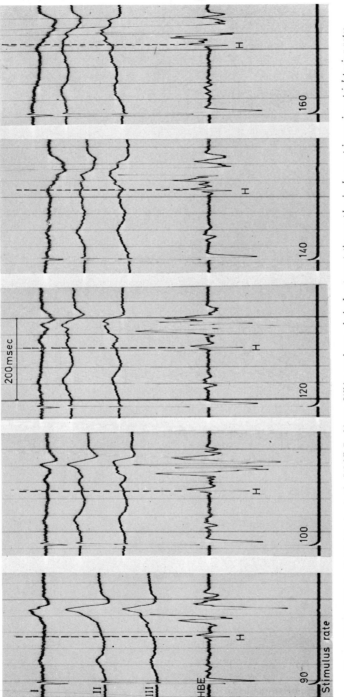

Figure 11.10—*Effects of atrial pacing in the Wolff–Parkinson–White syndrome. A single representative complex is shown at increasing atrial pacing rates (90–160 per minute). Note the His deflection is progressively delayed and merges with the QRS complexes at faster rates. Also the QRS morphology alters as the contribution of the anomalous pathway to total ventricular depolarization increases*

septum, and when functioning may bypass the bundle of His and its two main divisions. In *Figure 11.11* (after Ferrer), is illustrated diagrammatically how various combinations of these three bypass tracts can explain the three variations of anomalous A.V. conduction in the Wolff–Parkinson–White syndrome. In (*a*) a bundle of Kent results in a short P–R interval and a prolonged QRS with a delta wave. As described earlier, the H–V interval is

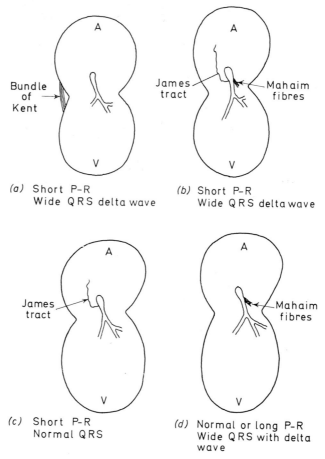

(*a*) Short P–R
    Wide QRS delta wave

(*b*) Short P–R
    Wide QRS delta wave

(*c*) Short P–R
    Normal QRS

(*d*) Normal or long P–R
    Wide QRS with delta wave

Figure 11.11—Diagrammatic representation (after Ferrer) of the varying combinations of bypass tracts which explain the variants of A.V. conduction in the Wolff–Parkinson–White syndrome

reduced and will be further shortened by atrial pacing until the His deflection is lost within the QRS complex. In (*b*) the presence of James' tract with Mahaim fibres will also produce a short P–R interval, prolongation of the QRS and a delta wave. The His bundle electrogram will demonstrate a short H–V time, but also a reduced low right atrium to His interval (LRA–H), as the A.V. node is bypassed. This interval will not increase with atrial pacing and the QRS complexes will not be affected. In (*c*) if James' tract is acting as the only A.V. nodal bypass, the short P–R interval will be due entirely to shortening of the LRA–H time and the H–V interval and QRS complexes will be normal. Atrial pacing will have no effect on these relationships. In (d) if there are functioning Mahaim fibres only, the P–R interval may be normal or even prolonged but the H–V interval will be reduced and the QRS prolonged with a delta wave. As the pacing stimuli which are delivered to the atrium will be conducted through the A.V. node, LRA–H

TABLE 11.1

Conduction Intervals and Effects of Atrial Pacing in the Variants of the Wolff–Parkinson–White Syndrome

Intervals	Kent	James + Mahaim	James	Mahaim
P–R: SR	Short	Short	Short	Normal
LRA–H: SR	Normal	Short	Short	Normal
AP	Increases	No change	No change	Increases
H–V: SR	Short	Short	Normal	Short
AP	Decreases	No change	No change	No change
Pre-excitation: SR	Present	Present	Absent	Present
(δ wave) AP	Increases	No change	Absent	No change
QRS: SR	Widened	Widened	Normal	Widened
AP	Increases	No change	Normal	No change

SR, sinus rhythm; AP, progressive increase in atrial pacing rate

will progressively increase at higher rates but the shortened H–V and the QRS complexes will be unaffected. This information is summarized in Table 11.1. These concepts are important for they not only explain the variations of anomalous A.V. conduction in the Wolff–Parkinson–White syndrome but, as will be seen later, they provide a rational basis for the mechanism of the arrhythmias which form so important a part of the clinical picture.

Arrhythmias in the Wolff–Parkinson–White Syndrome

Arrhythmias in the W.P.W. syndrome are of interest since it is usually for this reason that the patient seeks medical help. The commonest arrhythmia is extrasystoles which occur more frequently than in the general population and while they may be atrial, A.V. junctional or ventricular in origin, the commonest form is supraventricular. It is estimated that about 80 per cent of patients with the W.P.W. syndrome are subject to recurrent attacks of ectopic tachycardia. According to Newman, Donosco and Friedburg (1966), 80 per cent of such attacks are atrial tachycardia, 16 per cent are atrial fibrillation and 4 per cent are atrial flutter. There is considerable doubt whether attacks of ventricular tachycardia ever occur. The underlying mechanism of the attacks of supraventricular tachycardia was first postulated by Butterworth and Poindexter (1942) in the experimental animal. They connected the atria to the ventricles through an artificial circuit containing a simple amplifying valve. When atrial electrical activity was thus conveyed to the ventricles, bypassing the A.V. junction, the electrocardiogram recorded typical Wolff–Parkinson–White complexes. On the other hand, when ventricular electrical activity was passed to the atria through the

177

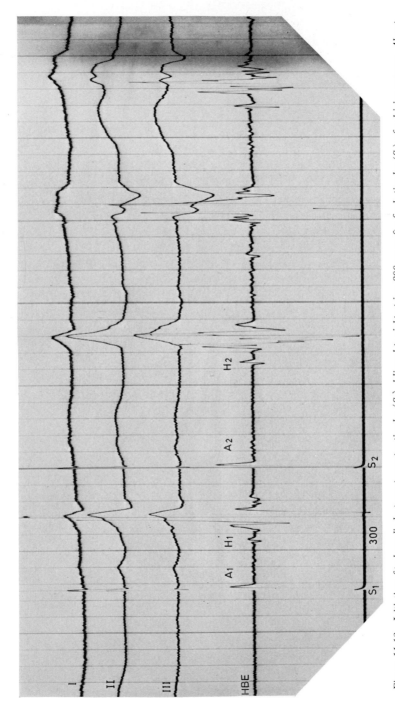

Figure 11.12—Initiation of tachycardia by premature extrastimulus (S₂) delivered to right atrium 300 msec after final stimulus (S₁) of a driving sequence. Absent delta wave in second QRS indicates block in the anomalous pathway with pure His–Purkinje conduction. Re-entry establishes supraventricular tachycardia with aberrant conduction (note His deflection preceding QRS)

artificial circuit, they produced atrial tachycardia with a rate of 300 per minute. They suggested that the cause of recurrent tachycardia in the Wolff–Parkinson–White syndrome was that the stimulus having reached the ventricles through the normal A.V. conduction pathway, would return through the bypass to the atria and elicit a second atrial contraction. If the stimulus then re-entered the normal A.V. conduction pathway, a circus movement would be set up, producing a so-called 'reciprocating tachycardia'. There is a good deal of clinical evidence to support the view that this mechanism operates in patients with the Wolff–Parkinson–White syndrome. When the onset of an attack is recorded, it is quite common for the last sinus beat before the tachycardia not to show pre-excitation, thus indicating that the anomalous pathway was not activated. It would therefore be in a non-refractory phase and could conduct that impulse in a retrograde direction back to the atria, thus precipitating a reciprocating tachycardia. This can be produced repeatedly by extrastimulus testing, as previously described. *Figure 11.12* demonstrates the initiation of a tachycardia by an appropriately timed testing stimulus after a series of regular paced atrial beats. There is no evidence of pre-excitation in the QRS complex following this stimulus and A.V. conduction is entirely through the bundle of His. Re-entry is then established. The retention of the H deflection during tachycardia confirms this to be supraventricular with aberration. In the majority of cases, supraventricular tachycardias in the Wolff–Parkinson–White syndrome do not show pre-excitation. Durrer and colleagues (1967) showed that premature beats electrically induced through a pacing catheter, either in the atria or the ventricles, if accurately timed, were capable both of initiating attacks of supraventricular tachycardia or conversely of terminating such attacks in patients with the Wolff–Parkinson–White syndrome. This has been considered in detail by Wellens (1971). It has already been mentioned above that further strong support for the existence of this circus pathway was obtained by Cobb and colleagues (1968) by the successful surgical interruption of a bundle of Kent in a patient with the Wolff–Parkinson–White syndrome, resulting in immediate cessation of anomalous conduction and cure of recurrent supraventricular tachycardia. Dreifus and colleagues (1968) produced strong evidence for the part played by the normal A.V. conduction pathways in the tachycardia by relieving a patient with the Wolff–Parkinson–White syndrome of attacks of recurrent supraventricular tachycardia by ligation of the bundle of His.

The occurrence of atrial fibrillation or flutter is attributed to the retrograde conduction of an impulse from the ventricles via the anomalous bypass, reaching the atria during their vulnerable phase.

The record of an attack of atrial fibrillation in a patient with the Wolff–Parkinson–White syndrome is shown in *Figure 11.13*. Ventricular excitation is predominantly via the bypass though occasionally complexes are normally conducted without pre-excitation. The QRS complexes of the anomalously conducted beats are wide, slurred and superficially resemble a ventricular tachycardia. This arrhythmia has sometimes been referred to as 'pseudoventricular tachycardia'.

Theoretically there is no reason why tachycardia should not develop due to an impulse travelling in the opposite way, that is, down the bypass from the atria to the ventricles, returning in a retrograde direction up the A.V. junction. If this happened the electrocardiogram would then show wide QRS complexes at a perfectly regular rate with retrograde P′ waves between them. Durrer and colleagues (1967) reported that a search of the literature revealed only one reported case which would fulfil these criteria.

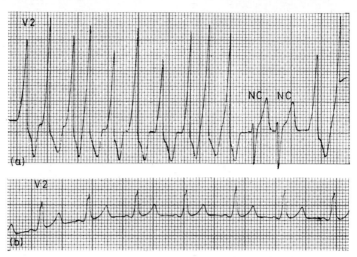

Figure 11.13—Atrial fibrillation in the Wolff–Parkinson–White syndrome. Both records are extracts from lead V2. In (a) atrial fibrillation is present with predominant conduction over the bypass. Two beats marked NC are conducted over the normal pathway without pre-excitation. Compare these beats with (b) recorded from the same patient in sinus rhythm, showing W.P.W. Type A

Clinical Features of the Wolff–Parkinson–White Syndrome

Patients with the Wolff–Parkinson–White syndrome may present with an attack of ectopic tachycardia or may give a history of recurrent episodes of palpitation. Occasionally, pre-excitation is an incidental finding in a routine electrocardiogram. Less commonly, the pre-excitation pattern may appear for the first time during some acquired cardiac illness, such as active rheumatic carditis or an acute myocardial infarction.

Although one would expect that pre-excitation would result in asynchronous contracture of the ventricles, studies of the mechanical consequences of pre-excitation have given contradictory results. In some patients with Type B Wolff–Parkinson–White, it has been demonstrated that the right ventricle contracts before the left and in several patients with the Type B variety I have noted clinically an accentuated first sound (due to the short P–R interval) and a paradoxical splitting of the second heart sound (due to late excitation of the left ventricle).

Prognosis

Although the Wolff–Parkinson–White syndrome is generally regarded as a benign electrocardiographic finding, the warning is usually added that occasional patients die suddenly and unexpectedly. Fatalities have been recorded during atrial fibrillation with wide QRS complexes due to preferential conduction over the anomalous pathways, often with very high

180

ventricular rates. Sudden and unexpected death is presumably due to the onset of ventricular fibrillation. This could result if an impulse reaches the ventricles down either conducting pathway during its vulnerable phase. It is reported that some life assurance companies in the United States of America who require an electrocardiogram as part of their routine medical examination find that candidates with the Wolff–Parkinson–White pattern have a 300 per cent higher mortality than normal subjects.

Treatment of the Wolff–Parkinson–White Syndrome

Treatment of the Wolff–Parkinson–White syndrome will be discussed in Chapter 13, page 214.

CHAPTER 12

TREATMENT OF ARRHYTHMIAS

GENERAL PRINCIPLES

The introduction of external, synchronized direct-current electric shock has revolutionized the treatment of sustained ectopic tachycardias during the past few years. Provided certain precautions are taken, this technique enables the majority of patients with atrial fibrillation, atrial flutter or other ectopic tachycardia to be safely reverted to sinus rhythm. Despite the frequency of relapses, particularly in atrial fibrillation due to rheumatic heart disease, the spectacular success of this technique has largely replaced the use of drugs in the treatment of sustained arrhythmias. Electric shock, however, is absolutely contra-indicated if the arrhythmia is due to digitalis intoxication, for irreversible ventricular fibrillation may be induced. It has, moreover, little application in the management of paroxysmal tachycardias, and none in the treatment of extrasystoles.

More recently electrical pacing has sometimes been used not only in the treatment of heart block with a slow ventricular rate but also in the management of fast arrhythmias which have proved resistant to anti-arrhythmic drugs and direct current shock. This technique will be considered on pages 205–208.

In this chapter, various anti-arrhythmic measures available will be considered, and their application in the therapy of individual forms of ectopic dysrhythmia will be described in Chapter 13. Anti-arrhythmic measures fall into three groups: (1) vagal stimulation, (2) anti-arrhythmic drugs and (3) electrical methods.

VAGAL STIMULATION

Supraventricular tachycardias can often be terminated by vagal stimulation. An increase in vagal tone may be effected either by certain simple manoeuvres or by drugs. Valsalva's or Muller's manoeuvre is occasionally successful in supraventricular tachycardia; the patient is instructed to take a deep breath and hold it as long as possible. Other measures include eyeball pressure and carotid sinus stimulation. Simultaneous pressure applied on both eyeballs by the physician's thumbs is occasionally successful, but to be effective the pressure is painful for the patient and the method is not recommended. Carotid sinus stimulation, if correctly carried out, is a much more effective technique which may be of both diagnostic and therapeutic value. Since effective carotid sinus stimulation can cause temporary hypotension or even transient cardiac arrest, it should always be carried out with the patient recumbent. Stimulation of the right carotid sinus is more frequently effective than of the left and should be carried out first. The carotid sinus is located at the division of the common carotid artery. It is often possible to identify it by palpation, but if not, stimulation should be applied to the artery just below the angle of the jaw at the upper border of the thyroid cartilage. Two or three fingers of the physician's left hand are placed over the artery and stimulation effected by an up and down vertical movement, pressure being directed backwards and medially, avoiding, if possible, obliteration of the arterial lumen. It is very useful to have the patient connected to a direct writing electrocardiograph during the procedure. Simultaneous auscultation of the heart is essential so that any change in rhythm can be noted immediately. Stimulation should be continued for approximately half a minute. If no effect is produced, after a minute's rest, the left carotid sinus should be tried. If the ventricular rate slows abruptly, stimulation should be stopped. The cardiogram may reveal reversion to sinus rhythm. If the slowing is only transient, the diagnosis is probably atrial flutter and this will be readily apparent on the cardiogram. In that event, further stimulation is pointless. If no effect on the cardiac rhythm is apparent, this may be evidence in favour of ventricular tachycardia.

It is well known that the carotid sinus reflex is enhanced by digitalis, and it used to be recommended that, if carotid sinus stimulation failed to revert a supraventricular tachycardia, the procedure should be repeated after digitalization. This, however, would be contra-indicated today since digitalis would preclude electrical reversion if it failed.

Vagal stimulation may also be achieved by drugs and they are always worth trying in supraventricular tachycardias. Drugs directly stimulating the vagus, such as acetylcholine, or mecholyl (a synthetic derivative) or prostigmine, have been employed successfully, but they are associated with such disagreeable side effects that the 'cure' may be worse than the 'disease'. Indirect stimulation of the vagus by pressor drugs is a much more pleasant mode of treatment. The rationale of the method is that a rise in arterial pressure will directly stimulate the baroceptors in the aortic arch and carotid sinuses and thus reflexly increase vagal tone. Experience shows that the efficiency of the method depends on a rapid increase in arterial pressure. The resulting reflex increase in vagal tone is probably not the whole explanation, for experimentally induced tachycardias in animals have been terminated after prior denervation of the heart. An improved coronary circulation following a rise in blood pressure may well be a contributory factor.

Experience in the coronary care unit indicates that this method for terminating supraventricular arrhythmias is contra-indicated in patients with recent myocardial infarction. It is rarely effective under these circumstances and often precipitates or aggravates left ventricular failure. The method, however, can be very useful in patients in whom a diagnosis of recent myocardial infarction can be excluded.

In order to achieve a rapid effect, the intravenous route should be used. Noradrenaline or metaraminol (Aramine) are suitable pressor agents; 8 mg of noradrenaline or 10 mg of metaraminol are dissolved in 500 ml. of 5 per cent glucose and are run in at a rate of 16–32 drops per minute. A careful watch is maintained on the blood pressure in the opposite arm. A systolic blood pressure of 160 mmHg should be aimed at; pressure in excess of 180 mmHg should be avoided because of the danger of precipitating pulmonary oedema. In the majority of cases, reversion to sinus rhythm will occur with a blood pressure of 150 mmHg in patients with supraventricular tachycardia. If reversion fails to occur, the drip should be adjusted to maintain a systolic pressure of 160 mmHg, and manoeuvres like carotid sinus stimulation may now prove effective. This method of treating supraventricular tachycardias has much to recommend it. The reversion rate is high —17 out of 19 attacks terminated (Gross and Jezzer, 1956)—and if it fails, it has not prejudiced electrical reversion which can be resorted to immediately if necessary.

ANTI-ARRHYTHMIC DRUGS

The dramatic success of electrical methods for reversion of ectopic tachycardias tended for a time to eclipse the use of anti-arrhythmic drugs. Indeed with the exception of digitalis in the treatment of chronic atrial arrhythmias, anti-arrhythmic drugs fell temporarily into disrepute; their toxic effects tended to be emphasized and the potential hazards of their administration were stressed. Today, however, anti-arrhythmic drugs are being increasingly used both for the prophylaxis of arrhythmias in such conditions as acute myocardial infarction and following open-heart surgery, and also for the reversion of ectopic tachycardias in these and other situations.

The number of anti-arrhythmic drugs now available to the physician has rapidly increased in the past decade. In the present state of our knowledge it is difficult to classify them in any simple logical manner. It would clearly be clinically valuable to group them according to the specific indications for their use but unfortunately this is not yet possible. Inevitably, moreover, individual clinicans have their own preferences for certain drugs and divergencies of opinion are bound to exist. For the purpose of the present discussion, anti-arrhythmic drugs will be classified as follows: (1) those with a 'quinidine-like action'; these include quinidine, procainamide, lignocaine, certain anti-malarial agents and some anti-histamine drugs (for example, antazoline); (2) drugs which block beta-adrenergic receptors; (3) drugs whose mode of action is at present uncertain, such as phenylhydantoin and bretylium tosylate; (4) other agents which have been used include potassium salts, calcium, magnesium and alkalinizing agents, such as molar sodium lactate; (5) digitalis.

Drugs with a 'Quinidine-like Action' on the Heart

The best known member of this group is quinidine itself which is the dextro-isomer of quinine and is one of the alkaloids extracted from the bark of the cinchona tree.

Pharmacology and Administration of Quinidine

Since many modern anti-arrhythmic drugs have an action very similar to quinidine, its pharmacological properties, mode of administration and toxic effects will be considered in some detail although indications for its use have now become fairly restricted.

The anti-arrhythmic action of quinine was first noted by Wenckebach (1914) who described a patient from the tropics who reported that quinine taken for malaria cured his attacks of paroxysmal atrial fibrillation. Frey (1918) described quinidine as having a more potent anti-arrhythmic action than quinine and this was confirmed by numerous investigators who found it to be five to ten times more active.

The action of quinidine on the fundamental physiological properties of heart muscle may be summarized as follows.

(1) Excitability — decreases
(2) Conductivity — slows
(3) Refractoriness — effective refractory period prolonged
(4) Rhythmicity — pacemakers slowed
(5) Contractility — tends to be reduced

Quinine alkaloids in addition have an 'atropine-like action' and reduce vagal tone. The slowing of conduction is due to a direct effect on the trans-membrane action potential.

In considering the effect of quinidine on the refractory period of heart muscle, it is necessary to distinguish between the absolute refractory period and what has been termed the 'effective refractory period'. The absolute refractory period of heart muscle is known to correspond approximately with the duration of the action potential. It has, however, been established that a propagated response may be evoked in cardiac muscle when it has been repolarized to about two-thirds of the normal resting potential. A local response may be obtained a little earlier than this but it will not be propagated because the rate of rise of the action potential will be too slow; thus the absolute refractory period is a little shorter than the 'effective refractory period'. The latter may be defined as the time interval before a second stimulus will effect a propagated response following a first stimulus. For a propagated response to occur there must be a certain minimal rate of rise of the depolarization phase of the action potential. It is known that when a stimulus is applied to heart muscle before it is repolarized, the rate of rise of the ensuing action potential is critically dependent on the transmembrane potential at the time, that is, on how far repolarization has proceeded. It has already been mentioned that in normal conditions the rate of rise of depolarization is sufficient to provoke a propagated response when the transmembrane potential during repolarization has reached two-thirds of its normal resting value (that is, about 50 mV for mammalian atrial muscle).

Vaughan Williams (1958) investigated the effect of quinidine on the action potentials of single atrial muscle fibres. He expected to find that prolongation of the refractory period resulted from prolongation of the phase of repolarization. Instead he found that the main effect was a reduction in the rate of rise of the action potential with reduction in its 'overshoot' and a slowing of conduction. The duration of the action potential was unchanged or prolonged by only a few milliseconds and the level of the resting potential was unaltered. Since, as shown above, a propagated response depends on the rate of rise of the action potential, it is necessary, in the presence of quinidine, for repolarization to proceed further than to two-thirds of the resting value for the critical rate of rise to be reached. The absolute refractory period is unaltered, for a local non-propagated response occurs at the usual point of repolarization, but the effective refractory period is prolonged. This work has been fully confirmed and forms the basis for modern views on the pharmacological action of quinidine and similar drugs. Their antiarrhythmic properties depend on prolongation of the effective refractory period, slowing of conduction, reduction in the rate of discharge of pace-makers, reduction in excitability and probably (in atrial fibrillation) on their vagolytic action.

Administration of Quinidine

In the majority of instances, quinidine is given by mouth in the form of its sulphate. Quinidine sulphate is available in tablets containing 0·2 g or 0·3 g. Before the advent of d.c. shock, it was occasionally given intravenously in the therapy of ventricular tachycardia, when the need to restore sinus rhythm was urgent, that is, in moribund patients. Quinidine hydrochloride (or the gluconate or lactate) was used and 0·6 g was dissolved in 200 ml of 5 per cent glucose and given by slow intravenous drip over about one hour. The electrocardiogram was continuously monitored so that the infusion could immediately be stopped when sinus rhythm was restored. The intravenous administration of quinidine was hazardous and was later replaced by procaine amide.

The oral route of administration is the one most generally employed. When used for the treatment of sustained tachycardias, it was found that reversion to sinus rhythm occurred when the blood level was about 6–8 mg per cent. Studies of the blood level of quinidine following oral administration provided a rational basis for dosage, and since the use of this drug is still occasionally indicated, the principles involved are worth re-stating. Following single oral doses, the blood level shows considerable variation in individual cases. However, in two-thirds of patients, a peak level is reached within 2 hours, after which it slowly declines to about 15 per cent of the peak after 24 hours. To attain maximal blood concentrations, it was therefore a common practice to give oral quinidine at 2-hour intervals for 6 or 7 doses. If the same dose were given on successive days, the peak level achieved increased each day for the first few days. In the remaining third of patients, the peak level following a single dose was delayed for as long as 10 hours. This individual variation explains why restoration of sinus rhythm (or the occurrence of toxic effects) was occasionally delayed for several hours after administration of the last dose. In attempting to restore sinus rhythm with oral quinidine, the drug should be given at 2-hour intervals for 6 or 7 doses (that is, from 8 a.m. to 8 p.m.), and the individual dose should be increased every two days. A usual commencing dose (in the non-urgent case) is 0·2 g of quinidine sulphate, increasing to 0·4 g on the third day and to 0·6 g on the fifth day. A maximal dose is 0·8 g, 2-hourly, on the seventh day. Ideally, an electro-cardiogram should be recorded and inspected for toxic effects before each dose is given. As soon as sinus rhythm is restored, the dose of quinidine is reduced to 0·4 g, 4-hourly, as a maintenance dose, in the hope of maintaining normal rhythm

Sustained Quinidine Release

Recently a new oral preparation of quinidine has been introduced, which is designed to achieve a more uniform blood concentration than is obtained with conventional tablets. The preparation is known as Kinidin Durules. These are porous, insoluble tablets containing quinidine bisulphate. They release 40 per cent of their quinidine content during the first hour and the remaining 60 per cent in the course of the next 8 hours. Each Durule contains 0·25 g of quinidine bisulphate which is equivalent to 0·2 g of quinidine sulphate. Plasma concentration curves of quinidine, following this preparation, show a delayed peak at about 4 hours, followed by a substantially unchanged concentration up to 12 hours. It is, therefore, possible to achieve a virtually constant blood level with twice daily administration. Clearly, this preparation should be ideal for maintenance therapy.

Toxic Effects of Quinidine

There is considerable individual variation in susceptibility to the toxic effects of quinidine, and serious or even fatal toxicity may follow quite modest dosage. Gastro-intestinal effects, including nausea, vomiting and diarrhoea, are usually due to idiosyncrasy. Allergic manifestations, including rashes, may occur. A fairly common and relatively innocuous side effect is headache, which is occasionally sufficiently troublesome to necessitate abandoning maintenance therapy. The most important side effects are cardiotoxic and are reflected in the electrocardiogram. The Q–T interval is often prolonged with depression of the S–T segment and inversion of a previously positive T wave. Such changes are not necessarily an indication for stopping the drug. A more serious indication of toxicity is impairment of conduction. This may be manifest by prolongation of the P–R interval or widening of the QRS complex. The latter may resemble a bundle branch block pattern, or increase in duration of the QRS may occur without any change in direction of the QRS forces. An increase in duration of the QRS complex of 50 per cent (that is, from 0·08 to 0·12 second) is an absolute indication for withholding the drug, and it is wiser never to allow more than 25 per cent widening to occur.

In common with many drugs which suppress ectopic beats, quinidine may also provoke them. It used to be thought that ventricular arrhythmias due to quinidine intoxication were rare, but it has recently become clear that they are probably the commonest hazard of quinidine therapy. Electrocardiographically, there may be frequent, multiform ventricular extrasystoles, ventricular tachycardia or repetitive ventricular fibrillation. The latter arrhythmia is by no means rare and is manifest clinically as recurrent attacks of syncope, sometimes with convulsions and incontinence. The clinical picture is sufficiently characteristic to have been named 'quinidine syncope'. The episodes of ventricular fibrillation last from a few seconds up to three or four minutes. Typically, they occur without premonitory symptoms; there is almost immediate loss of consciousness with intense pallor, or pallor and cyanosis. The incidence has been estimated as 3–4 per cent with high dosage quinidine therapy, although blood levels of the drug, where they have been estimated, have been within the therapeutic range, suggesting that the arrhythmia represents hypersensitivity. In the past, sudden deaths during quinidine therapy have been vaguely attributed to 'quinidine shock', but it seems much more likely they are due to ventricular fibrillation. *Figure 12.1* shows a typical example in which the first attack occurred eight hours after the last dose of quinidine. Between the attacks there were frequent, multiform ventricular extrasystoles.

Treatment of Quinidine Syncope

Individual episodes of ventricular fibrillation should be treated with external cardiac massage and artificial ventilation. This will rarely be necessary for more than two to three minutes, for most attacks cease spontaneously. The period of ventricular irritability is generally over in six hours. There is some evidence (Seaton, 1966) that intravenous propranolol may be specific in controlling the arrhythmia.

Systemic Embolism and Quinidine Therapy

It is well known that systemic embolism in heart disease is far more common in patients with atrial fibrillation than in those in sinus rhythm. It has, moreover, always been recognized that when the fibrillating atria are reverted to sinus rhythm, a clot may be dislodged from the left atrial

II

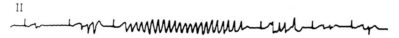

Figure 12.1—Quinidine syncope due to recurrent ventricular fibrillation

appendage, resulting in systemic embolism. This has resulted in somewhat paradoxical recommendations in the literature. Some authorities recommend reversion to sinus rhythm of patients with a history of embolus, as a prophylactic measure, whereas others have regarded a history of embolus as a contra-indication to reversion. This point is relevant to electrical reversion and will be discussed more fully later. Embolism following reversion with quinidine appears to have been very uncommon, but I have seen one fatal case.

Thompson (1956), in a review of the relevant literature, estimated that the mortality from quinidine therapy of chronic atrial arrhythmias was 3–4 per cent. In most instances it is likely that ventricular fibrillation was the cause, and this should not prove fatal in patients who were being monitored by modern techniques. It would, therefore, seem unreasonable to discard quinidine therapy altogether and, as will be seen, there are occasional indications for its use.

It is customary to recommend that before quinidine therapy is started, a test dose of 0·2 g should be given. In my experience, this seems pointless, for serious toxic effects only seem to occur with higher dosage, and even such benign symptoms as headache are never provoked by a single small dose. The place for low dosage quinidine for prophylaxis of arrhythmias is discussed below.

Other Drugs with a Quinidine-like Action on the Heart

Since 1946, a number of compounds with a quinidine-like action on the heart have been described. These include procaine, procainamide, lignocaine, atebrin and chloroquine. Up to the present, the most widely used of these has been procainamide (Pronestyl).

Procainamide

Procaine was originally introduced for the control of ventricular ectopic rhythms occurring during cardiac surgery. Such arrhythmias are often provoked during intubation and as a result of manipulation of the heart during surgery. Periods of anoxia are particularly liable to provoke arrhythmias. It was first found that topical application of procaine to the heart reduced its excitability, and later found that procaine was effective, both prophylactically and for treatment, when given intravenously. The duration of its action was short, and it proved unsuitable for use in unanaesthetized patients because of its stimulating action on the central nervous system. Investigation of allied compounds showed that procainamide had a more powerful and more prolonged anti-arrhythmic action and had little stimulatory effect on the central nervous system when given to conscious patients. Its cardiac actions are qualitatively very similar to quinidine, both in therapeutic and toxic doses. Although a number of cases have been reported which responded to procainamide after quinidine had failed, the converse is probably more frequently true. It may be given by the oral, intramuscular or intravenous routes. Prolonged oral administration has occasionally resulted in agranulocytosis, which necessarily limits its use. It is issued in tablets containing 0·25 g which correspond closely to 0·2 g of quinidine sulphate.

The main advantage of procainamide has been its relative safety when given intravenously. Its use by this route has largely replaced quinidine which tends to have a profound hypotensive action. By the intravenous route, it is recommended that it should be given at about 50–75 mg per minute up to a dose of 1–2 g. Continuous monitoring of the electrocardiogram is essential so that the drug can be immediately discontinued if sinus rhythm is restored or toxic effects appear. Since it also has a hypotensive action, a continuous watch should be kept on the blood pressure. In resistant ventricular tachycardia, the drug is occasionally more effective if given in 'boluses' of 100 mg every two minutes.

Lignocaine

It has recently been shown that another local anaesthetic, lignocaine (Xylocaine) may have many advantages over procainamide. Procainamide has both a hypotensive effect and impairs cardiac contractility, whereas lignocaine is free from these unwanted effects and has an equally potent anti-arrhythmic action. Harrison, Sprouse and Morrow (1963) reported on its use during cardiac surgery. Whereas they had previously been reluctant to use procainamide on account of its hypotensive effect, they found lignocaine to have at least equal anti-arrhythmic properties, with no hypotensive effect, and to cause no reduction of cardiac contractility. The duration of its action is relatively short, lasting 10–20 minutes, but it can be safely repeated. The dose is 1–2 mg per kg of body weight, intravenously. The average adult patient may be given 50 mg which can be repeated in 10–20 minutes.

The main value of lignocaine is for the suppression of ventricular ectopic beats and rhythms. It has little, if any, effect on supraventricular arrhythmias. If a dose of 25 or 50 mg intravenously is effective in suppressing ventricular ectopic beats, the drug should then be given by continuous intravenous infusion dissolved in 5 per cent dextrose solution, at a rate of 1 mg to 3 mg per minute. This is now a common practice for the suppression of ventricular

189

ectopic beats occurring following acute myocardial infarction or cardiac surgery.

It has been reported that an excess dose of lignocaine may produce drowsiness, euphoria or other mental disturbance, blurred vision, numbness and sweating. With large doses, as with procaine, fits may be produced.

In my experience, side-effects from continuous intravenous infusion of lignocaine in a dose of 1 mg to 3 mg per minute have been relatively uncommon. It seems to represent a major advance in the control of acute ventricular ectopic arrhythmias. Its use in the coronary care unit will be discussed in detail in Chapter 16.

Other Anti-malarial Agents

The anti-malarial agents, atebrin and chloroquine, have also been shown to have a quinidine-like action on the heart, but their practical therapeutic value seems to be small, and they have no particular advantages over more orthodox preparations.

Antazoline

Antazoline is an anti-histamine drug which has been shown by Kline and colleagues (1962) to have anti-arrhythmic properties. They found that in patients with atrial or ventricular extrasystoles the intravenous injection of antazoline was followed by a sharp reduction in the incidence of ectopic beats. They were also able to control recurrent ventricular tachycardia in three patients and were able to terminate an attack of supraventricular tachycardia which had been provoked in a child during right heart catheterization. No significant toxic or side-effects were noted. However, this drug has not come into general use as an anti-arrhythmic agent.

Beta-Adrenergic Receptor Blockade

A new approach in the medical treatment of arrhythmias followed the description by Black and Stevenson (1962) of a specific beta-adrenergic receptor blocking drug called pronethalol. Although this drug is no longer used, its introduction stimulated numerous pharmacological and physiological studies on the relationship between catecholamines and arrhythmias. Pharmacological studies had previously established that there were two types of sympathetic receptor in the tissues, the alpha receptors and the beta receptors. While several effective drugs existed which would block the alpha receptors, for example, phenoxybenzamine (Dibenyline), phentolamine (Rogitine), these compounds did not block sympathetic action on the heart which is mediated through beta receptors. Sympathetic action on the heart is mediated by catecholamines and is complex. An important action of catecholamines is to increase the rate of early spontaneous diastolic depolarization of pacemaker fibres. Sympathetic stimulation therefore increases the rate of the sinus node and also that of subsidiary pacemakers. There is also evidence that sympathetic stimulation results in a non-uniformity in repolarization of ventricular muscle fibres. There is good evidence that this non-uniformity of repolarization rather than a decreased refractory period lowers the threshold of the heart to ventricular fibrillation. Another important action of catecholamines on the heart is to increase the force of myocardial contraction.

In the experimental animal, beta receptor blockade is associated with slowing of the heart rate and this suggested that beta-blocking drugs might be of value in the management of arrhythmias.

Pronethalol proved to have troublesome side-effects and was found to be carcinogenic to mice. It was soon replaced by propranolol (Inderal). Numerous studies on the anti-arrhythmic action of both these drugs have now been published and most observers are in substantial agreement about their action.

In the present stage of our knowledge it is convenient to consider the effects of beta-blocking drugs on cardiac rhythm under three headings: (a) depression of automaticity (that is, rhythmicity), (b) depression of conduction and (c) suppression of digitalis induced ectopic beats and tachycardias.

Depression of Automaticity

Depression of automaticity is manifested in sinus rhythm by slowing of the heart rate. Extrasystoles, whether of atrial, junctional or ventricular origin, are frequently reduced in number or abolished, but this effect is unpredictable. (This action of beta-blocking drugs is not necessarily due to reduction in automaticity; other explanations are possible.) The rate of ectopic pacemakers, again irrespective of their site, is almost invariably slowed, and slowing is occasionally sufficient to restore sinus rhythm. In rare cases, following intravenous injection, there may be a total suppression of all pacemaker activity in the heart which stops in asystole. Depression of automaticity probably accounts for the value of these drugs prophylactically in paroxysmal tachycardia.

Depression of Conductivity

In sinus rhythm this is manifested by prolongation of the P–R interval and occasionally by widening of the QRS complex. In atrial fibrillation, slowing of the ventricular rate is a striking finding. Occasionally, depression of conductivity is manifested by second-degree sino-atrial block. (It is theoretically possible that suppression of extrasystoles and termination of ectopic tachycardias is due to depression of conduction producing exit block around the ectopic focus.)

Suppression of Digitalis Induced Ectopic Beats and Tachycardias

Mendez, Aceves and Mendez (1961) showed that in sympathectomized animals, overdosage of digitalis did not produce ventricular fibrillation. This finding led Vaughan Williams and Sekiya (1963) to investigate the protective action of pronethalol in experimental digitalis intoxication. They found that it doubled the lethal dose of ouabain. In man, pronethalol, intravenously, was found to abolish ectopic beats and tachycardias due to digitalis intoxication (Stock and Dale, 1963). Propranolol has been shown to have a similar action. Beta-adrenergic receptor blocking drugs are also effective in other drug-induced arrhythmias, particularly those occurring during halothane or cyclopropane anaesthesia. It is possible that they are effective in quinidine induced arrhythmias. Although this action of beta-blocking drugs is of considerable interest, its practical application is limited. This will be further discussed under digitalis intoxication (Chapter 15).

Negative Inotropic Action of Beta Blockade

An early disturbing clinical finding was that heart failure could be precipitated or aggravated by beta blockade. It is presumably due to weakening of the contractile force of the heart following removal of the catecholamine drive. Use of the drug often results in a fall in cardiac output with a prolongation of systole. This unwanted effect becomes increasingly marked in patients with advancing myocardial disease. Probably associated with the reduced cardiac output, quite severe hypotension is occasionally seen. Mendel (1966) has shown with a differential manometer that beta blockade reduces the dp/dt of the ventricular pressure curve.

This unwanted effect of propranolol seriously restricts its clinical value. To some extent, this weakening of myocardial contraction can be offset by simultaneous administration of digitalis and this will be discussed later under the therapy of individual arrhythmias.

Broncho-constrictive Action of Propranolol

Since the sympathetic receptors in bronchial smooth muscle are beta in type, propranolol may give rise to broncho-constriction in asthmatics or patients with chronic bronchitis (McNeill, 1964). Its use is therefore contra-indicated in patients with asthma or chronic obstructive airway disease.

Effect of Propranolol on the Action Potential

Vaughan Williams (1966) has investigated the effect of beta-blocking drugs on the action potentials of single rabbit atrial fibres. He found that there was no change in the resting potential, that the phase of repolarization was not prolonged (it is actually slightly shortened), and that, like other anti-arrhythmic drugs, propranolol and pronethalol greatly reduce the height and rate of rise of the action potential.

Thus, the effect of propranolol on the action potential is closely similar to that of quinidine and allied compounds. This led Vaughan Williams to anticipate that pronethalol and propranolol should also prove to be local anaesthetics. He has shown that in fact they have a local anaesthetic activity approximately twice that of procaine. One of the most important actions of all anti-arrhythmic drugs, therefore, appears to be interference with the sudden explosive increase in sodium conductance which follows stimulation.

Lucchesi (1965) reported that the dextro-isomer of pronethalol had not beta-blocking properties but appeared to have equal anti-arrhythmic action. Howitt and colleagues (1968) found the same to be true of the dextro-isomer of propranolol; d-propranolol has very little beta-blocking activity but is effective in arrhythmias due to digitalis intoxication. This finding is certainly contrary to expectations.

The anti-arrhythmic effects of propranolol would appear to be at two different levels. It has been known for some time that catecholamines may precipitate arrhythmias, and this effect is enhanced by sensitizing drugs like digitalis or the halogen anaesthetics. Arrhythmias provoked by exertion or emotion are almost certainly catecholamine induced, and it is in the prophylaxis of these that beta receptor blockade finds a valuable clinical application (*vide infra*). In addition, these drugs have a quinidine-like action in prolonging the effective refractory period and in slowing conduction. They differ, however, from quinidine in their action on the vagus. Quinidine is vagolytic, but beta-sympathetic blockade must necessarily accentuate vagal tone.

Administration of Propranolol

Pronethalol has now been withdrawn, but propranolol is available in solution for intravenous administration and in 10 mg and 40 mg tablets for oral therapy.

In our personal experience of approximately 100 intravenous injections of beta-blocking drugs, there were three deaths from cardiac arrest with suppression of all pacemaker activity in the heart. All three patients were seriously ill, but the drug was undoubtedly contributory to the fatal outcome. Similar cases have been encountered by others. A medical therapeutic measure with a 3 per cent mortality is clearly not one to be undertaken unless it is potentially life saving. In our opinion, the drug should not be given in an attempt to revert a sustained ectopic tachycardia not due to digitalis; the reversion rate is low (about 1 in 4) and if sinus rhythm is not restored, the clinical state of the patient may be worsened. On the other hand, many anaesthetists frequently give this drug intravenously to suppress any arrhythmias that may arise during surgical procedures. Clearly these injections must be free of any side effects and since presumably the patients so treated have normal hearts this does suggest that the danger of intravenous propranolol may be confined to patients with diseased hearts.

Other Beta Receptor Blocking Drugs. Practolol (Eraldin)

During the past few years a number of new beta receptor blocking drugs have been introduced. Perhaps the most important of these is practolol (Eraldin, I.C.I.). A most important property of practolol is that it is cardioselective. At first sight therefore it does not appear to be a beta-blocker for it produces only a small reduction of tachycardia caused by isoprenaline infusions unless given in a high dosage. This is probably because although cardiac receptors are blocked the reflex effect of peripheral vasodilatation is unhindered. Another important effect of practolol is that it has no negative inotropic action. In consequence it can be safely used in the coronary care unit or the post-operative recovery room for the suppression of any arrhythmias. A further advantage of practolol over other beta receptor blocking drugs is that it does not increase airway resistance and can therefore be safely used in patients with chronic obstructive airways disease. It has moreover less effect on the heart rate than the other beta blocking drugs. Its main value appears to be in supraventricular arrhythmias rather than ventricular. An initial dose of 5 mg is given slowly intravenously over a period of about three minutes. This dose can be repeated every five minutes until either the arrhythmia has been suppressed or a total dose of 25 mg has been reached.

Other beta receptor blocking drugs include oxprenolol (Trasicor, Ciba) which in practice is claimed to be rather more effective than practolol and Tolamolol (Pfizer). The number of drugs now available with beta receptor blocking properties is steadily increasing and each manufacturer claims special advantages for their product. It would clearly require extensive and complex controlled clinical trials to sort out the value of different claims and it is therefore wisest to stick to one or two preparations of proven value and to become familiar with their clinical use.

Anti-arrhythmic Drugs: Mode of Action Uncertain

There are now numerous anti-arrhythmic drugs whose mode of action is at present uncertain. These include diphenylhydantoin (Epanutin); bretylium tosylate (Darenthin, Burroughs Wellcome); verapamil (Cordilox, Pfizer); disopyramide (Rhythmodan, Roussel) and acebutolol (Spectral, May and Baker).

Diphenylhydantoin

Since the heart and central nervous system show a similar response to some drugs and since attacks of ventricular tachycardia following myocardial infarction might be regarded as analogous to post-traumatic epilepsy, Harris and Kokenot (1950) investigated the action of diphenylhydantoin (Epanutin) on ventricular tachycardia induced in dogs by coronary artery ligation. Considerable experimental work on animals has shown that the drug has appreciable anti-arrhythmic properties although its mode of action is not yet fully understood.

Conn (1965) described the immediate effects of intravenous injection of diphenylhydantoin in 24 patients with cardiac arrhythmias. He reported it to be particularly effective in abolishing both atrial and ventricular arrhythmias due to digitalis intoxication; it was also of benefit in controlling paroxysmal atrial and ventricular arrhythmias, not due to digitalis.

Helfant and colleagues (1967) studied the electro-physiological properties of diphenylhydantoin and compared it with procainamide in both the normal and digitalis-intoxicated heart of the dog. They found that it depresses ventricular automaticity and at the same time it enhances A.V. conduction while having little or no effect on intraventricular conduction or sinus rate. Procainamide, on the other hand (and presumably quinidine) caused depression of both A.V. and intraventricular conduction as well as slowing the sinus rate. They found, moreover, that when diphenylhydantoin was given prophylactically it increased the dose of digitalis necessary to produce toxicity by 72 to 224 per cent. They demonstrated that at constant heart rates, pre-treatment with diphenylhydantoin did not alter the elevation of rate of rise of left ventricular pressure produced by acetylstrophanthidin. It therefore seems that the inotropic and toxic actions of digitalis can be dissociated and that diphenylhydantoin may significantly widen the 'toxic therapeutic' ratio of digitalis. It certainly appears to be the drug of choice for the immediate treatment of toxic digitalis rhythms. It also sometimes proves of value in the management of ventricular arrhythmias following myocardial infarction. A dose of 250 mg diluted in 5 ml solvent is given slowly intravenously over one to three minutes. Maintenance oral therapy in a dosage of 200 to 400 mg daily may be given following intravenous therapy in divided dosage.

Bretylium Tosylate

Bacaner (1966) reported that bretylium tosylate (Darenthin, Burroughs Wellcome) substantially increased the threshold to electrically-produced ventricular fibrillation. The drug had previously been introduced in 1959 as a hypotensive agent but was rapidly supplanted by other preparations because tolerance to its hypotensive action developed rapidly. Its use has been recommended both for the prophylaxis and treatment of ventricular arrhythmias following myocardial infarction or open heart surgery. It is usually given by intravenous or intramuscular injection. Good results have been reported by Bacaner (1968) using the intravenous or intramuscular route in a dose of 5 mg/kg, occasionally increasing as high as 15 mg/kg. My personal experience in 6 cases of ventricular arrhythmias following myocardial infarction has been unimpressive. Allen, Shanks and Saidi (1969) moreover have failed to confirm in dogs the elevation of threshold to electrically-induced ventricular fibrillation. The same authors (1969) found that in catecholamine-induced experimental ventricular arrhythmias in dogs that bretylium in high dosage had some protective effect but that the arrhythmias were potentiated during the first hour after the drug was administered. The mode of action of bretylium on arrhythmias is obscure as it does not appear to possess quinidine-like or local anaesthetic activities (Papp and Vaughan Williams, 1969). Watanabe, Josipovic and Dreifus (1968) have suggested that its antifibrillatory action may be related to hyperpolarization and improved conduction.

Verapamil

Verapamil (Cordilox, Pfizer) was originally introduced for the treatment of myocardial ischaemia (Hoffman, 1964; Sandler and colleagues, 1968) and has now been shown to have anti-arrhythmic properties. The properties of this very useful drug may be summarized as follows. It will slow a sinus tachycardia. In atrial fibrillation it always slows the ventricular response and often makes this regular. It occasionally reverts atrial fibrillation to sinus rhythm. It reverts junctional rhythm to sinus rhythm and when given during attacks of paroxysmal atrial tachycardia, according to Schamroth it invariably terminates them, producing sinus rhythm. According to Schamroth, Krikler and Garrett (1972) it reverted 4 cases out of 15 of atrial flutter to sinus rhythm and this was sometimes preceded by an increase in the atrioventricular block. According to them there was no effect in a single case of paroxysmal ventricular tachycardia. They stated that these anti-arrhythmic effects were not associated with any side effects. They found no fall in blood pressure or precipitation or aggravation of cardiac failure. However, we have noticed that in some patients with left ventricular failure it has had a significant negative inotropic effect. Its use in this situation clearly requires caution. Verapamil, 10 mg, is injected intravenously over 15–30 seconds. The response to intravenous verapamil is only transient, lasting from 30 minutes up to an hour. By the oral route it often proves disappointing.

Disopyramide (Rhythmodan)

We have had no personal experience in using this new anti-arrhythmic drug. It is claimed to be a valuable anti-arrhythmic drug in both supraventricular and ventricular arrhythmias and it has a largely anti-cholinergic effect.

Acebutolol (Spectral)

At the time of writing, this new anti-arrhythmic drug has been released for clinical trials but is not yet generally available. It is claimed to be a beta receptor blocker and in a limited experience we have found it to be a promising drug, abolishing atrial and ventricular extrasystoles and suppressing repetitive tachycardias of both supraventricular and ventricular origin. It appears to have some negative inotropic action which may limit its use.

Treatment and Prevention of Cardiac Arrhythmias with Combined Propranolol and Quinidine

As long ago as 1966, Stern of Israel first pointed out that when propranolol and quinidine were used in combination in relatively small doses their anti-arrhythmic action appeared to be synergistic. The great advantage of using this combination in low dosage was that although the anti-arrhythmic actions were additive the toxic effects of the two drugs were not. Both drugs are known to reduce the height and rate of rise of the action potential in isolated preparations of myocardium (Vaughan Williams, 1966). Quinidine in high dosage tends to provoke ventricular arrhythmias whereas propranolol does not, but simultaneous administration allows a much smaller dose of quinidine to be used.

A further factor in the successful use of this combination may be that the negative inotropic action of quinidine at fast heart rates may be converted into a positive inotropic action at slow heart rates induced by propranolol.

Results of and Indications for Combined Therapy

According to Stern (1971) the combination may be used for the elective conversion of chronic atrial fibrillation to sinus rhythm. He treated 51 patients with this regime and 36 were successfully converted to sinus rhythm even though many had failed to convert with direct current shock. He also recommends the combined therapy for early post-operative conversion of atrial fibrillation following mitral valve replacement. Other indications for this technique include atrial flutter, supraventricular and ventricular extrasystoles and recurrent ventricular tachycardia.

Very few, if any, side effects have been encountered and it is clear that this combination should be tried first of all in all but extremely urgent cases before using d.c. shock.

Method

Propranolol, 10 mg, is given three to four times daily for three days and then quinidine, 0·2 g, three to four times daily is added. Once sinus rhythm is restored it would seem wise to continue the two drugs as a maintenance dose to prevent recurrence. Similar results have been claimed for the combination of practolol and quinidine.

Other Agents in Arrhythmias

Other drugs which have been used in ectopic arrhythmias include potassium salts, calcium, magnesium and alkalinizing agents, such as molar sodium lactate.

Potassium

It has long been appreciated that the action of potassium salts on cardiac rhythm is complex and dependent on many factors. Experimental work has established that potassium salts may abolish, as well as precipitate, ectopic arrhythmias. Potassium depletion from the body, not necessarily reflected in the serum level, sensitizes the heart to the toxic action of digitalis. This will be more fully considered in Chapter 15.

Following open heart surgery, it is now a common practice to give isoprenaline by intravenous infusion because of its potent inotropic and chronotropic effects. Unfortunately in some patients this leads to increased ventricular irritability with frequent ventricular extrasystoles, ventricular tachycardia and even ventricular fibrillation. Hoffman and colleagues (1969) have shown that ventricular arrhythmias induced in this way occur more readily in digitalized patients, particularly if the patient has hyperkalaemia or hypokalaemia. They found that giving 2 mg of isoprenaline dissolved in 500 ml of 5 per cent dextrose was much safer if 40 mEq potassium chloride were added to the solution. No ventricular arrhythmias developed in 40 of 46 of their patients and in the 6 in whom they did, the addition of a further 20 mEq of potassium chloride to the infusion successfully abolished the arrhythmias. They also found that hyperkalaemia had a similar effect in producing ventricular arrhythmias in patients receiving isoprenaline. These isoprenaline-induced arrhythmias in hyperkalaemic patients were also commonest in patients receiving digitalis. In these circumstances they found that these arrhythmias could be abolished by the administration of insulin in a dose of 0·03 units per kg.

It seems clear that post-operative hypokalaemia can be avoided by the post-operative administration of intravenous potassium chloride. Paradoxically hyperkalaemia may have the same effect and the arrhythmias may then be abolished by insulin.

Calcium

This has little use in the therapy of arrhythmias except when these are associated with a low serum calcium level. In resuscitation from cardiac arrest, calcium is sometimes of value in helping to restore contractility.

Magnesium

The intravenous administration of magnesium sulphate has been reported to be effective in atrial tachycardias and in digitalis-induced ventricular arrhythmias. It is given as 20 ml of a 20 per cent solution. It is rarely, if ever, used today.

Alkalinizing Agents

When arrhythmias are associated with acidosis, alkalinizing agents such as sodium bicarbonate and molar sodium lactate may prove of value. Their principal indication is in Stokes–Adams attacks due to heart block and following cardiac arrest; they will be discussed in Chapter 14. It has been claimed that molar sodium lactate may be of value in the treatment of cardio-toxicity due to quinidine or procainamide, particularly in cases with widened QRS complexes and hypotension.

Some Principles Governing the Choice of Anti-arrhythmic Drugs and their Route of Administration

The treatment of individual arrhythmias will be considered in more detail in Chapter 13. It will be useful here to consider some principles governing the choice of individual drugs and their route of administration. The treatment of arrhythmias may be considered under two main headings: (1) the immediate termination of an individual episode, and (2) maintenance therapy to prevent recurrence. In order to accomplish this intelligently the physician must clearly be familiar with the mode of action, the duration of action and the optimum route of administration of the various anti-arrhythmic drugs.

Immediate Termination of an Arrhythmia

The indications for the rapid termination of an arrhythmia must be largely clinical. Until recently, apart from digitalis, the principal anti-arrhythmic drugs available were quinidine and procainamide. For rapid action the intravenous route is essential. Intravenous administration of quinidine was hazardous and procainamide was the drug usually used. This was often effective in both supraventricular and ventricular arrhythmias. When it failed, however, conversion by direct current electric shock was usually employed, necessitating a general anaesthetic. Today, however, the choice of drug is much wider and more specific agents are available.

For the termination of supraventricular arrhythmias verapamil and practolol intravenously are now the drugs of choice and lignocaine intravenously for ventricular arrhythmias. Of these drugs only practolol is effective by mouth; the others cannot be given by the oral route and therefore cannot be used as maintenance therapy to prevent recurrence.

Maintenance Therapy

The object of maintenance therapy is to prevent recurrences and the drugs effective by the oral route must be used. The combination of quinidine and propranolol is very appropriate for maintenance therapy. Alternatively in difficult cases combinations of other anti-arrhythmic drugs may be necessary.

The duration of action of the various anti-arrhythmic drugs differs widely. For example, the duration of action of lignocaine is very short but of quinidine is fairly long. It is destroyed fairly slowly in the body. The main site of its destruction is the liver and Conn (1966) states that the liver can metabolize about 300 mg quinidine every four hours. Oral quinidine is thus a suitable drug for maintenance therapy and is available in long-acting form as Kinidin Durules. As we have seen, it seems to be even more effective when combined with propranolol which also has a long action when given by mouth.

Use of Digitalis in Arrhythmias

Digitalis holds a unique place in the therapy of cardiac disease. During the present century, three entirely different views have been held about its mode of action. It was believed by Lewis (1933) that its only effect was to slow the ventricular rate in atrial fibrillation and he forbade its use by his registrars for patients in sinus rhythm. McMichael and Sharpey-Schafer (1944), following studies by cardiac catheterization, suggested that its main effect was to reduce venous pressure by an extra cardiac effect on systemic veins. Today it is universally acknowledged that its main pharmacological action is to increase the force of contraction of the failing myocardium. In atrial fibrillation, it slows the ventricular rate, and the heart rate then forms a convenient indicator against which to titrate dosage. Some authorities maintain that even the slowing of the ventricular rate in atrial fibrillation is due primarily to the action of the drug in improving myocardial contraction, the rapid rate of the undigitalized patient being a manifestation of cardiac failure. This is almost certainly an oversimplification, and there seems little doubt that the action of digitalis is complex. Slowing of the ventricular rate in atrial fibrillation is due to two factors: direct stimulation of the vagus (which can be abolished by atropine) and in fuller doses it directly impairs conductivity in the A.V. junction, an effect only partly antagonized by atropine. Patients with mitral stenosis are particularly intolerant of a fast ventricular rate, and the onset of atrial fibrillation may lead rapidly to the development of acute pulmonary oedema. The dramatic improvement which follows digitalization in these cases is entirely attributable to the slowing of the ventricular rate by the combination of vagal stimulation and impairment of A.V. conduction. A direct effect on contractility can hardly be a factor.

In therapeutic doses, digitalis does not slow the normal heart; when given to patients in heart failure with sinus rhythm, slowing of the heart may follow restoration of compensation, but this is not a direct effect but is secondary to improvement in myocardial function. Digitalis has no effect on the tachycardia of fever, thyrotoxicosis or anxiety.

Since digitalis stimulates the vagus, it will shorten the refractory period of atrial muscle and will tend to perpetuate fibrillation. In atrial flutter, it is often more difficult to slow the ventricular rate with digitalis, but its effect of shortening the refractory period often converts atrial flutter to fibrillation and then the ventricular rate is more readily controlled.

It is often said that the two main pharmacological actions of digitalis are the increased force of contraction of the failing myocardium and the slowing of the ventricular rate in atrial fibrillation. In addition, however, digitalis unquestionably has an anti-arrhythmic action of its own which tends to be forgotten. The careful observations of Otto and Gold (1926) showed that digitalis would often abolish extrasystoles of both atrial and ventricular origin, and this is irrespective of whether organic heart disease is present or not. Rapid digitalization is often effective in terminating supraventricular tachycardia, and it still remains the treatment of choice in atrial tachycardia in infancy and childhood. For many years, ventricular tachycardia was regarded as an absolute contra-indication to digitalis. It was said that not only was it of no benefit, but there was a risk of precipitating ventricular fibrillation. This idea probably arose from the fact that, in toxic doses, digitalis may induce ventricular tachycardia, and further administration may be followed by ventricular fibrillation. There are, however, numerous reports in the literature of successful reversion of ventricular tachycardia to sinus rhythm following large doses of digitalis. There is still insufficient information available concerning the mode of action of digitalis on the heart for a clear understanding of its anti-arrhythmic action to be formulated. The correct use of digitalis is a clinical art which can only be learned at the bedside. The optimum therapeutic dose of any digitalis preparation is about 60 per cent of the toxic dose. This relatively narrow margin makes digitalis an unsuitable drug to utilize for the termination of arrhythmias, except in special instances. The use of digitalis will be further discussed later under the management of atrial fibrillation.

ELECTRIC TREATMENT OF ECTOPIC TACHYCARDIAS

The use of anti-arrhythmic drugs for the reversion of ectopic tachycardias to sinus rhythm has many disadvantages. It is by no means always successful and it requires high doses which are frequently associated with undesirable side effects, such as depression of cardiac contractility, often with hypotension, and prolongation of atrioventricular or intraventricular conduction times. These drawbacks have been appreciably reduced by the introduction of the newer anti-arrhythmic drugs and it seems likely that the indication for direct current shock may be appreciably lessened in the future by newer anti-arrhythmic drugs. However, the innovation of direct current shock treatment did represent a substantial advance in the therapy of ectopic tachycardias for the method was safe, rapid and largely free of side effects. The newer electrical techniques represent a dramatic advance in the therapy of ectopic tachycardias. Not only is the method safe, rapid and free from side effects, but the success rate is substantially higher.

Historical Background

Sudden death from electric shock is generally due to the development of ventricular fibrillation. It has been known for some time that a second electric shock, if given in time, may terminate ventricular fibrillation and restore sinus rhythm. Presumably the use of this second shock gave rise to the name 'countershock' and this term has been applied to the use of electric shock for the reversion of any ectopic tachycardia, whatever the aetiology. It was found that an electric shock would terminate ventricular fibrillation however it had been produced, and 'defibrillators' were designed for this purpose, initially for use in the operating theatre. In 1936, Beck reported successful treatment of ventricular fibrillation which was responsible for cardiac arrest during a surgical operation. He used 60 cycle a.c. at 110 volts with a current of 1–2 amperes for 0·1 second and delivered through electrodes applied directly to the heart. This technique gradually became universally adopted for the treatment of cardiac arrest due to ventricular fibrillation occurring in the operating theatre. It was, however, rarely possible to use this method outside the operating theatre, since it necessitated an immediate thoracotomy. It was recognized, however, that ventricular fibrillation was a common cause of sudden death following myocardial infarction or in Stokes–Adams syndrome, and in 1956 Zoll and colleagues described an external a.c. defibrillator which could be used without opening the chest. A substantially higher voltage was necessary—from 200 to 700 volts for 0·15 second—to defibrillate the heart with the chest closed.

It is considered that electric shock is effective by producing simultaneous depolarization of the whole heart and thus enabling the sinus node to resume control. Since the method is successful in ventricular fibrillation, it seemed reasonable to assume that it might also be effective in other arrhythmias. In 1961, Alexander, Kleiger and Lown reported the successful reversion of ventricular tachycardia using external a.c. shock. In 1962, Lown and Newman described synchronized d.c. shock for the treatment of various arrhythmias. This work was the culmination of a painstaking experimental study of various forms of external electric shock in dogs. A.C. shock applied to dogs in sinus rhythm resulted in the production of numerous and serious arrhythmias. Ventricular fibrillation occurred once in every five shocks and atrial fibrillation in 70 per cent of test shocks. Repeated a.c. shocks given to normal dogs was followed by the electrocardiographic pattern of acute antero-lateral myocardial infarction. During a week's follow up study, there was a 35 per cent mortality and it was concluded that external a.c. shock carried a substantial hazard to the heart.

Direct-current Shock

Apparatus was devised for administering a direct shock from a 16 micro-farad capacitor discharging through an inductance in 2·5 milliseconds. The energy used was calibrated in watt-seconds (joules). External d.c. shock was 100 per cent successful in reverting 550 episodes of ventricular fibrillation in 20 dogs. It was, moreover, frequently successful when a.c. shock had failed to restore normal rhythm and none of the dogs died. The experimental findings made it clear that d.c. shock was both more effective and safer than alternating current.

Vulnerable Period

The effect of d.c. shock on normal dogs was studied. Lown and Newman found that ventricular fibrillation was produced in about 2 per cent. It has been known to physiologists for some time that susceptibility to ventricular fibrillation is confined to a definite period in the cardiac cycle corresponding to the T wave. Lown developed an electronic synchronizer which enabled d.c. shock to be delivered through a time delay circuit triggered by the R wave of the electrocardiogram. The precise timing of the shock in the cardiac cycle could be varied at will. A systematic exploration of the cardiac cycle at 10-millisecond intervals was carried out with d.c. shocks across the closed chest. Analysis of 3,500 test shocks established that the vulnerable period of the cardiac cycle occupied 30 milliseconds just preceding the apex of the T wave. Shocks applied during this period invariably produced ventricular fibrillation. Shocks applied at any other time in the cardiac cycle never resulted in ventricular fibrillation. A similar vulnerable period for the atrium was demonstrated on the downstroke of the R wave or the S wave.

Shocks given during this phase produced atrial fibrillation. Thus, synchronized d.c. shock can be arranged to depolarize the whole heart without any danger of producing either ventricular or atrial fibrillation.

This technique of synchronized d.c. shock applied across the closed chest gained rapid acceptance as the simplest, safest and most effective method for terminating a variety of ectopic arrhythmias. D.C. defibrillators have now replaced a.c. machines in the cardiac operating theatre, since d.c. is found to be more consistently effective than a.c. in terminating ventricular fibrillation. When restoring sinus rhythm in ventricular fibrillation, there is no need for the shock to be synchronized and a switch on the machine enables the synchronizing device to be put out of the circuit. In a recent publication, Kreus, Salokannel and Woris (1966) have suggested that synchronization of the shock to avoid the vulnerable period is unnecessary in any arrhythmia. The evidence they present is not statistically significant and, in view of Lown's careful experimental work, seems a dangerous claim.

Terminology

This technique has already acquired a number of technical terms to describe it. D.C. countershock has been widely employed. The prefix 'counter' was presumably derived from the use of a second electric shock to counteract the effect of a first. It seems hardly suitable for routine use. The term 'conversion' has often been applied to techniques for restoring normal rhythm in arrhythmias. 'Conversion' of arrhythmias by synchronized direct current has been termed 'cardioversion', a neologium which has little to commend it. Perhaps the best term, which is applicable to any technique, electrical or pharmacological, is 'reversion' which implies restoration of a normal mechanism. The term then requires a qualifying phrase to indicate the method used, that is, one should speak of 'reversion with quinidine' or 'a.c. reversion' or 'synchronized d.c. reversion'.

Indications for Synchronized D.C. Reversion

Synchronized d.c. reversion is indicated for the termination of any sustained ectopic tachycardia, provided it is not due to digitalis or other drugs. There is now, moreover, ample evidence that digitalis intoxication, even in mild form, is an absolute contra-indication to the method, for even successful reversion is liable to be followed by dangerous ventricular arrhythmias. In using the method for the reversion of non-urgent cases, it is probably wisest to omit digitalis for 24–48 hours beforehand. In urgent cases it is extremely important to have accurate information about any recent digitalis administration. More detailed description of the indications for, and results of, synchronized d.c. shock will be found under the treatment of the individual arrhythmias in the next chapter. The equipment should always be ready when any procedure is undertaken which entails the risk of provoking an arrhythmia. It should, for example, always be at hand in the cardiac catheter room and thoracic surgical theatre. Ideally, a machine should be permanently installed in every operating theatre, x-ray department or casualty receiving room, ready for emergency use.

The Apparatus

The first piece of equipment available was the Lown 'cardioverter'. This is a table model which delivers synchronized d.c. shocks from a capacitor. It incorporates a cathode-ray oscilloscope for monitoring the electrocardiogram and has a built-in pacemaker for dealing with asystole, and a ratemeter which sounds an alarm if the heart rate should rise above or fall below predetermined values. This equipment is expensive, costing around £1,000. In this country, Cardiac Recorders Ltd. have produced a piece of equipment which is substantially cheaper and equally effective. They manufacture a console model which includes a ratemeter and pacemaker, but these additions are unnecessary for routine use and increase the size and cost of the machine considerably. In its simplest form, Cardiac Recorders produce a synchronized d.c. defibrillator with a separate cathode-ray oscilloscope for monitoring the electrocardiogram. These two pieces of equipment are essential for using synchronized d.c. shock. Pacemakers and ratemeters are sold as separate units; the combination of all these separate devices into one unit is both unnecessary and extravagant. The equipment required for monitoring patients will be discussed in Chapter 16.

All machines for delivering d.c. shocks are necessarily heavy, since the large capacitor has to contain oil. They cannot be made 'portable' but are readily 'transportable' on a suitable trolley. The meter on the front panel records the energy to which the capacitor is charged in watt-seconds (joules). The equipment can be used for delivering shocks in closed-chest or open-chest patients. A simple arrangement ensures that if the electrodes are applied direct to the heart, for example, at operation, only low-energy shocks can be given. For external shocks, large electrodes are used with heavily insulated handles. One of these electrodes has a button switch which can be conveniently operated by the thumb when the shock is to be given.

The shock is normally triggered from the R wave of the electrocardiogram. Occasionally, patients are encountered whose main deflection in each available lead is negative (that is, an S wave). There is a tumbler switch on the front panel which is marked R+ when the switch is up and R− when the switch is down. When the main deflection is an S wave, the switch is turned down and the shock will now be triggered by the downward deflection.

The precise moment in the cardiac cycle at which the synchronized shock will be given is indicated on the cardioscope (oscillograph) by a short vertical line. The position of this in the cardiac cycle can be varied by a screw on the front panel marked 'trigger delay'. Once this has been set to the correct position, it can be locked by a nut, and rarely, if ever, requires subsequent readjustment. The visible indication on the cardioscope of the time of the triggered shock is accompanied by an audible signal. This enables the physician to be continually aware of the heart rate when not looking directly at the monitor.

Recently Cardiac Recorders have produced a small d.c. defibrillator weighing only 20 lb. It is powered by two packs of small dry batteries (HP2) and the capacitor is of the electrolytic type instead of a heavy one containing oil. The equipment is essentially portable and eminently suitable for emergency treatment of ventricular fibrillation. Each pack of batteries is capable of delivering 20 shocks at a level of 400 watt-seconds and when both packs have 'run down', combining them enables a further 4 to 6 shocks to be obtained at 400 watt-seconds.

Technique of External Synchronized D.C. Reversion

The application of an electric shock to the closed chest of sufficient energy to depolarize the heart is far too painful to be carried out in the conscious patient. Light anaesthesia with sodium methohexitone or pentothal is essential. Just sufficient to put the patient to sleep is all that is required. For this reason, it may be convenient to do a 'list' of several non-urgent cases in one session.

It is probably wise, when possible, to have the patient on a wooden couch, rather than a metal bedstead. The electrocardiograph electrodes are applied to the limbs in the usual way. The monitor should be inspected to ensure that the trigger signal is falling in the correct place in the cardiac cycle. The two areas on the chest where the electrodes are to be applied are well rubbed with electrode jelly which is liberally applied to the electrodes themselves.

Electrode Position

Initially the electrodes were applied on either side of the chest, one in each axilla. It was later found that less electrical energy was required if one electrode was placed anteriorly and the other posteriorly. It is a little inconvenient to turn an anaesthetized patient on to his side, and there is now available a 'scapular' electrode on which the patient can lie. This is positioned overlapping the lower border of the left scapula, and the second electrode (with the firing switch) is positioned with its centre over the third right intercostal space. The operator must press firmly with this electrode to ensure good electrical contact.

Energy Level

It is customary to start with an energy level of 100 watt-seconds. If reversion fails to occur, the energy level should be increased in 100 watt-second steps up to 400. If 400 watt-seconds fails to restore sinus rhythm, the attempt should be abandoned. It is important to see that no one is touching the patient when the shock is given. When the trigger switch is pressed, contraction of the patient's chest and arm muscles is usually evident by slight movement. An electronic device in the machine automatically disconnects the cardioscope $\frac{1}{10}$ second before the shock is delivered. The electrocardiographic trace immediately disappears from the monitor but can be immediately restored with the 're-set' control. Successful reversion should be immediately apparent from the presence of P waves preceding each QRS complex.

Results

It is now universally acknowledged that synchronized external d.c. shock is the most consistently successful method yet available for the reversion of ectopic tachycardias to sinus rhythm. The vast majority of ventricular tachycardias revert easily. The same is true of supraventricular arrhythmias.

The widest application of the method has been in atrial fibrillation which is the commonest sustained arrhythmia. This will be further discussed in Chapter 13.

Complications

A few deaths following external synchronized d.c. shock have been recorded in the literature. From a perusal of the published accounts of fatal cases, it is clear that they were all suffering from digitalis intoxication, which is now accepted as an absolute contra-indication to the method.

Further details of the use and indications for synchronized d.c. shock will be given in Chapter 13.

Other Electrical Methods of Controlling Arrhythmias

Paired Pacing

Electrical pacing of the heart was primarily introduced to increase the rate in patients with severe bradycardia due to complete A.V. block. The usual duration of the stimulus from an artificial pacemaker is 3 milliseconds. In 1963, Lopez, Edelist and Katz demonstrated that if the duration of the stimulus was prolonged to 150–250 milliseconds in the paced dog heart, the rate of the heart was immediately slowed. They showed that the prolonged stimulus acted both at 'make' and 'break' and that an identical result could be produced by paired stimuli, each of 3 milliseconds duration, the second stimulus being given immediately at the end of the refractory period of the first. The second stimulus is analogous to a very premature extrasystole. It results in a second depolarization of the heart but, if accurately timed, there is no associated mechanical response; it is, however, followed by a second refractory period, so that the total refractory period from 'paired pacing' is substantially prolonged. There are two important consequences from this manoeuvre: paired pacing by prolonging the refractory period slows the heart below its natural rate, and the second stimulus acts as an 'extrasystole', so that the following mechanical beat manifests post-extrasystolic potentiation. The positive inotropic effect of paired stimulation is considerable and greatly exceeds that produced by any pharmacological agent.

Paired pacing has been employed in severe heart failure to increase the force of contraction of the heart. It has also been used in ectopic tachycardias which have proved resistant to drugs and electrical reversion, to control the heart rate.

Coupled Pacing

An alternative method of achieving the same result is to utilize the R wave of the electrocardiogram to 'trigger' the stimulus, timed to fall at the end of the refractory phase. This technique will exactly halve the heart rate. These methods are still in their infancy and are rarely required for the control of ectopic tachycardias. They are not free from risk, since the second stimulus (or the coupled stimulus) must fall very close to the vulnerable period of the preceding depolarization. Ventricular fibrillation has often occurred in the experimental dog and has been recorded at least once in the human. Despite the early promise of paired pacing and 'coupled' pacing, there have been few recent reports of the use of this technique, presumably because of the hazard of producing ventricular fibrillation.

Long-term Control of Drug Resistant Ectopic Tachycardia by Electrical Pacing

Occasionally patients are encountered who have recurrent ectopic tachycardias which prove resistant to anti-arrhythmic drugs. It has been shown that even in the absence of heart block, artificial electrical pacing of the heart can play an important role in the management of these cases. Sowton, Leatham and Carson (1964) first described the suppression of recurrent arrhythmias by artificial pacing in patients without heart block.

In patients in whom a sustained or recurrent ectopic arrhythmia proves resistant to drug therapy, artificial pacing, often combined with anti-arrhythmic drugs, may prove successful in controlling the arrhythmia and enable the patient to lead a normal life. Sowton and colleagues (1969) recommend that pacing should be from the ventricle, using a ventricular-triggered pacemaker, so that anti-arrhythmic drugs may be added to the regimen in increasing doses to suppress ectopic activity without requiring an unduly rapid pacing rate (that is, more than 100 per minute). If a trial of this technique proves successful, a permanent pacing system can then be implanted. Sowton and colleagues used propranolol as the anti-arrhythmic drug in a dose varying from 80 to 360 mg daily.

Patient-controlled Pacing for Supraventricular Tachycardia

Cardiac pacing may also be used to terminate episodes of tachycardia, either by overdrive suppression or by competitive pacing at a slower rate when a re-entry mechanism is responsible. This is particularly valuable in those patients who suffer frequent paroxysms of tachycardia which are resistant to long-term drug therapy. The inductively coupled cardiac pacemaker is ideally suited for treatment in this way, as it may be removed from the body when not required and the external control permits variation of rate and stimulus intensity. One of us has successfully treated two patients with resistant re-entrant supraventricular tachycardia with this technique. Epicardial leads were sutured to the atrium at operation and connected to the buried subcutaneous coil. At the onset of tachycardia, the patient applies the external coil to the overlying skin and turns on the pacemaker for 10 seconds to achieve competitive atrial pacing. During this period one of the stimuli is delivered at the appropriate moment to capture the atrium, enter the A.V. node and block the self-perpetuating re-entrant stimulus. The termination of an episode of tachycardia is shown in *Figure 12.2*. Leads I, II, III and a right atrial electrogram are recorded simultaneously during competitive atrial pacing. The pacing stimuli have been highlighted and numbered for clarity. Stimuli 2, 3 and 5 are delivered when the atrium is refractory and are ineffective. Stimuli 1 and 4 are able to achieve atrial depolarization as evidenced by the premature A, but do not affect the tachycardia. Stimulus 6, however, is delivered fractionally earlier and is able to

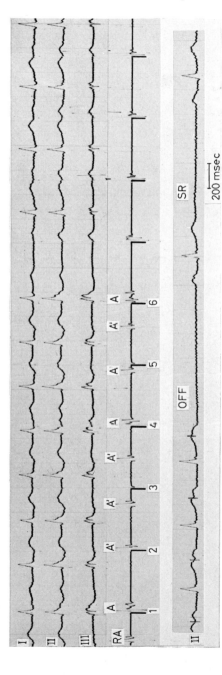

Figure 12.2—Competitive right atrial pacing during re-entrant supraventricular tachycardia. Lead II below is continuous. Pacing stimulus numbered 1–6. A' represents atrial depolarization due to tachycardia and A depolarization due to pacing captive. Stimulus 6 terminates the arrhythmia (see text)

enter the antegrade A.V. nodal pathway before the re-entrant impulse has reached it, and thus abolishes the tachycardia. Atrial pacing continues, in this example with a Wenckebach conduction sequence, until the pacemaker is turned off when sinus rhythm is regained. One of our patients has successfully terminated over 200 such episodes in this way.

CHAPTER 13

MANAGEMENT OF INDIVIDUAL ARRHYTHMIAS

The satisfactory management, specific therapy and prognosis of individual arrhythmias is still largely dependent on accurate diagnosis. While it is true that the majority of sustained tachycardias can be terminated by synchronized d.c. shock, whether they are supraventricular or ventricular in origin, the differentiation between them is still important, both for planning immediate treatment and particularly for prognosis, since the outlook in ventricular tachycardia is usually not good, while an attack of supraventricular tachycardia is relatively innocent. The importance of recognizing digitalis as the cause has already been stressed. It is, moreover, of great importance to be able to differentiate between benign arrhythmias which may be disregarded and those due to heart disease which require treatment.

Treatment of Sinus Tachycardia

Sinus tachycardia, which is secondary to heart failure, is a compensatory mechanism which is attempting to make up for a reduced stroke volume. No treatment for the tachycardia itself is indicated; therapeutic measures should be directed to the heart failure. Sinus tachycardia, occurring in nervous subjects with normal hearts, occasionally presents as a problem in symptomatic treatment. It is conventional to manage these cases with explanation, reassurance and sedation. An alternative to non-specific drugs is propranolol (Inderal). This at least is specific in removing the symptom of which the patient complains and, provided they are reassured that no organic disease is present, the symptomatic relief afforded can be of value in restoring confidence and is at least a rational approach.

Sinus Bradycardia

In normal subjects this requires no treatment, though it is important to appreciate that it may result in cardiac enlargement in a normal heart. It is occasionally an important therapeutic problem following acute myocardial infarction and will be discussed in Chapter 16.

Escape Beats and Rhythms

Escape beats and rhythms do not of themselves require treatment unless due to organic sino-atrial or A.V. block. This will be discussed in Chapter 14.

Treatment of Extrasystoles

It has been said that more patients change their doctor because of extrasystoles than for any other condition (Scherf and Schott, 1953). The first step in the correct management of extrasystoles is to establish the presence or absence of heart disease. If no heart disease is present, a cause for the extrasystoles should be investigated, such as excessive consumption of coffee, tobacco or alcohol. If these are excluded, a careful explanation to the patient of the nature of the disorder should be given, together with reassurance that the heart is normal. It is important to avoid drug therapy since this will only confirm the patient's fears that something is wrong. Successful reassurance of the patient is a test of the doctor's therapeutic skill and, in this sense, the administration of an anti-arrhythmic drug is a confession of failure. Extrasystoles can be very alarming to the patient and should never be lightly dismissed by the physician. If they can be abolished by light exercise, such as walking about the room, instruction to do this to terminate an 'attack' in itself helps to reassure the patient that his symptoms are benign. Occasionally the physician is driven in self-defence to prescribe an anti-arrhythmic drug for benign extrasystoles which are causing the patient undue discomfort or distress. The choice of drug is then important. Although digitalis is known often to abolish extrasystoles, even in the normal heart, it should never be used for this purpose because of the implications of the name to the patient. Most patients in whom it is necessary to suppress benign extrasystoles are anxious and introspective and it is likely that the rhythm disturbance is catecholamine induced. The use of a beta-adrenergic receptor blocking drug is therefore rational and propranolol, one 40 mg tablet 3 times daily, is usually effective. It can be discontinued after extrasystoles have disappeared for a few weeks. If propranolol proves ineffective in suppressing extrasystoles, quinidine sulphate 0·2 to 0·3 g four times daily may be tried, or procainamide up to 0·5 g, if quinidine is not well tolerated, or one of the newer anti-arrhythmic drugs may be used.

When extrasystoles are associated with organic heart disease, no special treatment apart from that of the underlying condition is necessary. In many cases extrasystoles disappear following digitalization. If they persist, it may be necessary to decide whether specific drug therapy is indicated. It is, of course, essential to be satisfied that the ectopic beats are not digitalis induced. If they are not, and they are occurring frequently, or in pairs, or in short runs of tachycardia, treatment may be necessary for two reasons. First, frequent ventricular extrasystoles may substantially reduce cardiac output and aggravate heart failure. Secondly, they may presage the development of more serious arrhythmias such as ventricular tachycardia or even fibrillation. This is particularly true following acute myocardial infarction or cardiac surgery. The subject will be discussed further in Chapter 16.

Treatment of Paroxysmal Tachycardia

Many cases of paroxysmal tachycardia seen in out-patient practice occur in patients without evidence of structural heart disease. Very often the attacks are of brief duration, lasting 2–3 minutes, and are relatively infrequent, occurring once or twice a week or even less often. The use of drug therapy in such cases is obviously to be avoided. Simple explanation and reassurance alone is required in most instances, coupled with simple instructions for some manoeuvre at the onset of an attack, such as taking a deep breath and holding it as long as possible. When attacks are more frequent or prolonged, and particularly if associated with distressing symptoms, such as dyspnoea, syncope, polyuria or even anginal pain, more positive treatment will be required. Knowledge of the nature of the abnormal rhythm may be useful. If there is good reason to believe that the attacks are due to paroxysmal atrial fibrillation, then permanent digitalization of the patient is probably the simplest measure. There is then a good chance that, when an attack occurs, the ventricular rate will be automatically controlled by the digitalis; the patient should then have no distressing symptoms and may even fail to notice the attack. Full digitalization is essential for this purpose, followed by a regular maintenance dose. This is certainly the best treatment in patients with rheumatic heart disease and paroxysmal atrial fibrillation.

In the past, quinidine was regarded as the drug of choice in the long-term prophylaxis of other forms of paroxysmal tachycardia. In our experience, however, the most generally effective drug now available is propranolol. The evaluation of any drug for the treatment of paroxysmal tachycardia, which is normally so capricious in its behaviour, is necessarily difficult and would require large scale double blind control trials. We are, however, satisfied that propranolol is of considerable value in three varieties of paroxysmal tachycardia: in those cases whose attacks are provoked by exertion or emotion (tachycardie parosystique à centre excitable), in patients with the Wolff–Parkinson–White syndrome, and in those cases with almost continuous paroxysmal tachycardia (Stock, 1966). There is no danger in using propranolol in these cases, even in the presence of organic heart disease, provided the patient is not in heart failure between attacks. In elderly subjects, however, or in those with ischaemic heart disease, it is a wise precaution to digitalize the patient as well. Relatively large doses of propranolol are necessary, 40 mg three or four times daily being an average requirement. In the absence of heart disease I have occasionally used up to 320 mg daily. If propranolol fails to prevent attacks, either practolol should be tried or one of the newer anti-arrhythmic drugs, or perhaps some combination such as practolol and quinidine or the electrical techniques referred to on pages 205 208.

Treatment of Sustained Ectopic Tachycardias

In the past either digitalis or quinidine was used, but there are now a large variety of anti-arrhythmic drugs of proven value which may be tried; either beta receptor blocking drugs or one of the newer drugs without beta blocking properties such as verapamil. It is wiser to avoid digitalis, for, if drug therapy fails, d.c. electric shock can be used with impunity.

Treatment of Paroxysmal Tachycardia in Infants

In paroxysmal tachycardia in infants, particularly the 'sustained' variety, digitalis appears to be specific. Nadas and colleagues (1952) recommend the following dosage scheme, using digitoxin (Nativelle's Digitaline): for children under 2 years of age, 0·03 mg per 0·5 kg body weight, and 0·02 mg per 0·5 kg body weight for children over the age of 2 years. This total amount is divided into 3 doses given over 24 hours. (If digoxin is preferred, the corresponding doses would be 0·07 mg per 0·5 kg body weight for infants under the age of 2 years and 0·05 mg for children over 2 years.) It is likely that with increasing experience, d.c. electric reversion may be used in infants, and in that case digitalis should be avoided for fear that, if it failed, electric methods would be contra-indicated.

General Management of the Individual Case

It is a common cardiological emergency, both in hospital and domiciliary practice, for a patient to present with a rapid heart rate of recent onset. The correct management of these cases depends on an accurate history and clinical examination in conjunction with an electrocardiogram. The following points in the history must always be obtained. It is first necessary to know if the patient has had similar attacks before. In the majority of patients, attacks of ectopic tachycardia tend to follow the same pattern and, if there is no evidence of heart failure or undue distress, and previous attacks have terminated spontaneously and uneventfully, the wisest plan is to do nothing apart from reassurance and sedation; in most of these cases, spontaneous reversion to sinus rhythm will occur within a few hours.

A second vital point in the history is to have precise details about any recent digitalis medication. This information is best obtained from the patient's general practitioner and should be asked for as routine whenever a request is made for the admission of a patient with an arrhythmia. If the patient has been treated with digitalis for some time, the possibility of digitalis intoxication must be considered and this subject will be discussed in detail in Chapter 15. If treatment with digitalis has been started for the present episode, it is very important to know how much has been given, since this will determine how soon d.c. shock can safely be used should this be considered necessary. Quite often only a small dose will have been given, for example, digoxin 0·25 mg b.d. without an initial loading dose. If this has been administered for less than a week, there would be no need to delay electrical reversion, whereas full digitalization would entail a delay of at least 24 hours.

A careful clinical evaluation of the case should be made in conjunction with the cardiogram. If the patient is not in heart failure and is free from dyspnoea or cardiac pain, there is no indication for urgent action. The differential diagnosis between ventricular and supraventricular tachycardia has already been discussed in previous chapters. Precise diagnosis is more important from the point of view of prognosis than treatment. However, if the cardiogram reveals QRS complexes of normal duration, a confident diagnosis of supraventricular tachycardia can be made and d.c. shock can be postponed until the effect of vagal stimulation has been tried. When the site of origin of the tachycardia is uncertain, vagal stimulation should certainly be tried as a preliminary measure; if it fails to revert the arrhythmia, the timing of d.c. shock must be determined by the digitalis status of the patient.

Vassaux and Lown (1969) emphasize that it is often difficult to identify with certainty when digitalis intoxication is responsible for a supraventricular arrhythmia. They suggest that when the possibility of digitalis intoxication is entertained, treatment should be started with such drugs as diphenylhydantoin, lignocaine or procainamide. If these drugs prove ineffective they recommend trying d.c. shock, starting with very low dosage, for example, 1 watt-second, and observing the effect on the monitor. They quote a case with an atrial rate of 204 per minute and 2:1 A.V. block, which was given a trial dose of 5 watt-seconds. This resulted in a ventricular extrasystole following each normal QRS complex and acceleration of the atrial rate from 204 to 330 per minute, establishing digitalis toxicity as the cause of the arrhythmia. They recommend titration of the shock energy in small increments of energy level, commencing with one 1 watt-second, increasing to 5, then 10 then 25 watt-seconds. They conclude that the employment of low energy discharges with d.c. shock may not only provide a definite therapeutic result but at times may afford otherwise unobtainable evidence of the presence of digitalis intoxication.

A difficult problem is presented by a seriously ill patient with a rapid tachycardia who has already been treated with large doses of digitalis. Such patients may be in heart failure, with weak peripheral pulses and low or unrecordable blood pressures. D.C. shock should not be used until at least 24 hours after the last dose of digitalis. In the meantime an intravenous dose of frusemide (Lasix) should be given and an infusion of a pressor drug set up. The clinical condition of the patient may well be improved by these measures and a few may even revert to sinus rhythm. If no improvement follows the use of pressor drugs and the patient's condition remains grave, the use of an anti-arrhythmic drug will require consideration. In these circumstances the drug of choice would probably be verapamil.

If, when the patient is first seen, the rhythm of the heart is manifestly irregular and if the cardiogram confirms that the arrhythmia is atrial fibrillation, no attempt at electrical reversion should be made; the patient should first be digitalized and, when the ventricular rate has come under control, electrical reversion should be undertaken after digitalis has been withdrawn for 24 hours. Details about digitalis dosage will be given later in the section on treatment of atrial fibrillation.

The treatment of ectopic tachycardias occurring during the course of acute myocardial infarction will be discussed in Chapter 16.

Provided proper precautions about digitalis medication are taken, synchronized d.c. electric shock is a simple and almost uniformly successful treatment for sustained ectopic tachycardias. Ventricular tachycardia, which used to present such an anxious therapeutic problem, is now almost invariably reverted to sinus rhythm with a single shock of 100 watt-seconds. Supraventricular tachycardias, which have failed to revert by vagus stimulation, show a similar high reversion rate. Occasional failures occur, particularly with ventricular tachycardia. This arrhythmia is not very common and it may be several years before there is sufficient experience to state the percentage failure rate with any precision.

Treatment of Atrial Flutter

Before the introduction of synchronized d.c. shock, atrial flutter was frequently a difficult arrhythmia to manage. It was unusual to obtain satisfactory control of the ventricular rate by digitalis, and even when digitalization produced 4:1 A.V. block, with a ventricular rate of 75 per minute at rest, the rate commonly doubled on light exertion. Attempts to revert flutter to sinus rhythm with quinidine frequently failed. It used to be recommended that flutter be initially treated with large doses of digitalis.

Since this drug shortens the refractory period of the atria, it often converted flutter to fibrillation. It was then suggested that digitalis was stopped and a few cases would then revert to sinus rhythm. In general, however, atrial flutter proved a most resistant and unsatisfactory arrhythmia to treat with drugs. Fortunately the majority of cases revert very easily to sinus rhythm with synchronized d.c. shock and this is the immediate treatment of choice without any initial drug therapy. If digitalis has already been given, it should be withdrawn for 24 hours before reversion is carried out. In my experience, and that of others, flutter reverts easily, usually with one shock of relatively low energy. Very occasionally, a resistant case may be encountered and Lown (1967) has described one. By altering the timing of the shock in the cardiac cycle so that it fell on the 'T' portion of the flutter wave, he was able to convert it to atrial fibrillation, which is much more readily controlled by digitalis therapy. Today the first approach to the management of a case of atrial flutter would be the trial of one of the newer anti-arrhythmic drugs such as verapamil, disopyramide or acebutol. Cases which prove drug resistant, provided digitalis has not been given, will usually revert easily with d.c. shock.

Treatment of Wolff–Parkinson–White Syndrome

Since pre-excitation in the absence of recurrent attacks of tachycardia is entirely symptomless, no treatment is required for this finding alone, though it may perhaps be wise to warn the patient of possible attacks of palpitation. In patients who are subject to recurrent attacks of ectopic tachycardia, treatment is much the same as for other cases of paroxysmal tachycardia and this has already been described (page 210). If the attacks are relatively infrequent and short, the patient may find some simple manoeuvre, such as breath-holding, to be immediately effective in terminating an attack. In such cases, of course, no drug therapy is necessary. When drug therapy is required, one might expect that quinidine would be most effective in those cases in which it abolishes the pre-excitation pattern, since it presumably acts by blocking the accessory pathway. Many patients, however, are intolerant of long-term quinidine and in our experience the most effective drug has been propranolol in a dose of 40 mg three or four times daily.

If the patient presents with a sustained attack of ectopic tachycardia, vagal stimulation should be tried first and if this fails the attack should be terminated by direct current electric shock. If the mechanism of the tachycardia is atrial fibrillation, it is almost certainly wiser to avoid using digitalis since this may serve only to block the normal conduction pathway, without having a similar effect on the anomalous bypass.

In the occasional case with almost continuous ectopic tachycardia which proves resistant to drug therapy, the question of surgical treatment may arise. In some patients with Type B Wolff–Parkinson–White syndrome, the anomalous pathway is a bundle of Kent in the right atrio-ventricular sulcus. To establish its presence it is necessary to demonstrate pre-excitation of the right ventricle, in sinus rhythm, close to the right atrio-ventricular groove. Cobb and colleagues (1968) achieved this by plotting iso-potential lines on the body surface. This was accomplished by recording the electrocardiogram from 50 different points on the thorax and analysing the records with the aid of an analogue computer. An alternative surgical procedure, as already mentioned above, is ligation of the bundle of His. This procedure, however, would necessarily have to be associated with implantation of a demand pacemaker since the anomalous pathway cannot be guaranteed to conduct continuously. It would be necessary moreover to ensure that the anomalous pathway was not in the A.V. junction itself, since it could well be simultaneously ligated with the bundle of His.

Treatment of Atrial Fibrillation

Whatever the underlying aetiology, the initial treatment of atrial fibrillation should be digitalis. When the ventricular rate has come under control, consideration may be given to the use of d.c. shock to restore sinus rhythm as an elective measure. It should again be emphasized that the onset of atrial fibrillation in a patient with mitral valve disease of rheumatic origin ought always to be regarded as a medical emergency. Even if the patient is not unduly distressed by the arrhythmia, stasis of blood in the left atrial appendage may quickly result in clot formation and a disastrous systemic embolus may follow. Rapid digitalization to control the ventricular rate and intravenous heparin to prevent clot formation are indicated. Although the majority of cases probably do well without such heroic measures, these are certainly justifiable to prevent the occasional irremediable catastrophe.

Occasionally, patients are seen with atrial fibrillation, associated with organic heart disease, whose ventricular rates are normal. The low ventricular rate is probably due to partial A.V. block and these patients are often very sensitive to digitalis. The drug is probably best withheld under these circumstances unless there is evidence of heart failure.

Choice of Digitalis Preparation

There are numerous preparations of digitalis on the market today and it is a sound rule to become familiar with the use of only a few and not to change preparations without some clear indication. It is now well established that the qualitative action of all digitalis glycosides is the same; they differ only in their speed of action and rate of dissipation. These two factors are closely linked, the rapidly acting preparations being rapidly dissipated; the converse is similarly true. It has long been known that the initial dose of the drug, the digitalizing dose, must be substantially larger than the maintenance dose. Once the optimum therapeutic effect of digitalis has been obtained, the maintenance dose should be designed to offset exactly the rate of dissipation so that a constant state is achieved. It is important to appreciate that individual patients vary widely in their response to different doses, so that only average digitalizing and maintenance doses for different preparations can be given. When digitalis is used for the treatment of heart failure in patients in sinus rhythm, correct dosage is a matter of careful and skilled clinical assessment. Fortunately, in the treatment of atrial fibrillation, the ventricular rate provides a simple and reliable guide to dosage.

There are four preparations of digitalis with which it is useful to be familiar. For oral administration, a relatively slow acting and slowly dissipated preparation is indicated. Digoxin is the most generally useful but, as will be mentioned below, an occasional patient is intolerant of digoxin and then digitoxin (Nativelle's Digitaline) may be substituted. Both these preparations can also be given intravenously.

When rapid digitalization is required, a rapidly acting preparation should be chosen and should be given intravenously. There are two preparations which can be used for this purpose. Lanatoside C (Cedilanid) is a rapidly acting cardiac glycoside and, following intravenous injection, it takes effect in 10–20 minutes and is maximal in about two hours. It is quite unsuitable for oral administration for it is impossible to maintain digitalization with it, partly because of rapid dissipation and partly because of poor absorption. A still more rapidly acting glycoside is ouabain. This is given intravenously and takes effect in 2–4 minutes, becoming maximal in half an hour. It is unsuitable for oral administration for it is destroyed in the gastrointestinal tract.

These four preparations are all purified glycosides of definite composition and uniform potency. They have now largely replaced the older preparations such as Tab. Digitalis Folia which is made from the dried powdered leaves of *Digitalis purpurea* and contains a mixture of glycosides. Although relatively cheap, Tab. Digital. Fol. has the disadvantages that it is biologically standardized and cannot be given intravenously. Each tablet contains 60 mg and is equivalent to one tablet of either digoxin or digitoxin.

Only one of the four purified preparations discussed above is obtained from the ordinary *Digitalis purpurea*. This is digitoxin which is available in tablets containing 0·1 mg. Lanatoside C is extracted from a particular variety of foxglove, the *Digitalis lanata*. Digoxin is prepared from lanatoside C by a chemical process which removes glucose and acetic acid. Ouabain is a pure crystalline substance which is obtained from the seeds of *Strophanthus gratus*.

Table 13.1 shows the usual route of administration, the speed of action, the average digitalizing and maintenance doses, and the duration of toxicity of these four purified cardiac glycosides.

Digoxin is the most useful cardiac glycoside and is the preparation of choice in the majority of cases. Occasionally patients are encountered who develop nausea and vomiting on digoxin, due to a local irritant effect on the gastric mucosa. This must be distinguished from the nausea and vomiting of digitalis intoxication which is central in origin. Differentiation is not usually difficult, for the former appears very early in treatment before intoxication could have occurred. When this local irritant action is encountered, digitoxin may be substituted, since it is free from this effect. This is probably the only indication for digitoxin which has the disadvantages of being slow in action and slow in dissipation. The slow dissipation is a serious drawback for, if digitalis intoxication should occur, it may take 3 or more weeks to disappear after the drug is withdrawn. It should be used with great caution in elderly subjects.

Of the two intravenous preparations, lanatoside C is the safest and is very reliable. Ouabain is still more rapid in action and is very rapidly dissipated, although, paradoxically, the slowing of the ventricular rate in atrial fibrillation often lasts up to 4 days following a single dose. These valuable properties tend to be offset by a relatively narrow gap between its therapeutic and toxic doses. Since individual patients vary widely in their susceptibility to

TABLE 13.1

Preparations of Cardiac Glycosides

Preparation	Content of tablet	Usual route of administration	Time of onset of action	Time of maximal effect	Average digitalizing dose	Average maintenance dose	Duration of toxicity
Digoxin	0·25 mg	Oral, but can be I.V. or I.M.	30 min.	1–2 hours	3·5 mg	0·5 mg per day	3–4 days
Digitoxin	0·1 mg	Oral, but can be I.V.	1–2 hours	6–9 hours	1·7 mg	0·2 mg per day	3 weeks
Lanatoside C	—	Intravenous	10–20 min.	$\frac{1}{2}$–1$\frac{1}{2}$ hours	1·6 mg	—	1 day
Ouabain	—	Intravenous	5 min.	30 min.	0·7 mg	—	2–6 hours

Although tablets of lanatoside C are available, it is unsuitable for oral administration. Digoxin can be given by the intravenous (I.V.) route. This is rarely necessary and should only be done if the patient's digitalis status is known. Digitoxin is so slow in action that there is little point in giving it intravenously. The figures given in this table should only be regarded as approximate.

digitalis, it is unwise to give a full digitalizing dose (0·7 mg) straight away. Lown and Levine (1955) recommend two doses of 0·25 mg with an interval of half an hour, followed by 0·1 mg at half-hourly intervals. If the patient should require 0·7 mg, little time is saved compared with lanatoside C. It is suggested that ouabain is reserved for dire emergencies, that is, moribund patients with acute pulmonary oedema. It should never be used unless the patient's digitalis status is known for certain.

Management of Atrial Fibrillation of Recent Onset

The choice of digitalis preparation and the route of its administration should be determined by the urgency of the case. The following recommendations are based on the assumption that the patient has not received any digitalis preparation during the preceding 2 weeks.

If there are no urgent features and the patient has no evidence of mitral valve disease, oral digoxin is the drug and route of choice. Theoretically the whole digitalizing dose can be given at once. This, however, is unwise for 2 reasons. First, there is no safe way of calculating the dose for an individual patient. Secondly, a single large oral dose of digoxin is very liable to cause vomiting and this may well antagonize the patient to the tablets he may require to take for the rest of his life. An initial dose of 0·75 mg (three tablets) followed by 0·5 mg at six hour intervals, until the ventricular rate has fallen to between 70 and 80 per minute, is a satisfactory routine. The average maintenance dose is then 0·25 mg b.d., but some patients require more (up to 1 mg daily) and some less (0·25 mg once daily).

If urgent symptoms are present, or if the patient has mitral valve disease, a rapidly acting intravenous preparation should be employed. Lanatoside C is safe and reliable; the full digitalizing dose varies from 1·2 to 3 mg. Lown and Levine recommend an initial dose of 1·2 mg intravenously, followed by 0·4 mg every two hours until adequate ventricular slowing is achieved. If the patient has mitral valve disease, heparin, 12,000 units, should be given intravenously with the first dose of lanatoside C and should be repeated in 12 hours time. At the same time, oral digoxin should be started, giving 0·5 mg at six hour intervals for 24 hours and thereafter according to the ventricular rate. The digoxin will become effective by the time the action of the lanatoside C is wearing off. The majority of patients with atrial fibrillation can be safely and satisfactorily managed in this way. Ouabain should be reserved for the dire emergency and should be given in the dosage mentioned above.

Difficulties sometimes arise if the patient is vomiting. Vomiting may be due to the development of congestive heart failure with onset of atrial fibrillation. If, when first seen, no digitalis has been given, lanatoside C intravenously is indicated and oral digoxin should not be started until the vomiting has ceased. On the other hand, a more common problem is the patient who has already been started on digitalis before admission. The question must then be decided as to whether the vomiting is due to heart failure or to digitalis. In atrial fibrillation the ventricular rate is a reasonably reliable guide. If this is still fast, heart failure is probably responsible for the vomiting. Intravenous digitalis is probably best avoided in this situation, when it is impossible to know how much digitalis has been absorbed.

Digoxin by the intramuscular route may be safely employed in the same dosage as if given by mouth.

From time to time, patients with atrial fibrillation are encountered whose ventricular rates fail to slow satisfactorily on apparently adequate digitalis dosage. One of the commonest causes for this is underlying thyrotoxicosis. It is a common experience that the ventricular rate in thyrotoxic atrial fibrillation will not be slowed appreciably by digitalis until the thyrotoxicosis is controlled. 'Masked' thyrotoxicosis is not uncommon in middle-aged or elderly patients and may be associated with other forms of organic heart disease, particularly rheumatic. The thyrotoxicosis may then be overlooked. When, therefore, the ventricular rate in atrial fibrillation fails to slow with adequate digitalis therapy, thyrotoxicosis must first be excluded. A few cases remain in which no explanation can be found for the failure of adequate slowing of the ventricular rate. If these cases are unsuitable for electrical reversion to sinus rhythm, or if electric shock fails, consideration should be given to the addition of a beta-adrenergic receptor blocking drug. Although these drugs by themselves will slow the ventricular rate in atrial fibrillation, they may well precipitate heart failure and, in our opinion, should never be used for this purpose in undigitalized patients. The combination of a beta-blocking drug and digitalis seems to have its greatest value in mitral stenosis with atrial fibrillation. It can be shown that, for a given cardiac output, the left atrial pressure will vary inversely as the square of the diastolic filling time. This is why patients with mitral stenosis are particularly intolerant of tachycardia. If, for any reason, mitral valvotomy is contra-indicated, patients with mitral stenosis and atrial fibrillation can often be considerably improved by adding propranolol to their treatment. This is particularly true if the resting heart rate on digitalis alone exceeds 80 per minute, or if there is reason to believe that the ventricular rate rises unduly on exercise. One should aim at achieving a resting ventricular rate of 60 per minute or even less. This usually requires about 20 or 30 mg of propranolol 3 times a day in addition to digitalis. This combination is particularly useful in patients who have re-stenosed following mitral valvotomy, for it often enables a second operation to be postponed, at least for a while (Stock, 1966).

In other forms of organic heart disease with uncontrolled atrial fibrillation, the addition of propranolol will always slow the ventricular rate, but this is not necessarily followed by clinical improvement. It rarely proves helpful in mitral regurgitation or aortic valve disease but may be always worth trying.

It seems likely that the addition of practolol in these circumstances might well be of equal value to propranolol and would at least be free from the negative inotropic action of the latter.

Every effort should be made to restore patients to sinus rhythm when the ventricular rate in atrial fibrillation is not controlled by digitalis. For example, a patient with thyrotoxic atrial fibrillation failed to revert to sinus rhythm when the thyrotoxicosis had been controlled by therapeutic [131]I. Her ventricular rate persisted at 120–130 per minute, despite digitalis being increased to the point of toxicity. After reversion to sinus rhythm with d.c. shock, her heart rate fell to 72 per minute.

In patients who have been in atrial fibrillation for some time with a satisfactory control of the ventricular rate by digitalis, the development of a fast heart rate should always raise the question of digitalis intoxication. This problem will be discussed more fully in Chapter 15.

Reversion of Atrial Fibrillation by Synchronized D.C. Shock

There is no doubt whatever that synchronized d.c. shock is at present the safest and most effective method available for the reversion of atrial fibrillation to sinus rhythm. Now that the first flush of enthusiasm for this technique is over, it is pertinent to ask several questions. First, is restoration of sinus rhythm beneficial for the patient? Secondly, how long does sinus rhythm persist and what measures will help to maintain it? Thirdly, which patients should be selected for reversion?

There is ample evidence now that reversion of atrial fibrillation to sinus rhythm is beneficial in the majority of patients. Subjective improvement is usually considerable. This may be due partly to abolition of the uncomfortable palpitation associated with atrial fibrillation. That at least some of the beneficial effect is psychological is suggested by patients who claim to be improved at follow up, but who are found to have relapsed into atrial fibrillation. Physiological studies, however, have demonstrated that restoration of sinus rhythm leads to an increased cardiac output, though this may not be demonstrable until a week after reversion. Moreover, the abnormal response of the heart rate to exercise is abolished. A further benefit of sinus rhythm is a greatly reduced incidence of both systemic and pulmonary emboli. All observers are agreed that the benefits of sinus rhythm compared with atrial fibrillation are considerable.

There are three main contra-indications to restoring sinus rhythm. Patients with a long history of recurrent episodes of supraventricular tachycardia who have developed atrial fibrillation are probably best left alone. Restoration of sinus rhythm would almost certainly lead to recurrence of their attacks. It is well known that patients with ischaemic heart disease may lose their angina if they develop atrial fibrillation. Restoration of sinus rhythm in these patients would be likely to lead to recurrence of angina. Thirdly, patients with atrial fibrillation due to organic heart disease, whose ventricular rates are slow without digitalis, should not be reverted. Restoration of sinus rhythm in these patients may result in sinus bradycardia or junctional rhythm and subjective deterioration. A further group of patients in whom the indications for reversion are at best equivocal are those with lone atrial fibrillation. This group is very resistant and difficult to revert; they normally have no symptoms and require no treatment and the risk of systematic embolus is very low. The combination of propanolol and quinidine may be tried or one of the newer anti-arrhythmic drugs.

Maintenance of Sinus Rhythm

The initial high percentage of success of d.c. shock in restoring sinus rhythm is to some extent offset by a disappointing number of subsequent relapses. Halmos (1966) reported on 175 patients followed for a minimum of 9 months. His initial reversion rate was 78 per cent. At 9 months follow up only 42 per cent remained in sinus rhythm. Morris, Peter and McIntosh (1966), on the other hand, reverted 88 per cent of 108 patients and 52 per cent of these were still in sinus rhythm at follow up 20 months later. However, a number of these had relapsed and been re-reverted in the meantime. These authors appear convinced that drug therapy is necessary to maintain sinus rhythm and their patients were maintained on quinidine gluconate in sufficient dosage to maintain a serum level of 4 mg per cent. Halmos, on the other hand, maintained his first 56 patients on quinidine sulphate (5 grains 4 times daily), his next 41 on effervescent potassium (2 tablets 4 times daily), while his last 40 patients had no maintenance therapy. There was no significant difference in the relapse rates of the three groups. Although no well designed controlled trial of maintenance therapy with quinidine has been reported, it seems unlikely from these figures that it has any striking value. A well controlled trial of propranolol revealed no protective effect.

Our present information indicates that, following successful reversion of atrial fibrillation, there is a disappointingly high relapse rate and that only about half or rather less will still be in sinus rhythm a year later. These disappointing long-term results may well be improved by the use of the newer anti-arrhythmic drugs.

Complications of D.C. Reversion of Atrial Fibrillation

Transient supraventricular arrhythmias are fairly common during the first few minutes following successful reversion. The sinus node may be slow in resuming control of the heart with resulting sinus bradycardia, junctional escape beats or junctional rhythm. Occasionally there are single or multiple atrial extrasystoles, sometimes with short runs of atrial or junctional tachycardia. These arrhythmias are quite benign and generally settle to regular sinus rhythm within 5 minutes. Another type of picture has been termed by Lown the 'sick sinus node'. It is characterized by 'chaotic atrial activity with continual changes in P wave contour and bradycardia interspersed with multiple and recurring ectopic beats with runs of atrial or nodal tachycardia' (Kleiger and Lown, 1966). This type of picture almost always reverts to atrial fibrillation. It seems that in these cases, following depolarization of the heart, there is no stable pacemaker to take over control.

Ventricular arrhythmias following electrical reversion are less common and appear to be always due to digitalis intoxication.

Occasionally, successful reversion is followed by acute pulmonary oedema. This is unusual and always transient, responding quickly to conventional treatment.

Systemic emboli following reversion are rare, occurring in less than 1 per cent of cases. In patients with a history of recent embolus it is probably wise to give anticoagulants for 2 weeks before reversion is attempted, for there is good evidence that emboli are always composed of recently formed clots. Otherwise, there is no indication for the use of anticoagulants.

Indications for D.C. Reversion

When the technique was first introduced, the only indication for attempting reversion was the presence of atrial fibrillation. With growing experience, a rational selection of cases has become increasingly possible. The contra-indications have already been discussed. It should be emphasized again that any evidence of digitalis intoxication is an absolute contra-indication. All observers agree that the duration of atrial fibrillation is a very important factor, both in determining immediate reversion rate and for subsequent maintenance of sinus rhythm. The highest rate of success, both for reversion and maintenance, is in patients with a history of less than 6 months. When atrial fibrillation has been present for more than a year, attempts at reversion should only be made with good reason.

An exception to this general rule is when atrial fibrillation develops during mitral valvotomy. Initially, reversion was attempted at the comple-tion of the operation. Experience quickly showed that many patients failed to revert, and those who did, very often relapsed in the immediate post-operative period. Reversion should be postponed until about two months after operation.

The high relapse rate during the first few months following successful reversion of atrial fibrillation to sinus rhythm, particularly in patients with rheumatic heart disease, has made some authors question whether reversion is worth attempting at all. However, the following three circum-stances, when present, make attempt at reversion well worth while. (1) If atrial fibrillation is of recent origin, (2) if radiologically the heart is shown to be small and (3) if the cause for atrial fibrillation has been successfully treated.

A high success rate of reversion is seen in patients with uncomplicated thyrotoxic atrial fibrillation who have not reverted spontaneously after the thyrotoxicosis has been controlled. Surprisingly enough, a number of these patients will later revert to atrial fibrillation without any recurrence of thyrotoxicosis. Atrial fibrillation is not uncommon in patients with alcoholic cardiomyopathy and in 4 patients who had been persuaded to become teetotallers we have been able to convert all 4 to sinus rhythm, so far without relapse, after periods varying from 2 to 7 years.

A NOTE ON THE MANAGEMENT OF ARRHYTHMIAS FOLLOWING CARDIAC SURGERY

Arrhythmias following cardiac surgery, particularly open heart surgery with bypass, are common. Potentially fatal arrhythmias may compromise otherwise technically satisfactory surgical procedures. These arrhythmias have many similarities to those following acute myocardial infarction with the main difference that many of the surgical patients have already had prolonged medical treatment with digitalis and diuretics. This may well have resulted in electrolyte disturbance, particularly potassium depletion, although the latter may not necessarily be reflected in the serum level. Potassium loss moreover increases during the immediate post-operative period and since potassium depletion sensitizes the heart to the toxic action of digitalis it is important to assess the patient's potassium status immediately before operation. If the serum potassium is found to be low, this is good evidence that the patient is depleted. If, however, it is normal, the patient should be placed on a normal diet (that is, without sodium restriction) and without a dieuretic and the urine should be collected for 24 hours. If the 24-hour volume of urine contains less than 20 mEq of potassium, this is good evidence that the patient is potassium depleted and he should be given potassium supplements in the form of Slow K, 2 tablets 3 times a day, and 40 mEq potassium chloride should be added to the post-operative infusion as described on page 197. This is particularly true if the patient is on digitalis and if intravenous isoprenaline is used.

Beller, Frater and Wulfsohn (1968) described a useful technique in which electrical pacing could be readily instituted if necessary during the post-operative period. At operation, pacing wires were sewn into position in both the atria and ventricles choosing whichever side was operatively convenient and bringing the wires out through the pericardial drainage tube. As soon as they are no longer required, the wires can be removed at the same time as the pericardial drainage tube. The original article should be consulted for the details of the technique. The main purpose of these wires is that it enables the surgeon to pace the atria if, as not infrequently happens, brady-cardia develops, since these hearts are not usually capable of increasing their stroke volume. If atrio-ventricular block should develop the ventricle can be paced directly. Beller and his colleagues also used the technique to suppress ventricular ectopic beats. However, the main value of the technique is for accelerating the heart rate when this is slow due either to sinus bradycardia or heart block.

Ventricular arrhythmias should be treated with lignocaine, and supra-ventricular arrhythmias with practolol, as will be described in the manage-ment of acute myocardial infarction in Chapter 16 (pages 299–301).

CHAPTER 14

HEART BLOCK

ATRIOVENTRICULAR BLOCK

The term heart block in clinical medicine, when used without further qualification, is generally taken to refer to impaired conduction between the atria and ventricles. In Chapter 2 (page 23) some general features of disturbed impulse conduction were discussed and it was pointed out that the different types of block could generally be recognized at whatever site in the conduction system they occurred. It is suggested that this section (pages 23–31) should be re-read before continuing further. It should again be emphasized that the term A.V. dissociation is not synonymous with (complete) heart block; it should in fact be restricted to the arrhythmias discussed in Chapter 10, in which complete orthograde block is not the cause. Pathological orthograde A.V. block may be due to prolongation of the refractory period and be potentially reversible, or it may be due to an anatomical lesion interrupting the normal conduction pathway, in which case the refractory period would be infinity.

Physiological Considerations

It has long been traditional to classify A.V. block into three grades, according to its severity. In first-degree heart block, all atrial impulses are conducted to the ventricles, but conduction time is prolonged and this is recognized in the cardiogram by lengthening of the P–R interval. In second-degree heart block, some atrial impulses reach the ventricles, whereas others are blocked at the A.V. junction. The severity of second-degree A.V. block may be conveniently expressed as the ratio of the total number of atrial impulses (reaching the A.V. junction) to the number which are conducted and thereby elicit ventricular contractions. In the mildest forms of second-degree block, this ratio varies widely; for example, it may be 5:4 or 3:2, indicating that every fifth or every third atrial impulse is blocked. Usually a Wenckebach type of conduction anomaly is present, successive P–R intervals showing progressive lengthening until an atrial impulse is blocked (*see* page 25). Less frequently an atrial impulse suddenly fails to reach the ventricles without preliminary lengthening of the P–R interval. The more advanced stages of second-degree block show a 2:1, 3:1 or even a 4:1 A.V. conduction ratio.

First- and second-degree A.V. block are often referred to as partial heart block. In third-degree A.V. block, no atrial impulses reach the ventricles and complete heart block is said to be present. The atria and ventricles then beat independently, the ventricles being controlled by an escaping subsidiary pacemaker.

It is important to appreciate that the three degrees of A.V. block do not necessarily represent successive stages of a progressive condition. These terms were originally introduced by Gaskell (1881) to describe the rhythm-

produced by experimental, step by step severing of the junctional tissues of the tortoise heart. Progression through these three experimental stages has its counterpart in man only in acute conditions such as digitalis intoxication or acute myocardial infarction. It is, moreover, still not sufficiently widely appreciated that second-degree heart block occurs in two distinct forms which behave in quite different ways and in which the prognosis is entirely different. These two types were first recognized by Hay (1906) and were later differentiated more precisely by Mobitz (1924). They are known as Type I partial A.V. block (Wenckebach) and Type II partial A.V. block, or Mobitz Type II block.

Type I second-degree heart block is the more benign form. When mild, it is characterized by Wenckebach periods with progressive lengthening of the P–R interval until an atrial impulse is blocked. The A.V. ratio is a simple measure of its severity. The severest grade is 2:1 A.V. block and, when present, the P–R interval of the conducted beat is generally prolonged. This type of partial block is rarely associated with Stokes–Adams attacks and is generally transient. Common causes are active rheumatic carditis, digitalis intoxication and acute myocardial infarction. Its outstanding characteristic is that 1:1 A.V. conduction can usually be restored by any factor which increases the atrial rate, such as exercise, intravenous atropine or the inhalation of amyl nitrite. Conversely, slowing the atrial rate by vagal stimulation, for example, from the carotid sinus, usually increases the severity of the block.

Type II second-degree A.V. block forms a striking contrast. In its mildest form with intermittent 'dropped' beats, there is no preliminary lengthening of the P–R interval which remains normal up to the blocked beat. In more severe forms, a simple arithmetic A.V. ratio of 2:1, 3:1 or, occasionally, 6:1 is obtained; the P–R interval of the conducted beat is often normal. Contrary to the behaviour of Type I second-degree block, Type II tends to be persistent and, even if it resolves, this is usually only temporary, and insidious progression to complete heart block with recurrent Stokes–Adams attacks is the more general course. A fundamental feature of Type II partial block is that acceleration of the atrial rate by exercise, atropine or amyl nitrite, in contrast to Type I, immediately increases the degree of block. The change in the severity of the block occurs at precise atrial rates. *Figure 14.1* shows an example of Type II block. In (*a*) with an atrial rate of 70 per minute there is normal sinus rhythm; in (*b*) with an atrial rate of 96 per minute there is 2:1 A.V. block and in (*c*) with an atrial rate of 108 per minute, complete A.V. block is present. Conversely, as was first described by Wenckebach, carotid sinus stimulation, by slowing the atrial rate, may produce paradoxical acceleration of the ventricular rate, for example, when 2:1 block is converted to 1:1 conduction. These different responses to a change in atrial rate make the clinical differentiation between Type I and Type II partial A.V. block relatively simple. This will be discussed later in greater detail in the clinical section.

Katz and Pick (1956) suggested that the difference in behaviour between the two types of partial A.V. block could be explained in terms of the refractory period of the A.V. junction. In Type I block, the relative refractory period is prolonged but with far less change in the absolute refractory period. In Type II block, in contrast, it is the absolute refractory period which is prolonged, the relative refractory period remaining approximately normal. It will be remembered that the refractory period shortens with increasing heart rates. It was suggested that the relative refractory period shortens proportionately more than does the absolute refractory period. In Type I block with Wenckebach periods, acceleration of the atrial rate by shortening the relative refractory period will shorten the P–R interval and hence lengthen the next R–P interval. This lengthening of the R–P interval may be sufficient, despite the increase in rate to prevent a sinus impulse from

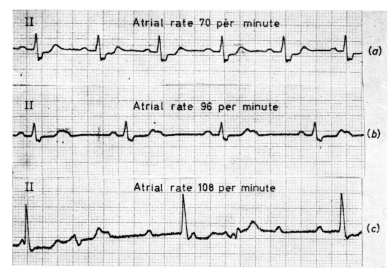

Figure 14.1—Mobitz Type II second-degree heart block. The three records were taken in immediate succession, the patient being lightly exercised by straight leg raising. The critical relation between atrial rate and the degree of block is well illustrated

reaching the A.V. junction in its absolute refractory phase so that persistent 1:1 conduction would then be restored.

In Type II partial heart block, it was suggested that it is the absolute refractory period which is primarily lengthened and this does not appear to shorten as the atrial rate increases. With increasing rates, therefore, a point is reached when the sinus impulse arrives at the A.V. junction during its absolute refractory phase and the degree of block will abruptly increase. However, while this mechanism will explain the difference in response of the two types of partial heart block to changes in atrial rate, it does not explain the intermittent block which appears in Type II without any preceding change in the P–R interval or in the heart rate. (*Figure 14.5.*)

Increasing evidence, both electrocardiographic and pathological, has accumulated in the past few years that the anatomical site of the block is different in the two types. Type I partial A.V. block is usually due to a lesion involving the A.V. node whereas in Mobitz Type II block the anatomical lesion is most frequently situated at a more peripheral site in the A.V. conduction system and in fact usually represents bilateral bundle branch block.

Electrophysiological studies by Watanabe and Dreifus (1967) strongly support this view.

These workers recorded simultaneously atrial and ventricular electrograms, together with the action currents from two micro-electrodes impaled in a cell in the A.V. node and in another cell in the bundle of His. In the isolated profused rabbit heart they demonstrated that in Wenckebach Type I partial A.V. block after preliminary lengthening of the P–R interval, failure of transmission of the atrial impulse to the ventricle occurred in the A.V. node.

In Mobitz Type II partial heart block, on the other hand, they found that failure of transmission of the atrial impulse to the ventricles occurred in or below the bundle of His. The precise mechanism was not always clear but in some experiments the block was caused by re-excitation in the A.V. node. Presumably due to the presence of a dual pathway in the A.V. junction, an atrial impulse was able to turn back from the lower portion of the bundle of His and to re-enter the A.V. node from below, thus rendering it refractory to the next sinus impulse. While the mechanism is still not entirely clear, the site of failure of transmission of an atrial impulse to the ventricles in Mobitz Type II block is invariably more peripherally situated in the conduction system. This is certainly in keeping with the electrocardiographic evidence to be presented later, that Mobitz Type II block is generally associated with bilateral bundle branch block.

Clinical His bundle electrography has largely confirmed these earlier observations, but over the last few years as the published literature has increased, exceptions have been documented. Thus Type I block within the bundle branches and Type II block at the A.V. node have been clearly illustrated. It would appear, therefore, that although in the majority the type of block is a valuable guide as to the level at which block occurs, it is not totally reliable and the definitive answer will only be given by the His bundle electrogram. This is of some practical importance, as it is now felt that the site of block may be a more important determinant of prognosis than the type of block. Rosen and colleagues (1971a) reported five patients with Type II block occurring proximal to the His deflection. In all cases this was not progressive. If such a mechanism occurred in patients with pre-existing bundle branch block an erroneous diagnosis of bilateral bundle branch disease might precipitate unnecessary pacemaker treatment.

Watanabe and Dreifus also suggested that in higher degrees of partial A.V. block, for example with a 3:1 A.V. ratio, there was unhomogeneous conduction in the A.V. node resulting in fractionation of the wave fronts. Progressive impairment of conduction in the more rapidly conducting fibres might allow gradual synchronization of advancing wave fronts which would finally summate and permit propagation of the impulse to the ventricles.

Aetiology

There are many well recognized causes of A.V. block. These include congenital A.V. block, digitalis intoxication, active rheumatic carditis, recent diaphragmatic myocardial infarction and chronic coronary artery disease. It used to be assumed that in the majority of patients with established chronic complete heart block, the cause was arteriosclerotic or hypertensive heart disease. It has recently been recognized that this assumption is unjustified. Complete heart block, complicating acute myocardial infarction, almost always resolves with a return of normal sinus rhythm in patients who survive. If these patients are excluded, the aetiology of complete heart block is, at present, largely obscure. It is however established that the majority of patients presenting with chronic complete heart block have bilateral bundle-branch fibrosis without involvement of the A.V. node or bundle of His or other apparent myocardial disease. Harris and colleagues (1969) have reported an adequate clinico-pathological correlation in 65 cases. Of these cases, 26, almost half, had selective loss of conduction fibres in both bundle branches at multiple sites with replacement fibrosis. Davies and Harris (1969) suggest that this bilateral bundle-branch fibrosis probably has several different aetiologies. They consider that some may represent ageing changes superimposed on a conduction system damaged by previous myocarditis and in others the morphological changes suggest a primary degenerative process of conduction tissue. Other causes of chronic heart block in this series included cardiomyopathy, coronary artery disease, myocarditis and calcification of the mitral or aortic valve or the valve rings. Rarer causes were collagen disease, amyloid deposits, transfusion siderosis, congenital heart block and syphilitic cardiovascular disease.

A rare but well recognized cause of A.V. block is involvement of the conduction system by metastatic growths. Complete heart block has been reported in lymphangio-endothelioma, hemangio-endothelioma, myeloblastoma, reticulum-cell sarcoma, bronchogenic carcinoma and leukaemic infiltration of the ventricular septum.

Other uncommon causes of chronic heart block include myxoedema, Paget's disease and, in South America, Chagas' disease.

During the past 12 years the cardiac surgeon has emerged as a new aetiological agent in producing complete A.V. block. Improved surgical techniques are rapidly reducing the incidence of this iatrogenic block which at one time was a serious cause for anxiety during open heart procedures.

Pathological Basis of Heart Block

In the majority of cases of primary complete heart block, the pathological basis is bilateral bundle-branch fibrosis. The histological changes have recently been fully described by Davies and Harris (1969) in 26 cases. In only 10 of the 65 cases described by Harris and colleagues (1969) was ischaemic heart disease considered to be the cause of A.V. block. In one of these patients there was occlusion of the A.V. nodal artery with complete destruction of the main bundle and A.V. node. In the remaining cases there were old thrombotic occlusions involving all three major coronary vessels and ischaemic scarring involving both bundle branches was found though the A.V. node in these cases was normal.

In acute myocardial infarction, heart block is much commoner when the site of the infarct is diaphragmatic (that is, inferior) than when it is anterior. There is usually occlusion of the right coronary artery or occasionally of a dominant left circumflex artery (Sutton and Davies, 1968). Block results from inflammation and oedema in the region of the A.V. node. When heart block complicates anterior myocardial infarction, there is usually occlusion of the anterior descending branch of the left coronary artery. This results in necrosis in the anterior part of the interventricular septum remote from the A.V. node. Block occurs only if both bundle branches are involved and for this to happen the area of muscle damage must be extensive, as will be seen later in Chapter 16. The prognoses in these two varieties of heart block in myocardial infarction are completely different.

In congenital complete heart block, few post-mortem studies are available. There is usually either interruption of the bundle of His or even its complete absence.

Clinical Signs

It is usually possible to recognize both the presence and degree of A.V. block at the bedside.

First-degree Atrioventricular Block

First-degree A.V. block with a prolonged P–R interval is not responsible for any symptoms. Its presence may be suspected clinically by finding a soft first heart sound and this suspicion may be confirmed by careful inspection of the jugular venous pulse when a delay may be observed between the A and the V waves.

Levine and Harvey (1949) emphasized that the intensity of the first heart sound depended on the position of the cusps of the A.V. valves at the onset of ventricular systole. If this follows closely on atrial systole, the A.V. valves are wide open and will be closed violently and abruptly by ventricular systole, causing a loud first sound. When the interval between atrial and ventricular systole is longer, the cusps will have tended to 'float' back towards the atria and will be moved a much shorter distance when closed by ventricular systole and the first sound will then be soft.

Second-degree Atrioventricular Block

Second-degree A.V. block with Wenckebach periods and dropped beats must be differentiated from the pause following an extrasystole. This is readily achieved with the stethoscope, and the trained ear may detect the ventricular acceleration before the pause. Occasionally a blocked atrial extrasystole may cause a pause in sinus rhythm. If the P wave is hidden in the T wave, an electrocardiogram may not be easy to interpret. Clinically, however, the atrial extrasystole will produce a cannon wave in the neck.

More advanced second-degree heart block with a 2:1 A.V. ratio results in a marked ventricular bradycardia which must be differentiated from complete A.V. block. The most reliable clinical signs are a first heart sound of uniform intensity and the absence of cannon waves in the jugular venous pulse. Confirmation may be obtained if the A wave of the blocked atrial impulse can be seen in the neck following each V wave of the conducted beat.

Complete Atrioventricular Block

In the majority of cases the clinical diagnosis of complete A.V. block is relatively easy. There is bradycardia with a ventricular rate usually between 30 and 50 per minute. There is marked, usually striking, variation in the intensity of the first heart sound. From time to time, when ventricular systole follows close on atrial systole, the first sound is extremely loud. The term 'bruit de canon' has been given to this very loud first sound which is particularly characteristic. It may sometimes be necessary to listen for up to one minute before hearing it, since its occurrence depends on a chance time relationship between the P wave and QRS complex. Inspection of the jugular venous pulse will reveal occasional large, abrupt waves, so-called 'cannon waves', when atrial and ventricular systole coincide. Finally, in many cases it is possible to hear atrial sounds occurring independently of the sounds of valve closure produced by the ventricle. They are best sought between the apex and left sternal edge. It should be remembered that patients in atrial fibrillation with complete heart block will show none of these signs, which are the result of the constantly varying time relationship of atrial and ventricular systole.

Before discussing the varied clinical picture of heart block, some description of one of its main complications, Stokes–Adams attacks, is necessary.

Stokes–Adams Disease

Patients suffering from A.V. conduction disturbances are liable to attacks of paroxysmal cerebral ischaemia due to sudden cessation of the circulation. Such episodes are called Stokes–Adams attacks. As will be seen later, several different mechanisms may be responsible for the abrupt cessation of circulation, but it is convenient to regard the attacks as due to cardiac arrest. The clinical symptoms vary with the duration of the arrest; if this lasts for only 2–5 seconds, the patient may only notice transient dizziness or faintness with a momentary sense of blankness and uncertainty. When arrest lasts from 5–10 seconds, consciousness is usually lost, particularly if the patient is standing. He will fall to the ground, just as in epilepsy, and injuries are frequently sustained. On recovery, he may remember nothing of the attack. If circulatory arrest persists for fifteen seconds or more, convulsive movements may occur with stertorous breathing and foaming at the mouth. After 30 seconds, the patient may appear dead, without evidence of cardiac or respiratory function. If the attack lasts 3 or more minutes, recovery is rare. A striking and important feature of Stokes–Adams attacks is the colour changes in the skin, which are very helpful in diagnosis. With the onset of circulatory arrest, the face becomes suddenly deathly pale. If convulsive movements occur, pallor may become replaced by cyanosis. Return of circulation is signalled by a sudden, vivid flush. This sequence of colour changes is contrary to those occurring in epilepsy. During an epileptic fit, the colour is plethoric and cyanosed and on recovery the skin is pale. When A.V. conduction is normal between Stokes–Adams attacks, the diagnosis should always be possible if a reliable observer has witnessed an attack and can describe the sequence of colour changes.

Mechanism of Circulatory Arrest in Stokes–Adams Attacks

In the majority of Stokes–Adams attacks, the immediate cause of circulatory arrest is ventricular asystole. It has been said that the term Stokes–Adams attack should be reserved for those instances of circulatory arrest when the atria continue to beat while the ventricles are still. This restricted use of the term is difficult to justify since it entails, for certain proof, an electrocardiographic record of the attack. The original descriptions of Stokes–Adams seizures were purely clinical and were written long before graphic methods were available for demonstrating the mechanism.

It has been recognized for some time that episodes of fast ventricular arrhythmia, rather than simple asystole, may be responsible for Stokes–Adams attacks. Parkinson, Papp and Evans (1941) analysed cardiographic records made from 64 patients during attacks and reported four different mechanisms. The most common was ventricular asystole without preceding ventricular tachycardia. In other cases, asystole was preceded by a run of ventricular tachycardia. They subdivided ventricular tachycardia into two groups, 'low' and 'high'. In 'low' ventricular tachycardia, the rate was about 160 per minute or less; this alone did not cause loss of consciousness, but it was followed by a period of asystole. In 'high' ventricular tachycardia, the rate was between 200 and 500 per minute, ranging from a fast ventricular tachycardia to ventricular flutter, or fibrillation. This 'high' ventricular tachycardia might itself be responsible for syncope, reverting to the previous rhythm without an intervening pause. In other cases, a 'high' ventricular tachycardia was followed by asystole prolonging the attack. A fourth, rare, cause of attacks was extreme slowing of the ventricular rate to under 20 per minute. In this series, Stokes–Adams attacks were caused or initiated by fast ventricular arrhythmias in 45 per cent. When an attack is initiated by a 'low' ventricular tachycardia preceding asystole, the patient may be conscious of palpitation preceding loss of consciousness. In some recent publications, the term 'ventricular tachyarrhythmia' has been introduced to denote the rhythm in attacks not due to simple asystole. This term is ugly, imprecise and seems a poor substitute for the simple phrase 'fast ventricular arrhythmia' which adequately describes what happens, although it perhaps lacks that touch of mysticism which is conveyed by a manufactured word.

Clinical Spectrum

Disturbances of A.V. conduction have a varied aetiology, clinical course and mode of presentation. In the present state of our knowledge, it is perhaps best to classify the varieties of A.V. block on clinical grounds. Table 14.1 shows a suggested classification of the clinical spectrum of A.V. block.

Acute Transient A.V. Block

Acute transient A.V. block is characterized by complete resolution of the conduction defect if the patient survives the causal illness. It may not progress beyond first-degree block, or progression through all degrees with subsequent regression may occur. Common causes of this variety of A.V. block are drugs, including digitalis, quinidine and procaine amide. Atrioventricular block in digitalis intoxication will be discussed in Chapter 15. Acute infections may also cause transient block, particularly active rheumatic carditis and (now rare) diphtheria. Other less common infective causes are measles, mumps and typhus. In active rheumatic carditis, first-degree heart block with a prolonged P–R interval is common and may help to

TABLE 14.1

Clinical Spectrum of Atrioventricular Block

Clinical variety	Degree of block and clinical course	Aetiology
Acute transient A.V. block	May be partial or complete May progress and regress through all 3 degrees Always resolves if illness is survived	Drugs—digitalis, quinidine Infections—active rheumatic carditis, diphtheria, Acute myocardial infarction
Persistent first-degree A.V. block	Does not progress	Chronic ischaemic heart disease Rheumatic heart disease Reiters syndrome
Chronic progressive A.V. block (Gilchrist)	May follow either course A or course B (Type II block)	Usually obscure
Cases presenting with complete A.V. block	Third degree Usually chronic; in rare cases conduction returns	Usually obscure; known causes include congenital, fibroelastosis, rheumatoid arthritis, metastatic tumour, valve calcification, cardiac surgery

confirm the clinical diagnosis. It often persists for some weeks after other evidence of activity has disappeared. Less often it progresses to second-degree block, usually manifested by 'dropped beats' with Wenckebach periods. Higher degrees of partial block or complete block are very rare. Recovery from the attack is always associated with a return to normal conduction. It is important to differentiate between antegrade A.V. block in active rheumatic carditis and A.V. dissociation with capture beats due to junctional tachycardia with retrograde block. This is a frequent transient manifestation of active carditis.

More advanced chronic A.V. block may occur in rheumatic heart disease in middle life. It is then not due to active carditis but may be associated with calcification of the mitral annulus.

An important cause of transient A.V. block is acute myocardial infarction. Contrary to previous teaching, this almost always resolves if the patient survives the attack. It is a serious complication of myocardial infarction and will be discussed in detail in Chapter 16.

Persistent First-degree Heart Block (Campbell, 1943)

Persistent first-degree heart block is a fairly common cardiographic finding in organic heart disease. It is seen in chronic rheumatic heart disease, chronic coronary artery disease, some cardiomyopathies and following bacterial endocarditis. In my experience, it rarely progresses and is an incidental finding of little significance.

Chronic Progressive Atrioventricular Block

Gilchrist (1958), in a classic and authoritative paper, described the clinical features of high-grade heart block based on his personal experience of 140 cases. His classification accords well with our own experience and will be closely followed. He describes 55 cases who, when first seen, had partial heart block, but who progressed ultimately to chronic complete block. They did so in one of two ways which separated them clearly into two different groups which he labelled course A and course B.

Course A (Gilchrist)—Patients in this group are usually in normal sinus rhythm when first seen but have a history of syncopal attacks recurring, as a rule, at long and irregular intervals. When a cardiogram is recorded during a syncopal episode, it reveals normal sinus rhythm changing suddenly without warning to complete block with ventricular standstill. There is no preliminary lengthening of the P–R interval or any change in atrial rate. There is apparently a sudden increase in the absolute refractory period of the A.V. junction. When the ventricles resume beating, complete A.V. block is usually present for a period of minutes or hours, followed by normal sinus rhythm, without an intervening period of second-degree block. The symptoms of an attack depend on the duration of ventricular standstill and may vary from transient dizziness up to syncope with convulsions or even death. If an attack is witnessed, the diagnosis may be suggested by the behaviour of the pulse. At the onset of the attack, the pulse disappears and on recovery there is bradycardia for a time due to complete block.

Such attacks may recur at irregular intervals over very long periods with normal cardiograms between attacks. (One of us has a patient who has experienced approximately 12 attacks each year for more than 11 years, but whose cardiogram between attacks remains normal.) In Gilchrist's experience, all patients with this syndrome, who do not die in an attack (or from any other cause), ultimately progress to complete block with perhaps a short intervening phase of second-degree block. With the onset of complete block, Stokes–Adams attacks may cease, but do not necessarily do so. The duration of the stage of paroxysmal heart block varies widely. It may be as short as a few weeks, but it is usually measured in years.

Unless the patient is seen during an attack, diagnosis in the paroxysmal stage has to be made on the history. It should always be suspected when a middle-aged or elderly patient has a history of recurrent, unexplained 'faints'. The diagnosis can be made with confidence if a reliable witness can recount the characteristic colour changes, deathly pallor in the attack, followed by a vivid flush heralding recovery. The diagnosis is probably often missed unless, as sometimes happens, the patient has a series of attacks close together and is admitted to hospital. It is necessary in all cases to exclude the carotid sinus syndrome.

Course B—Gilchrist described as course B, patients who have Type II partial block when first seen. These always progress to complete block, again after a variable interval which, as in course A, is often measured in years. For this reason it is very important to recognize Type II partial block and differentiate it from the much more benign Type I. If, when the patient is first seen, second-degree block with dropped beats is present, the

Wenckebach phenomenon is absent, and there is no preliminary lengthening of the P–R interval before an atrial impulse is blocked. If 2:1 A.V. conduction is present, a diagnosis of Type II block is suggested if the P–R interval of the conducted beat is normal. If the P–R interval of the conducted beat is prolonged, however, Type II block is not excluded since mixed forms of Type I and II may occur. Differentiation is most readily achieved by observing the effect of changes in atrial rate on the degree of block. The atrial rate may be accelerated by exercise, intravenous atropine or inhalation of amyl nitrite. In Type II block, acceleration of the atrial rate is associated with little change or actual slowing of the ventricular rate from an abrupt increase in the degree of block. The degree of block changes at a critical atrial rate which serves as a measure of the severity of the block. In individual patients, progression of the disease is marked by an increased block at lower atrial rates. Serial observations, however, may reveal spontaneous fluctuations in the relation between the atrial rate and the degree of block.

Conversely, slowing of the atrial rate may result in improved conduction. A characteristic feature of Type II block is a paradoxical acceleration of the ventricular rate in response to carotid sinus stimulation, first described by Wenckebach (1899). *Figure 14.2* shows 2:1 A.V. block at an atrial rate of 68 per minute. Right carotid sinus stimulation slows the atrial rate to 60 per minute and this is associated with 1:1 conduction and consequent ventricular acceleration. This may prove a useful rapid bedside test for establishing a diagnosis of Type II A.V. block. Differentiations between the two types of heart block may be made by recording a His bundle electrogram.

According to Gilchrist, syncopal attacks occur less commonly in course B than in course A progressive A.V. block. Exceptions, however, occur and Stokes–Adams attacks are common in the final stage of complete heart block. Common symptoms, in the early stages, are fatigue, exertional dyspnoea and angina pectoris. Fowler (1962) has particularly stressed angina of effort as a symptom of Type II block. He described four cases: two had normal cardiograms at rest, but developed 2:1 block on exercise; the other two had 2:1 block at rest, which became complete on exercise. In these patients the pain is characteristic of angina but is not relieved by nitroglycerine which may accelerate the atrial rate and increase the degree of block. These cases are probably not due to coronary artery disease and the mechanism of the pain is obscure; there is some reason to believe that it is associated with distension of the heart due to an increased venous return from the exercise, with abrupt slowing of the ventricular rate.

It has already been mentioned that paroxysmal tachycardia, induced by exertion, may be responsible for angina with a normal resting cardiogram (page 149). This is a second disturbance of cardiac rhythm, which may cause angina, in which the resting cardiogram is normal. Despite the fallacies inherent in recording cardiograms following exercise, in patients with angina (Friedberg and colleagues, 1962), it must be admitted that these types of cases could hardly be missed if it was done as routine.

Gilchrist believes that all cases of Type II partial block progress ultimately to chronic complete block, provided they survive long enough. The duration of the stage of unstable block may be difficult to estimate, complete heart block when it first occurs being often transitory. In Gilchrist's series, the

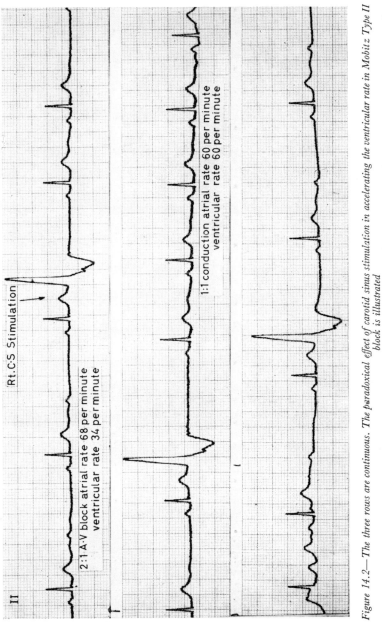

II

Rt.C·S Stimulation

2:1 A·V block atrial rate 68 per minute
ventricular rate 34 per minute

1:1 conduction atrial rate 60 per minute
ventricular rate 60 per minute

Figure 14.2— The three rows are continuous. The paradoxical effect of carotid sinus stimulation in accelerating the ventricular rate in Mobitz Type II block is illustrated

duration of the stage of partial block varied from 6 months to 12 years, but he regarded the estimates of the duration of unstable block to be, at best, an approximation.

It seems likely that most cases of chronic progressive atrio-ventricular block which follow Gilchrist's course B have bilateral bundle branch block. The electrocardiographic diagnosis of bilateral bundle branch block will be discussed later.

Complete Atrioventricular Block

In any series of cases of chronic heart block, complete block is seen more often than partial block. It seems reasonably certain that many cases of complete A.V. block develop suddenly without an intermediate stage of partial block. This syndrome is most often seen in the older age groups, over the age of 50 years; a few may be due to ischaemic heart disease, but usually the aetiology is obscure. Some patients give a history of syncopal episodes in the past, indicating that they have been through a stage of progressive heart block (course A), but in most patients no such history is obtained and, on first seeking medical advice, fully established complete A.V. block is found. About 70 per cent of these patients have syncopal attacks of varying frequency, and some cases present with frequent recurrent Stokes–Adams attacks, any of which may prove fatal. Other symptoms include dyspnoea on exertion, which may be severe, and congestive heart failure with peripheral oedema. Intellectual deterioration and mental depression are common features which disappear when heart block is treated by pacing. Attacks of circulatory arrest of short duration not causing loss of consciousness are common and result in episodes of dizziness which can be very distressing to the patient.

It used to be taught that the ventricular rate in heart block was fixed and unalterable. This is not so; the rate may increase in response to exercise or emotion, albeit within a very narrow range.

Congenital Heart Block

Congenital heart block may be an isolated lesion or it may occur in association with some other congenital cardiac anomaly. It used to be said to occur particularly in association with ventricular septal defect but, with the great increase in our knowledge of congenital heart disease in the past 20 years, it is now recognized that the most common associated defect is, in fact, corrected transposition of the great vessels. This may be associated with ventricular septal defect, but I have seen one case with pulmonary stenosis, an intact ventricular septum and complete heart block.

Congenital heart block is more usually an isolated lesion. The block is almost always complete, but partial block occasionally occurs, usually in the form of Wenckebach periods. It is relatively uncommon; in an electrocardiograph survey of 67,375 asymptomatic males, Johnson, Averill and Lamb (1960) found only one example.

Rosen and colleagues (1971b) demonstrated the lesion to be proximal to the bundle of His in six of the seven children they studied. The other patient demonstrated 'split' H potentials, the first (H_1) being associated with the P waves and the second (H_2) with the QRS complexes, suggesting disruption of the His bundle. The six children reported by Kelly and colleagues (1972) were also found to have block proximal to the bundle of His. The location of isolated congenital heart block is therefore consistent with discontinuity in the A.V. nodal approaches, in the A.V. node or in the A.V. nodal–His bundle connection.

In the majority of patients, congenital complete block is symptomless. It is commonly missed, since the ventricular rate is usually appreciably higher than in the acquired variety, often being 55–60 per minute. On exercise, the ventricular rate increases far more than in acquired block. In the case of Johnson, Averill and Lamb (1960), the rate in response to maximal exercise reached 140 per minute. One of the seven cases of Campbell (1943) was subject to recurrent bouts of Stokes–Adams attacks; clinically he was considered to have a ventricular septal defect. In general, the prognosis in isolated congenital complete block is very good and no restrictions need be placed on the patient's activities.

Iatrogenic Heart Block

The development of right bundle branch block following open heart surgery for congenital heart lesions is relatively common. It is symptomless and usually irrelevant to the successful outcome of the operation and it is usually permanent. A much more serious complication of open heart surgery is the development of complete A.V. block due to surgical damage to the common bundle. This complication has a high mortality rate, even in patients who are artificially paced. Fortunately, improved surgical techniques have considerably reduced its incidence.

Atrioventricular Block in the Carotid Sinus Syndrome

Middle-aged and elderly patients with hypersensitive carotid sinus reflexes are liable to syncopal attacks closely resembling Stokes–Adams seizures and this cause should always be excluded before a diagnosis of paroxysmal heart block is made. In a study of 16 cases, Hutchinson and Stock (1960) found the usual mechanism of the attack to be transient total cardiac arrest with a fall in systemic vascular resistance. We did not encounter a case who developed A.V. block. Gilchrist (1958), however, described three cases whose attacks were due to transient occurrence of complete A.V. block and published a very convincing illustration.

Spontaneous Recovery from Chronic Complete Heart Block

Spontaneous recovery from chronic established complete A.V. block is a rare but well authenticated event. Gilchrist (1958) described two cases from among 46 of chronic complete block. One was known to have been in complete block for 22 years; cardiograms then suddenly demonstrated partial block with Wenckebach periods, alternating with long runs of sinus rhythm with a prolonged P–R interval. One of my patients had Type II partial block when first seen. This progressed to complete block after 6 months, and 3 months later a pacemaker was implanted. After 4 months pacing she developed thyrotoxicosis and presented at follow-up with a sinus tachycardia of 120 and a normal P–R interval. Fortunately the cardiogram showed no evidence of pacemaker impulses, presumably owing to an electronic failure.

These cases are of interest, since they necessarily imply that complete A.V. block is not always due to an anatomical lesion completely interrupting the conducting tract. In some cases, at least, complete failure of conduction is a manifestation of disturbed function which is reversible.

Electrocardiography

Painstaking and elegant analyses of clinical electrocardiograms in A.V. block have contributed significantly to our knowledge of both the normal and abnormal physiology of conduction in the heart. Phenomena, like concealed conduction and conduction during a supernormal phase, were first recognized from studies of clinical records. The following account of the electrocardiographic changes in A.V. block is not intended to be comprehensive but to serve as an introduction to a complex subject.

First-degree Heart Block

The normal upper limit of the P–R interval is generally accepted as 0·2–0·21 second in the majority of healthy individuals. Mammoth studies of large numbers of normal subjects, such as that of Johnson, Averill and Lamb (1960), reveal that 0·5 per cent (that is, about 1 in 200) of normal individuals have P–R intervals in excess of 0·21 second, apparently as a physiological variant. Of their 67,375 asymptomatic subjects, 350 had P–R intervals, at rest, in excess of 0·2 second; the range was from 0·21 second up to 0·39 second, the majority lying between 0·22 and 0·26 second. There was no evidence that any of these 350 subjects were suffering from organic heart disease. Thus, the finding of a P–R interval in excess of 0·2 second, while unusual, does not itself imply the presence of disease.

All authorities agree that the P–R interval tends to lengthen slightly with age and shorten on exercise.

Scherf and Dix (1952) have shown that a prolonged P–R interval often shortens appreciably when the cardiogram is recorded with the patient erect. The change occurs after a delay of 10–15 seconds and is independent of the heart rate.

The P–R interval is measured from the commencement of the P wave to the commencement of the QRS complex. Since the initial forces of either the P wave or the QRS may be isoelectric in some leads, the lead with the longest P–R interval is chosen.

In first-degree heart block of organic origin, the P–R interval may be greatly prolonged so that at normal heart rates the P wave coincides with the preceding T wave. *Figure 14.3* shows an example from a patient with

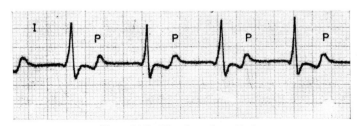

Figure 14.3—First-degree heart block

aortic regurgitation. This P–R interval measures 0·52 and remained constant in serial records over a 5-year period of observation.

The standard electrocardiogram gives no indication of the site of delayed conduction and this may occur at any point from the atrium to the peripheral ventricular conducting system. In *Figure 14.4a* selective increase in the A–H interval indicates A.V. nodal delay. In *Figure 14.4b* increase in the H–V interval in association with left bundle branch block localizes the delay in the right bundle branch. In *Figure 14.4c* both A–H and H–V intervals are increased. The normal QRS complexes would indicate either identical slowing in both bundle branch systems or delay within the bundle of His itself.

Second-degree Heart Block

In its mildest form, second-degree heart block is manifested by occasional 'dropped' beats. In the electrocardiogram, this phenomenon is seen in two forms. Usually there are Wenckebach periods with progressive lengthening of the P–R interval up to the dropped beat. This type of partial block characterizes Type I and is due mainly to prolongation of the relative refractory phase. The mechanism was discussed on page 25. In the experimental animal, Wenckebach periods which precisely obey the 'rules' given on page 26 can be readily produced. In clinical records, minor variations from these rules are very common in A.V. block. *Figures 14.5a* and *b* show typical Wenckebach periods from two patients. An example recorded with a His bundle electrogram is seen in *Figure 14.4d*.

Watanabe and Dreifus (1967) have drawn attention to an occasional variation of the typical Wenckebach period. In these cases progressive increments in the P–R interval, instead of becoming less, become greater so that in consequence the ventricular rate slows during Wenckebach periods.

Type II partial heart block with dropped beats is characterized by sudden failure of a P wave to elicit a ventricular contraction without preliminary lengthening of the P–R intervals (*Figure 14.6*). Sometimes the impulse reaches the A.V. junction in its absolute refractory phase; in other cases, an impulse is blocked unexpectedly without any change in atrial rate.

In more advanced second-degree heart block, the A.V. ratio is often fixed at 2:1, alternate sinus impulses being blocked (*Figure 14.7*). In Type II partial block, the P–R interval of the conducted beat is usually within normal limits (*see Figure 14.4e*). In 2:1 A.V. block, the spacing of the P waves often has a distinctive arrangement. The P–P intervals which enclose a QRS complex are often obviously shorter than the P–P intervals which do not. This irregularity of the P cycle is usually referred to as ventriculo-phasic sinus arrhythmia. It has been attributed to changes in coronary blood flow, the shortened P cycle resulting from improved coronary perfusion following a ventricular systole. An alternative explanation is that it reflects a baroceptor response to ventricular conduction so that the vagal tone is reduced following the QRS complex and the next P wave therefore appears slightly earlier. It is uncommon to see A.V. ratios higher than 2:1 when the atria are in sinus rhythm and the patient is at rest; 3:1 or 4:1 A.V. block would result in a very slow ventricular rate if the sinus rate were normal, and a subsidiary pacemaker would almost certainly escape. On exercise, however, 3:1 or 4:1 A.V. ratios may occur in subjects with Type II

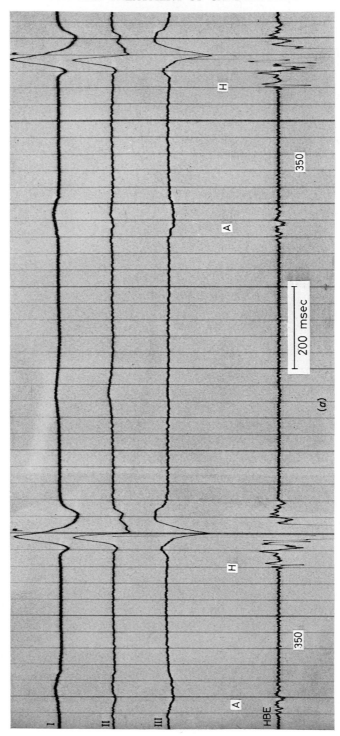

Figure 14.4—(a) First-degree heart block. P–R, 0·40 sec. Right bundle branch block (RBBB). A–H, 350 msec; H–V, 35 msec. Delay entirely at A.V. node

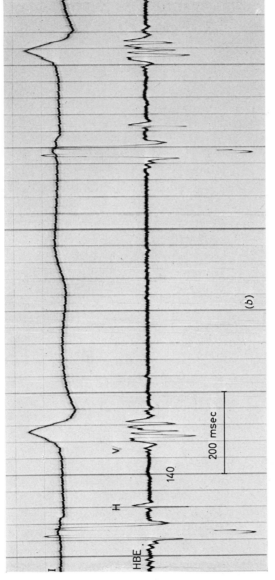

Figure 14.4—(b) First-degree heart block. P–R, 0·24 sec. Left bundle branch block A–H, 80 msec; H–V, 140 msec. Delay therefore entirely within right bundle branch

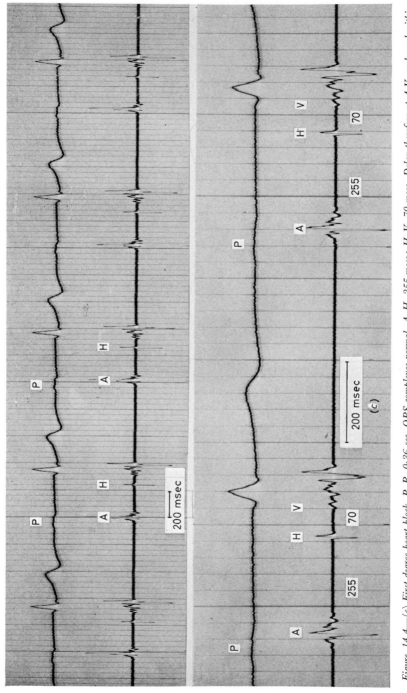

Figure 14.4—(c) First-degree heart block. P–R, 0·36 sec. QRS complexes normal. A–H, 255 msec; H–V, 70 msec. Delay therefore at A.V. node and within ventricle

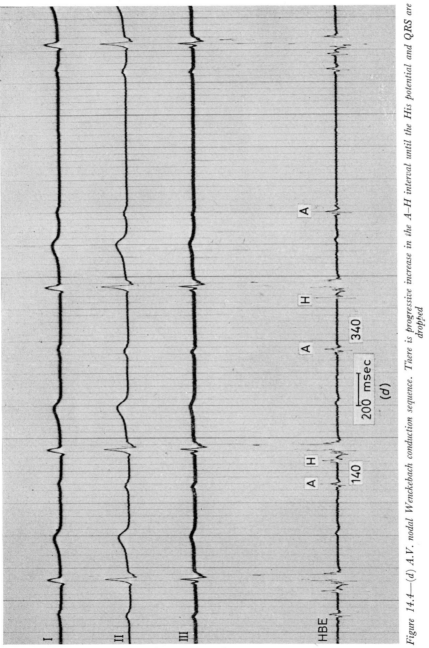

Figure 14.4—(d) A.V. nodal Wenckebach conduction sequence. There is progressive increase in the A–H interval until the His potential and QRS are dropped

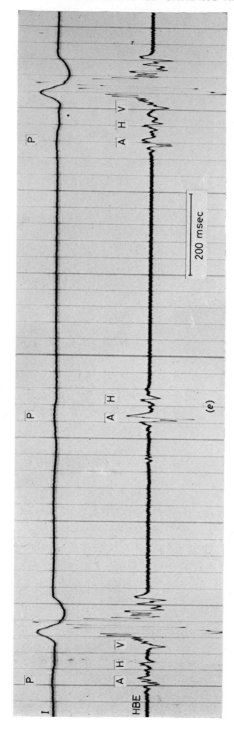

Figure 14.4—(e) Type II second-degree heart block. 2:1 A.V. ratio with conducted complexes exhibiting RBBB and normal P–R interval. HBE clearly reveals the block is below the level of the bundle of His

block, as the atrial rate accelerates. These higher A.V. ratios are commonly seen when partial heart block is associated with ectopic atrial tachycardias. *Figure 7.11* shows an example of atrial flutter with a 4:1 A.V. ratio in an undigitalized patient.

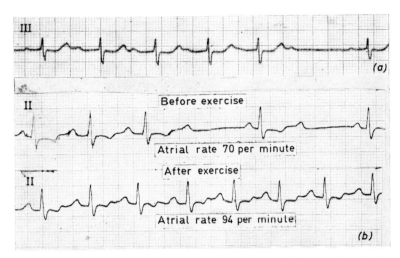

Figure 14.5—(a) This shows a typical Wenckebach period in a girl aged 16 years with active rheumatic carditis. (b) This was recorded from a patient with aortic valve disease. The upper row at rest shows an atrial rate of 70 per minute and a typical Wenckebach period with a 4:3 A.V. conduction ratio, followed by 2:1 heart block. The lower strip was recorded after light exercise, the atrial rate is now 94 per minute and conduction is virtually normal

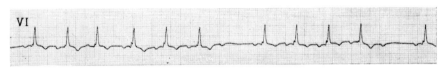

Figure 14.6—This shows periodic dropped beats without preliminary lengthening of the P–R interval. This is due to Type II block. The first part of the record shows 7:6 A.V. conduction and the second part 5:4

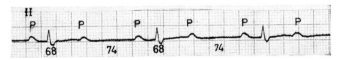

Figure 14.7—Second-degree A.V. block with a 2:1 A.V. ratio. The record illustrates ventriculo-phasic sinus arrhythmia

'Skipped' P waves

When in partial heart block, the P–R interval is so long that it exceeds the P–P cycle length, a non-conducted P wave may precede a (conducted) QRS complex. This is most often seen with fast atrial rates; *Figure 14.8* shows an example. The non-conducted P wave preceding a QRS is referred to as a 'skipped' P wave.

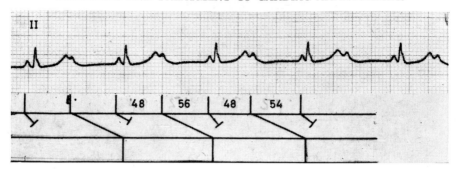

Figure 14.8—2:1 A.V. block with ventriculo-phasic sinus arrhythmia resulting in 'skipped' P waves. The P–R interval of the conducted beats exceeds the P–P cycle which enclosed a QRS complex

Third-degree Atrioventricular Block

In complete A.V. block, the ventricles are controlled by a subsidiary pacemaker and beat independently of the atria. Complete antegrade A.V. block must be differentiated from A.V. dissociation due to other causes (*see* Chapter 10). In most cases the distinction is readily made, for in A.V. block the atria beat faster than the ventricles, whereas in A.V. dissociation, without antegrade block, the ventricular rate is faster than the atrial. Occasional exceptions to this general rule were referred to in Chapter 10. In complete block, the contour and duration of the QRS complex depends on whether the ventricular pacemaker is situated above or below the division of the main bundle of His. If the new ventricular pacemaker is above the division, the QRS complex will be unaltered. If it is below the division, the QRS complex will have a bundle branch block pattern, for the excitation wave will have to spread to the other ventricle by the slow intramyocardial route.

The site of the new ventricular pacemaker is primarily determined by the site of the block. If this is in the upper part of the A.V. node, or even in the first part of the common bundle, the new pacemaker is likely to lie above the division of the common bundle. In many instances, however, the lesion involves either the bundle just above its division, or both bundle branches may be blocked; the site of the new pacemaker will then be in one or other ventricle. In most cases it is the left bundle, for when the QRS complex is widened it usually shows the pattern of right bundle branch block.

In complete heart block, the new ventricular pacemaker is often referred to as 'idioventricular'. There is, however, no consistency about this, for some writers reserve the term 'idioventricular pacemaker' for those situated below the division of the bundle of His. Strictly speaking, part of the common bundle is a ventricular structure, but it is convenient to restrict the term idioventricular pacemaker to cases of complete block with a widened QRS complex due to a new pacemaker below the division of the bundle. These pacemakers often have very slow rates and tend to be unstable, with more, or less, frequent spells of ventricular standstill.

Complete heart block can be recognized from the cardiogram at a glance when the ventricular rhythm is regular and slow, and the more frequent

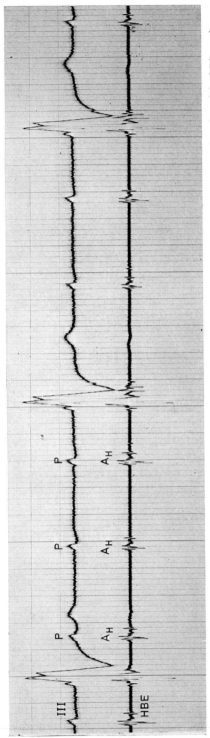

Figure 14.9—Complete heart block at intraventricular level. Atrial depolarization is constantly followed by a His deflection and both are independent of the QRS complexes

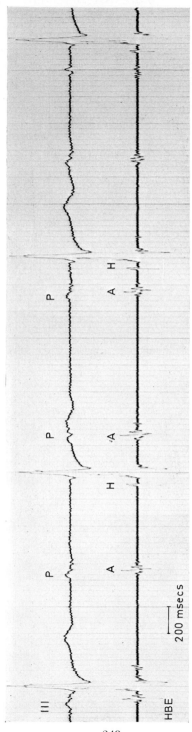

Figure 14.10—Complete heart block at A.V. nodal level. Each QRS is preceded by a His deflection indicating that the ventricles are controlled by a junctional focus below the A.V. node

P waves continually alter their time relationship to the QRS complexes. If the QRS complexes are normal in duration, it may be safely assumed that the ventricular pacemaker is situated above the bifurcation of the bundle of His. Such pacemakers are generally more stable and tend to have rather faster rates than idioventricular pacemakers situated below the division of the bundle.

In complete A.V. block with a ventricular rate of 40 or more per minute, the QRS complex is generally normal in duration and the rhythm is virtually regular. When the QRS complex is widened, it usually has the pattern of right bundle branch block and the rate is frequently less than 40 per minute. If the pacemaker is idioventricular, that is below the division of the main bundle, the right bundle branch block pattern indicates that it is situated in the left main bundle. This pattern is seen in about 70 per cent of cases of complete A.V. block.

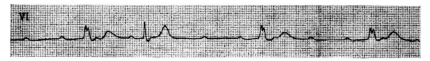

Figure 14.11—Third-degree A.V. block. The three main QRS complexes have the pattern of right bundle branch block, but the second complex is much more normal in configuration and appears to have been conducted. This might possibly have been due to a supernormal phase of recovery although its P wave is lying at some distance beyond the preceding T wave

Confirmation of the site of complete heart block is now possible. If a His potential follows each P wave and both are independent of the QRS complexes (*Figure 14.9*) the level of block is clearly distal to the bundle of His and within the bundle branches. If each QRS complex is constantly preceded by a His deflection (*Figure 14.10*), then the supraventricular impulse must have been interrupted at A.V. nodal level. This may be the only way to localize the site of block in some patients; for example, in those who demonstrate a bundle branch block whilst in sinus rhythm and who later develop third-degree A.V. nodal block, since the QRS widening will persist.

In many cases of complete A.V. block the ventricular pacemaker is regular, and successive QRS complexes are identical both in contour and timing. Occasionally, the ventricular rhythm is regular, but variations in QRS contour occur. This is presumably owing to variations in the path of the excitation wave in the ventricles, resulting from inequality in recovery in different parts of the conduction system. More often, variations in QRS contour are associated with irregularities in the ventricular rate. An irregular ventricular rhythm in complete heart block may pose a difficult electrocardiographic problem to solve. There are four main causes.

(1) The occurrence of occasional conducted beats may result in premature QRS complexes. On rare occasions, this is owing to the supernormal phase of conduction. *Figure 14.11* shows a possible example. Conduction during a supernormal phase is suggested when premature QRS complexes always follow P waves at the same interval, and the P waves fall in the same position on the T wave of the preceding QRS complex.

(2) Irregularity of the ventricular rhythm may be due to the occurrence of ventricular extrasystoles. These are recognized by their fixed coupling

time to the preceding QRS complex. Ventricular extrasystoles in complete A.V. block have been discussed in Chapter 6. *Figure 14.12* shows an example.

(3) It is not uncommon for 2 or even more idioventricular pacemakers to 'compete' for control of the ventricles. The cycle lengths of the 2 pacemakers

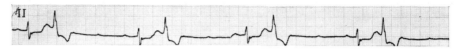

Figure 14.12—There is complete A.V. block and a ventricular extrasystole follows each beat of the dominant rhythm with a fixed coupling time

are usually different and a change from one to the other may result in a premature beat of different contour, followed by a run of new ventricular rhythm at a different rate. Sometimes measurements suggest that the new

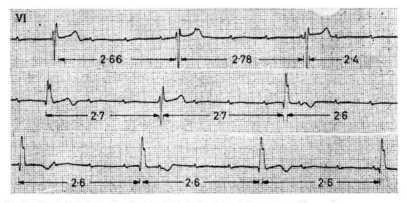

Figure 14.13—The three rows are continuous. There is complete A.V. block and the ventricles are controlled by two different idioventricular pacemakers. The overall ventricular rate is slow, averaging 26 per minute. Both pacemakers appear to be relatively unstable

pacemaker is an 'escape' rhythm taking over control when the other pacemaker has slowed or temporarily failed (*Figure 14.13*).

(4) A common cause of an irregular ventricular rhythm in complete heart block is an unstable idioventricular pacemaker. This is often seen with slow pacemakers which may transiently stop, resulting in asystole and a Stokes–Adams attack (*Figure 14.14*).

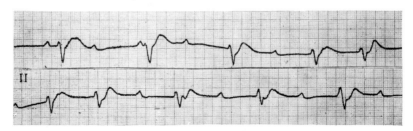

Figure 14.14—The two rows are continuous. There is complete A.V. block and the ventricular pacemaker is irregular with cycle lengths varying between 1·0 and 1·8 seconds

Atrial Fibrillation in Complete Atrioventricular Block

Atrial fibrillation may occasionally precede complete A.V. block. The occurrence of the latter may be recognized from a regular *slow* ventricular rate. This may be a manifestation of digitalis intoxication. It should be differentiated from A.V. dissociation with junctional tachycardia which is a more common effect of digitalis intoxication in atrial fibrillation (Chapter 15, page 275). Perhaps, more often, atrial fibrillation develops late in the course of complete A.V. block. Its occurrence then has little significance, except perhaps as a manifestation of advancing myocardial disease.

Retrograde Conduction with Atrial Capture in Complete A.V. Block

A rare occurrence in complete A.V. block is retrograde conduction of the ventricular impulse to the atria, with atrial capture. *Figure 14.15* shows an example. Such an event is of theoretical interest, since its occurrence clearly demonstrates that the block cannot be due to a complete anatomical severance of the conducting pathway.

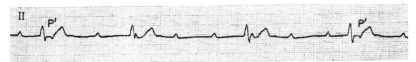

Figure 14.15—There is complete A.V. block with a ventricular rate of approximately 26 per minute. The first and last QRS complexes of the strip have a retrograde P wave at precisely the same point in their ST segments. The atrial cycle length is fairly constantly 0·8 second but is considerably prolonged following retrograde activation of the atria

Hemi-blocks

In Chapter 1 (page 5) the modern views on the anatomy of the intra-ventricular conduction system were reviewed. These new concepts were due in the main to the work of Rosenbaum and his colleagues in Buenos Aires. The same authors also described the appearances of isolated block of the anterior or posterior divisions of the left main bundle and they termed these 'left anterior hemi-block' and 'left posterior hemi-block' respectively. Left anterior hemi-block is the commoner lesion; isolated posterior hemi-block is relatively less common since the posterior division is a more robust structure than the anterior and has a richer blood supply. Isolated block of the more slender anterior division (left anterior hemi-block) is fairly common. When this occurs the initial QRS forces are directed downwards and to the right, due to normal conduction down the posterior fasicle. These are followed by the main QRS forces which are directed upwards and to the left. This results in a net QRS axis of −45° or even more leftward but without significant QRS widening. Left anterior hemi-block is now recognized as the commonest cause of left axis deviation in the electrocardiogram. In patients over the age of 40 years the most frequent cause of left anterior hemi-block is anterior myocardial infarction. *Figure 14.16* shows an example of the limb leads in left anterior hemi-block.

Some patients presenting with typical angina but without infarction show left anterior hemi-block in their electrocardiogram and this may be an indication of disease of the left anterior descending coronary artery which provides this conducting fasicle with blood. In younger patients the more common causes are aortic valve disease and the cardiomyopathies. Left anterior hemi-block is also recognized as occurring in some types of congenital heart disease, particularly the endocardial cushion defects. There is some evidence that this is due to relative hypoplasia of the anterior division of the left bundle branch (Feldt, DuShane and Titus, 1970). Left posterior

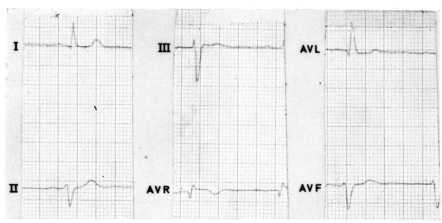

Figure 14.16—This shows the limb leads in left anterior hemi-block. There is left axis deviation with a mean frontal QRS axis of −60° and initial small Q waves in leads I and AVL

hemi-block is a very uncommon isolated lesion largely because of its robust structure and rich blood supply. This results in the main QRS forces being directed rightwards and anteriorly with an Â QRS of around +130°. This has to be distinguished from right ventricular hypertrophy and this can usually be done by the absence of evidence for this in the praecordial leads. *Figure 14.17* shows an example of isolated posterior hemi-block.

Right Bundle Branch Block Associated with Hemi-block of the Left Bundle

When anterior or posterior hemi-block is associated with right bundle branch block this provides very strong evidence for the presence of bilateral bundle branch block. The presence of either of these patterns in a patient with a history of syncopal attacks immediately indicates that these are Stokes–Adams attacks due to the transient onset of complete heart block with ventricular standstill.

Figure 14.18 shows an example of right bundle branch block with left anterior hemi-block from a patient who was having Stokes–Adams attacks. *Figure 14.19* shows right bundle branch block with left posterior hemi-block from a patient who was also having Stokes–Adams attacks. *Figure 14.20* shows right bundle branch block with 2:1 left anterior hemi-block, the alternate QRS complexes demonstrating left axis deviation.

Probably the commonest form of acute bilateral bundle branch block is anterior myocardial infarction with involvement of the septum and both bundle branches. In patients who survive the acute episode the complete heart block usually returns to sinus rhythm. Chronic bilateral bundle branch block is divisible histologically into two distinct groups. In one group there is bilateral bundle branch fibrosis of uncertain causation and Rosenbaum and

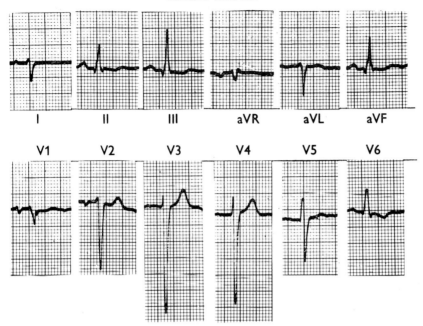

Figure 14.17—This illustrates left posterior hemi-block. (Reproduced by courtesy of Dr. D. A. Chamberlain)

his colleagues have termed this 'Lenegre's disease' since it was first fully described by Lenegre in 1964. There is a further group of elderly patients, usually over the age of 70 years, with right bundle branch block and left anterior hemi-block but with no other evidence of organic heart disease

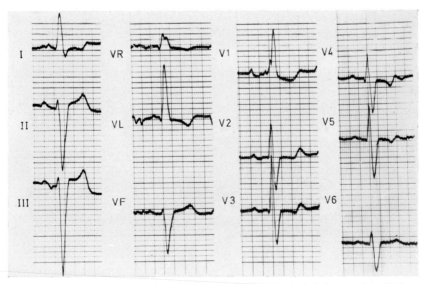

Figure 14.18—There is right bundle branch block with marked left axis deviation, that is −75 degrees. (Time markings 1/10 second.)

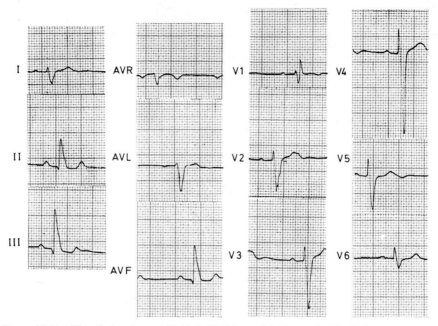

Figure 14.19—There is first-degree A.V. block (P–R interval 0·24 second). The QRS complexes show right bundle branch block with right axis deviation of the terminal portion of the QRS complex. In the absence of right ventricular hypertrophy this suggests block of the inferior division of the left main bundle. The record could be interpreted as right bundle branch block with block of the inferior division of the left main bundle and first-degree block of the superior division of the left main bundle. For further discussion, see text

who, unlike patients with Lenegre's disease, rarely develop complete A.V. block. The cause in this group is sclerosis of structures adjacent to the conduction system and since this was first described by Lev (1964) Rosenbaum and his colleagues have termed this group 'Lev's disease'. Precise differentiation between these two eponymous syndromes must clinically be largely retrospective.

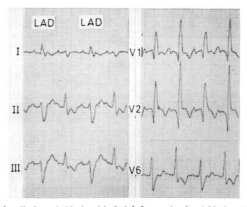

Figure 14.20—Right bundle branch block with 2:1 left anterior hemi-block. Alternate QRS complexes demonstrate left axis deviation (LAD)

In Rosenbaum and his colleagues' (1968) experience, about 5–10 per cent of patients with right bundle branch block and left anterior hemi-block eventually develop complete heart block, whereas the combination of right bundle branch block and left posterior hemi-block constitutes the QRS pattern most consistently heralding the development of complete heart block.

Treatment

A great advance in the treatment of A.V. block has been the development of electrical pacemakers for the treatment of third-degree block. Electrical pacing has enabled many patients who were completely disabled either by heart failure, or repeated Stokes–Adams attacks, to return to leading normal lives.

First-degree Heart Block

Since first-degree heart block is symptomless, no treatment is necessary unless it is drug induced, when withdrawal of the causal agent or a reduction in dosage is indicated.

Second-degree Heart Block

Partial heart block with Wenckebach periods is usually a benign condition with a good prognosis. It rarely requires treatment but can, if necessary, be abolished with atropine. More advanced partial block or paroxysmal complete block present difficult therapeutic problems. If the patient is having frequent Stokes–Adams attacks which are not controlled by drug therapy, he then requires electrical pacing using either a demand pacemaker or a ventricular triggered pacemaker. The most commonly used drugs today, in the treatment of A.V. block, are sympathomimetic amines. In the past, ephedrine was employed orally, and later isoprenaline was administered sublingually. More recently, a long-acting isoprenaline preparation, Saventrine (Pharmax) has become the preparation of choice. It is made up in 30 mg tablets and is given orally. The main action of sympathomimetic amines is to increase the heart rate; to a much lesser extent they may improve conduction. In Type I partial heart block, acceleration of the atrial rate may reduce the degree of block. In paroxysmal heart block (course A), Saventrine may be prescribed, but it is doubtful if attacks are significantly reduced in number. In Type II partial heart block, sympathomimetic amines may be harmful by accelerating the atrial rate and increasing the degree of block. Slowing the atrial rate by propranolol is occasionally useful to diminish the increased rate in response to exercise, thus preventing it from reaching the critical level at which an increase in block occurs. When used for this purpose, it is better, if possible, to avoid giving digitalis, since it tends to impair conduction. A dose of 40 mg of propranolol, three times daily, is well worth trying and may sometimes appreciably increase effort tolerance. On the other hand, occasionally an adverse effect on A.V. conduction is dominant so that the degree of A.V. block is increased at a slower atrial rate.

Complete Heart Block

Complete A.V. block may present as a dire emergency in acute myocardial infarction or in a patient having repeated prolonged Stokes–Adams attacks. It may also first present in elderly patients as a cause of congestive heart failure. Whatever the presentation, the physician is faced with the choice between drug therapy and electrical pacing. As a general rule, drug therapy should be tried first.

Pharmacological Agents

Numerous drugs have been used in the treatment of complete heart block; they include vagolytic agents (for example, atropine), sympathomimetic drugs, such as adrenaline, ephedrine and isoprenaline, alkalinizing agents (molar sodium lactate) and steroids.

The mode of action of atropine is not entirely clear, but when given intravenously, as an emergency measure, it sometimes appears to stop frequently recurring paroxysmal heart block and it may restore normal conduction in the heart block of myocardial infarction. The primary action of sympathomimetic amines is to accelerate the rate of discharge of the ventricular pacemaker, and this may terminate frequent Stokes–Adams attacks, whether they be due to asystole or fast ventricular arrhythmias. The latter action appears paradoxical, since ventricular ectopic beats and rhythms are so often the result of catecholamine action. The abolition of ventricular ectopics, however, is clearly related to an increase in heart rate and is presumably the result of increased coronary flow and reduction in ischaemia. This beneficial effect is not invariable, however, for sympathomimetic amines may only serve to precipitate or aggravate ventricular ectopic beats and may have to be discontinued.

Molar or half molar sodium lactate solution was found by Bellet, Wasserman and Brody (1955) to be of value in the treatment of frequent Stokes–Adams attacks. They reported acceleration of the ventricular rate with narrowing of the QRS complexes. In one case of complete A.V. block, with a ventricular rate of only 15 per minute and a state of shock, the intravenous infusion of molar sodium lactate increased the heart rate to 60 per minute, narrowed the wide ventricular complexes and raised the blood pressure to 120–140 mmHg systolic. Other workers have been less enthusiastic and, at present, isoprenaline is the most frequently used drug for accelerating the ventricular rate.

Steroids were first recommended for the treatment of heart block by Lown and colleagues (1955) on the basis of the following observations. In a group of 50 patients with Addison's disease, the mean P–R interval was 0·18 second, and 20 per cent exhibited heart block during some phase of their disease. In a group of 34 patients with Cushing's syndrome, on the other hand, the mean P–R interval was 0·14 second. A short P–R interval in this condition appeared to correlate with the urinary excretion of 17-ketosteroids. Administration of cortisone in Addison's disease shortens the P–R interval, whereas correction of Cushing's syndrome lengthens it. Finally, when cortisone is given to subjects with an endocrine disorder, the P–R interval is shortened. It was, therefore, suggested that adrenal steroids facilitated A.V. conduction. In practice, their use has proved disappointing.

Intravenous hydrocortisone is still employed in the treatment of complete heart block complicating acute myocardial infarction, mainly in the hope of reducing the inflammatory reaction believed to be involving the conduction tract (*see* Chapter 16).

Other drugs which have been used in the treatment of heart block include barium chloride and drugs with a quinidine-like action. Barium chloride was employed because it was found experimentally to increase cardiac excitability. It has proved valueless in practice.

Quinidine and procainamide have been tried in patients whose Stokes–Adams attacks were known to be due to ventricular tachycardia or fibrillation. It seems clear that in this situation they are not only valueless but dangerous and may, in fact, precipitate ventricular arrhythmia.

In the medical management of complete heart block, the choice of drugs and their route of administration is determined by the clinical presentation. The treatment in acute myocardial infarction will be discussed in Chapter 16. Other forms of complete heart block may present either as emergencies due to frequent Stokes–Adams seizures or as non-urgent cases, and a clear-cut programme of medical treatment should be followed in each case.

Treatment of the Urgent Case

The urgent case is the patient having frequent Stokes–Adams attacks or one who is semi-conscious with a heart rate of 25 per minute or less.

It is of the greatest value in the management of these cases if the patient's electrocardiogram can be continuously monitored on a cathode-ray oscilloscope, preferably one incorporating a rate meter which will sound an audible alarm if the heart rate falls below or rises above a predetermined level. The physician can then recognize at a glance the mechanism of any attacks which occur and can readily 'titrate' his treatment against the heart rate. Where possible, these cases are best nursed in a coronary care unit where all necessary equipment is available. There are two main objectives in treatment: the immediate restoration of circulation when this is arrested and the prevention of further attacks.

Restoration of circulation—If the circulatory arrest is due to asystole, the heart can often be restarted by a sharp blow on the praecordium. If this fails, external cardiac massage should be started, with artificial respiration. With these measures the heart will usually restart within a minute, but if it fails to do so, further action must be determined by the help and equipment available. When the patient is connected to a monitor and ventricular asystole is seen to be the cause of circulatory arrest, direct intracardiac injection of adrenaline should be tried (0·2–0·5 ml of 1 in 1,000 solution). On the other hand, if the mechanism of arrest is seen to be ventricular fibrillation, external d.c. shock (not of course, synchronized) should be used. When the mechanism is known to be asystole, if intracardiac adrenaline fails, external electrical stimulation with a pacemaker may be started as a temporary measure, but it is often unsuccessful.

If no monitor is available, it is unlikely that there will be a defibrillator and, in these circumstances (that is, when the cause of the arrest is unknown), intracardiac adrenaline should be tried and, if it fails, attempts at resuscitation should be abandoned after 10–15 minutes.

Prevention of further attacks—In complete heart block, the prevention of Stokes–Adams attacks may be achieved by accelerating the ventricular rate. This is true, irrespective of whether the attacks are due to asystole or a fast ventricular arrhythmia. An increased ventricular rate can nearly always be achieved by an intravenous drip of noradrenaline or isoprenaline. Both noradrenaline and isoprenaline have similar actions in accelerating slow ventricular pacemakers. The choice between them should be determined by the patient's blood pressure. If this is low (100 mmHg systolic or less) noradrenaline should be used for its pressor effect. If the pressure is not very low, isoprenaline is chosen, for it has little effect on blood pressure. Either drug should be given in a dilution of 4 mg per litre and the drip rate should initially be 15–30 drops a minute, corresponding to 4–8 μg of the drug. The speed of the drip should be increased every four minutes until a ventricular rate of about 60 per minute is achieved. If the drip speed necessary to achieve this appears excessive, more of the drug should be added to the vacolitre and the rate of infusion correspondingly slowed. It is of very great value in these cases to have an automatic drip counter as described in the section on coronary care (page 298). This method of accelerating the heart rate was originally described by Zoll and colleagues (1958) and they later showed it was effective in the prevention of Stokes–Adams attacks due to ventricular fibrillation (Zoll and colleagues, 1963). In cases whose attacks are due to recurrent ventricular fibrillation, ventricular ectopic activity tends to disappear abruptly when a critical ventricular rate is reached. Before this happens, the incidence of ventricular ectopic activity may temporarily increase, but with perseverance a rate will be achieved when ectopic activity will disappear. Admittedly, when doing this, it is reassuring to have a d.c. defibrillator at hand, should ventricular fibrillation supervene. Fortunately this rarely occurs with this technique; if it should, of course, the infusion should be stopped before defibrillation is carried out. It is impossible to lay down any hard and fast rule about how long the drip should be continued. If sinus rhythm returns, the drip may be stopped, though relapse into block would necessitate restarting. When complete block persists, attempts should be made to wean the patient on to oral Saventrine after 48 hours.

Treatment of the Non-urgent Case

Complete A.V. block is occasionally an accidental finding in an otherwise asymptomatic patient. This is particularly true of congenital block and such cases rarely require treatment. Patients presenting with complete A.V. block and non-urgent symptoms, such as dyspnoea on exertion, with or without attacks of dizziness, or evidence of congestive heart failure, should first be tried on medical treatment. The preparation of choice today is Saventrine. It is made up in tablet form, each tablet containing 30 mg. The tablets should be swallowed whole. Before starting oral therapy in these cases, it is probably wise first to admit the patient for assessment of his tolerance to isoprenaline. The drug should first be administered intravenously, simultaneously monitoring the electrocardiogram. If a ventricular rate of 60–70 per minute can be achieved without provoking ventricular ectopic rhythms, the drug can safely be given by mouth. If ventricular ectopic rhythms develop, although they may be overcome by increasing the drip speed, it would be unwise to give the drug by mouth, since there is no way of controlling the blood level. One of Harris and colleagues' (1966) patients developed a ventricular tachycardia and lost consciousness during a trial of oral isoprenaline.

If the response to the intravenous trial is satisfactory, long acting iso-prenaline may be started by mouth. The initial dose is 60 mg (2 tablets) 8-hourly, and dosage is increased both in amount and frequency until a satisfactory heart rate is achieved. The maximal dose is 720 mg daily, divided in 2-hourly dosage. Side effects are common, and even patients without extrasystoles may complain of disagreeable palpitation. Nausea is frequent and some patients are intolerant of an adequate dose. However, approximately 40–48 per cent of cases of complete A.V. block can be managed successfully on Saventrine.

Electrical Pacing

Although the development of electrical pacing for complete A.V. block represents a dramatic advance in the management of these patients, there are still a number of disadvantages which are not yet overcome. One important difficulty is that approximately 25 per cent of patients who are electrically paced revert to sinus rhythm. When this happens, the pacemaker impulses become a 'built-in' parasystole. Sowton (1965) reported that when this occurred, the risk of sudden death was greatly increased. Compared with other artificially paced patients who did not revert to normal conduction, the death rate was 53 per cent as opposed to 10·3 per cent. Sowton pointed out that the presence of parasystole could result in the pacemaker impulse falling during the vulnerable period of the cardiac cycle (that is, on the ascending limb of the T wave of a conducted beat), thus exposing them to the danger of pacemaker induced ventricular fibrillation. He calculated that this risk might occur about twice a minute, or 3,000 times a day.

Methods of artificial pacemaking—It is not proposed here to discuss in any detail the electronics of pacemaking, or the surgical techniques involved. However, a brief summary of the general principles is important. Electrical pacemaking was first achieved by placing electrodes outside the chest. Since excitable tissue is stimulated by the negative electrode (cathode) when the circuit is first completed, the negative electrode is placed on the chest at the site of maximal pulsation. The positive or 'indifferent' electrode may be placed almost anywhere else on the chest at a distance. Although this method is often successful in stimulating the heart, a large voltage, approxi-mately 120 volts, is required. In the conscious patient, this produces painful contraction of surrounding muscles and may cause skin burns. It is only applicable for brief periods to restart a heart which has gone into asystole.

Implantable electrodes—In this technique silver electrodes are sutured to the epicardial surface of the heart at thoracotomy and the leads are either brought out through the skin to an external portable pacemaker, or small transistorized pacemakers are implanted in the abdominal wall or axilla. The pacemaker is equipped with a mercury battery which should have a life of 2–3 years.

An alternative technique devised in Birmingham by Abrams, Hudson and Lightwood (1960) is known as the inductive method. The wires from the implanted electrodes are connected to a circular coil which is placed subcutaneously. An external pacemaker is then connected to a second coil which is placed on the skin over the coil connected to the implanted electrodes. Each pacemaker impulse then flows through the external coil and 'induces' a current in the buried coil.

The use of epicardial electrodes has many disadvantages; in the first place, their insertion requires a thoracotomy, which is a formidable experience for elderly patients. Inflammatory reaction develops round the electrodes so that the voltage necessary for stimulation may increase; 3 volts may be adequate initially but this may rise to 8 or 12 volts later.

Endocardial pacing—A considerable advance has been made by the introduction of the electrode catheter. This is introduced via a peripheral vein and the tip (with its electrode) is wedged at the apex of the right ventricle. At first this technique was introduced as an emergency measure, but it has been found safe to use an electrode catheter in the right ventricle for permanent pacing. The catheter may be introduced via the subclavian or external jugular vein. An indifferent (positive) electrode is left in any convenient subcutaneous position. Wires from each electrode may be connected to an external pacemaker unit, to an implanted unit in the axilla or to a coil, as in the Birmingham technique. The endocardial catheter has two main advantages: its insertion does not require a thoracotomy, and resistance does not seem to develop at its tip as it does with implanted epicardial electrodes.

Long-term endocardial pacing is remarkably free from complications. Occasionally the tip may perforate the right ventricle, but little harm results. The gloomy forecasts of thrombotic complications have not materialized in practice. Recent advances in the design of electrode catheters seem to have overcome the difficulties of fracture occurring.

Careful haemodynamic studies have shown that when patients in complete heart block with slow ventricular rates are electrically paced, the cardiac output increases, usually reaching a maximum at a rate of about 70 per minute. Not only are Stokes–Adams attacks abolished, but dyspnoea and congestive heart failure are relieved and patients may return to normal social activities. Increase in the rate above 70 per minute does not lead to a further increase in cardiac output, which may actually fall. The ideal pacing rate is probably that which achieves the maximum resting output and this may be judged fairly accurately from the atrial rate. As the rate is increased, the atrial cycle length increases, but shortens again when the ideal rate is passed. Although the ventricular rate is necessarily fixed, some increase in cardiac output on exercise is possible from an increase in stroke volume.

The main disadvantage of electrical pacing at a fixed rate is that if the patient returns to sinus rhythm the artificial pacemaker and the patient's own pacemaker will be in competition with all the dangers of parasystole.

Non-competitive Pacemakers

This difficulty has been overcome by modern pacemakers using sophisticated electronic techniques. It is arranged that the stimulating electrode in the ventricle also senses spontaneous electrical activity. In the demand pacemaker system, spontaneous ventricular activity inhibits the pacemaker which only stimulates the ventricle if a pause in spontaneous ventricular activity occurs. It therefore acts as an artificial escape rhythm. A second variety of non-competitive pacemaker is termed 'ventricular triggered' or 'ventricular synchronized'. In this model it is arranged that every spontaneous R wave of ventricular activity activates the pacemaker but its stimulus falls in the absolute refractory period of the ventricle. If, however, spontaneous activity falls below a predetermined rate of 70 per minute, the pacemaker automatically discharges at a rate of 70 per minute until spontaneous activity at this rate is resumed. These systems, of course, cannot be used with the Birmingham inductive technique.

Another modern electronic technique is to use the P wave of the patient's electrocardiogram to activate the pacemaker after an appropriate delay corresponding to the P–R interval. This technique has the advantage that it results in a fixed P–R relationship and a variation in ventricular rate correlates with variations in atrial rate.

More recently Chamberlain and Leinbach (1970) have described the use of a double electrode system which produces sequential pacing of the atria and ventricles. They claim that as the result of the restoration of the normal time relationship between atrial and ventricular contraction the cardiac output was significantly increased and the blood pressure was raised in patients with complete heart block following acute myocardial infarction.

SINO-ATRIAL BLOCK

Sino-atrial block, although occurring far less often than A.V. block, is a very real entity of considerable interest. It must be distinguished from S.A. inhibition, or arrest, in which the rate of formation of sinus impulses in the node either slows or temporarily stops. The distinction is not always possible and the two mechanisms may co-exist in the same patient.

As far as is known, there are no special conducting fibres between the sites of impulse formation in the sinus node and the surrounding atrial muscle, yet it is clearly established that a normal sinus impulse may fail to reach and excite the atrial musculature, or may do so after an abnormal delay. The evidence for this is necessarily indirect, since the electrocardiogram only records the excitation wave spreading over the atria; it cannot record either impulse formation in the node or conduction time between the node and the atria. Delay or failure of S.A. conduction can only be deduced from the time relationship of successive P waves.

There is clearly no method of recognizing first-degree S.A. block from the cardiogram, nor can third-degree S.A. block be distinguished from sinus arrest. However, partial S.A. block can be recognized in the cardiogram and occurs in 3 forms.

(1) When a slow heart rate *abruptly* doubles on exercise, or even on change of posture 2:1 S.A. block can be confidently diagnosed. Sometimes this may happen spontaneously.

(2) Less advanced partial S.A. block may be recognized when the atrial cycle lengths show the typical structure of Wenckebach periods as first described by Winton in 1948.

(3) Partial S.A. block also occurs in the form of occasional blocked

impulses without preliminary lengthening of the conduction time and is presumably analogous in this sense to the Mobitz Type II A.V. block.

Figure 14.21 shows an example of 2:1 S.A. block with a rate of 30 per minute, which abruptly doubles spontaneously to 60 per minute. Measured cycle lengths in S.A. block do not always conform precisely to mathematical rules, since some degree of sinus arrhythmia is usually present. In this case, the last cycle length of the slow rate is slightly shorter than the others, presumably owing to sinus irregularity.

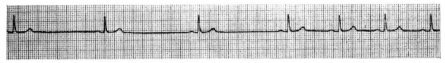

Figure 14.21—2:1 S.A. block illustrated by sudden spontaneous doubling of the heart rate from 30 to 60 per minute

Figure 14.22 shows an example of partial S.A. block with a Wenckebach type of conduction anomaly. Winton first described the criteria for recognizing Wenckebach conduction in S.A. block and they have been applied in other arrhythmias where conduction times cannot be measured on the record (that is, junctional tachycardias with block, *see* Chapter 15). The principles were fully discussed in Chapter 2 but Winton's criteria for Wenckebach conduction in S.A. block are worth re-stating.

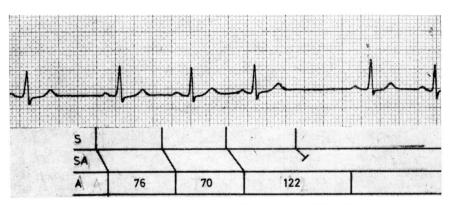

Figure 14.22—This illustrates the Wenckebach type of S.A. block

(1) The P–P interval including a blocked S.A. impulse is shorter than twice the length of the P–P interval preceding it.

(2) The P–P interval following the dropped S.A. impulse is longer than the P–P interval preceding it.

(3) There is progressive diminution of the P–P intervals (up to the pause).

It will be seen that these criteria are fulfilled by the record shown in *Figure 14.22*.

Schamroth (1966) has pointed out that Winton's first criterion is valid if there is only one blocked impulse. Sometimes more than one impulse is blocked in succession; the pause may then be considerably longer than twice the preceding cycle length. The combination, in the same record, of Wenckebach S.A. periods with more than one blocked impulse in succession and perhaps periods of regular 2 : 1 S.A. block may produce complex looking irregularities of rhythm.

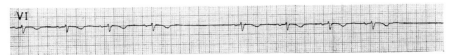

Figure 14.23—This shows 5:4 S.A. block without evidence of a Wenckebach type of conduction. This would presumably correspond to the Mobitz Type II dropped beat, illustrated in Figure 14.6

Figure 14.23 shows an example of periodic blocked sinus impulses without the Wenckebach phenomenon, that is, without preliminary increases in conduction time. There is 5 : 4 S.A. block with only slight sinus arrhythmia present.

Differential Diagnosis

The irregularities of rhythm produced by S.A. block have to be differentiated from sinus extrasystoles, sinus arrhythmia and sinus inhibition. Sinus extrasystoles are rare; they have been described on page 92. They can be recognized by the fact that the cycle following the premature beat is never compensatory but is equal to a normal sinus cycle. Sinus arrhythmia is usually recognizable by phases of progressive shortening and lengthening of successive P–P cycles. The distinction of sinus arrhythmia from S.A. block is not always immediately apparent, especially when a Wenckebach type of S.A. block is complicated by some sinus irregularity. However, the typical pattern of Wenckebach cycles can usually be recognized on measurement.

The terms 'sinus inhibition' and 'sinus arrest' should be reserved for that form of irregularity due to the slowing or cessation of impulse formation in the sinus node, in the absence of S.A. block. It is, of course, impossible to differentiate between the two mechanisms for certain with the electrocardiogram, but slowing of impulse formation and arrest is strongly suggested by progressive lengthening of P–P cycles preceding a pause. This type of irregularity is presumably a manifestation of excessive vagal action. It generally leads to escape beats or rhythms and is a common cause of the so-called 'wandering pacemaker' between the sinus and A.V. junctions.

Aetiology

Sino-atrial block may occur as a transient manifestation in active rheumatic carditis and acute myocardial infarction. It may also be a toxic effect of digitalis and less frequently of quinidine. In the absence of some obvious causal factor, it is usually a manifestation of organic disease involving the sinus node, usually ischaemic in origin. Such cases tend to run a chronic and progressive course and, for this reason, it is important to recognize them and to differentiate them from other causes of sinus irregularities.

Clinical Picture

Sino-atrial block may be entirely symptomless and discovered by chance. A sinus bradycardia which is found abruptly to double its rate on exercise may be the only finding in an asymptomatic patient.

Sick Sinus Syndrome

There is a definite group of patients who present with a history of attacks of dizziness and occasional syncope. On clinical examination there is usually marked bradycardia, often with some irregularity, and an electrocardiogram may show one of the varieties of S.A. block. Clinical differentiation from A.V. block is usually easy for there is no variation in intensity of the first heart sound and during pauses no venous waves can be seen in the neck. A characteristic feature of the attacks of dizziness and syncope is that they occur more commonly when the patient is lying down. This was noticed in a case described by Birchfield, Merefee and Bryant (1957) and attributed by them to an increase of vagal tone in the recumbent posture. Many of these patients are prone to attacks of paroxysmal tachycardia or atrial fibrillation which has led to the term tachy-bradycardia syndrome. The term 'sick sinus syndrome' was introduced by Ferrer (1967).

In 1970 Rokseth and colleagues described 14 patients with sin-oatrial block. Of these patients six were subject to attacks of supraventricular tachycardia. In four of them the supraventricular tachycardia was atrial fibrillation. In these patients atrial fibrillation was associated with a rapid ventricular rate varying from 140 to 180 per minute. It is of considerable interest that Rokseth and colleagues reported that they were able to relieve their patients of their attacks of dizziness and syncope and also of their episodes of supraventricular tachycardia by electrically pacing from the ventricle.

More recently Lloyd-Mostyn, Kidner and Oram (1973) have described 11 patients with this syndrome which they term 'sino-atrial disorder'. They class their patients, all of whom had attacks of paroxysmal tachycardia, into three categories: (1) chronic sinus bradycardia without S.A. block or junctional rhythm; (2) sinus rhythm with or without bradycardia and episodes of S.A. block, junctional rhythm or asystole; and (3) persistent junctional rhythm. In this last group reciprocal beats are frequent, episodes of asystole are also common. They felt that the most important indication for pacing was the occurrence of syncopal attacks.

Marriott (1972) prefers to call the syndrome 'double nodal disease' since he feels that both the sinus node and the A.V. node are involved.

The diagnosis of the sick sinus syndrome can usually be made from the electrocardiogram when assessed in the light of the clinical history. In those patients in whom there is some doubt as to whether their sinus bradycardia is related to their symptoms, a more objective assessment of sinus node function and sino-atrial conduction is valuable. Delayed intra-atrial conduction may not be apparent on the standard electrocardiogram and an increase in the P–A interval recorded from a His bundle electrogram may be found. In the more extreme examples, this increase alone may account for a prolongation of the P–R interval. During atrial pacing, a similar increase may be evident in the interval from the pacing stimulus to atrial depolarization. A short period of rapid atrial pacing has been found to significantly delay the sinus node recovery time in patients with this condition and constitutes a valuable diagnostic test (Narula and colleagues, 1972). The rate response to intravenous atropine also appears to be affected.

It is important to remember that a precisely similar picture may be produced by digitalis intoxication and thus must always be excluded. Moreover a similar picture may occur in the acute stage of myocardial infarction.

Treatment of Sick Sinus Syndrome

Digitalis intoxication must first be excluded. Drug therapy of the syndrome is not satisfactory: since tachycardia and bradycardia alternate, drugs suppressing either of these rhythms will tend to exacerbate the other. Each case must be judged on its merits but all cases with paroxysmal cerebral ischaemia should be paced from the ventricle. This seems to be effective in abolishing both the bradycardia and also the episodes of fast arrhythmia.

Treatment of S.A. Block

When S.A. block is due to digitalis or quinidine, the drug should be withdrawn. In acute myocardial infarction, the best treatment is probably atropine. This will be further discussed in Chapter 16. When occurring as an isolated manifestation with no symptoms, no treatment is required. In patients experiencing paroxysmal cerebral ischaemia, the correct treatment today is electrical pacing of the ventricles.

CHAPTER 15

DIGITALIS INTOXICATION

After nearly 200 years, digitalis still remains unchallenged as the most important single drug we possess for the management of many forms of heart failure. During the past few decades, improved preparations of digitalis, particularly the purified glycosides, together with a better understanding of the pharmacology of the drug, have enhanced its therapeutic efficacy. Like most potent therapeutic agents, there is a relatively narrow gap between the optimum therapeutic dose of digitalis and one which is toxic. There is now considerable evidence that the incidence of digitalis intoxication has risen considerably, largely as a result of potassium loss from the body due mainly to long continued therapeutic diuresis. Potassium depletion narrows the gap between the therapeutic and toxic dose of the drug.

FREQUENCY AND IMPORTANCE

Several recent studies have emphasized the frequency of digitalis intoxication. For example, Rodensky and Wasserman (1961), in a year's planned study of a hospital population, found an incidence of 20 per cent of patients taking digitalis who developed a toxic rhythm. Schott (1964) reviewed 2,000 consecutive electrocardiograms recorded in a group cardiographic department; 348 patients had received digitalis within a fortnight preceding an electrocardiographic recording and 42 (12 per cent) of these showed arrhythmias highly suggestive of digitalis intoxication. Of these patients, 13 died, and in 9 there was evidence that digitalis had been responsible for, or had contributed to, the fatal outcome.

I have no doubt myself that many lives are still needlessly lost through failure to recognize toxic digitalis rhythms. It is worth emphasizing that it is unusual for digitalis intoxication to be the result of a simple excess dosage of the drug; more frequently toxicity develops suddenly or insidiously on a dose of digitalis which had previously been beneficial to the patient whose tolerance to the drug has been reduced by some other factor.

PREDISPOSING FACTORS

The gap between the therapeutic and toxic dose of digitalis may be narrowed by many factors. These include variations in individual susceptibility, increasing age and advancing myocardial disease. Interference with the normal dissipation of the drug may result from renal or hepatic disease which may lead to the appearance of toxicity. The simultaneous administration of certain drugs, such as reserpine, has been shown to sensitize the heart to the toxic action of digitalis glycosides (Lown and colleagues, 1961). As already indicated, the most common cause of digitalis intoxication today is intracellular potassium depletion, not necessarily reflected in the serum level, which has followed the long continued administration of diuretics.

Goldsmith and colleagues (1969) recently claimed to have shown an increased concentration of digoxin in the myocardium of hypokalaemic dogs. Using tritiated digoxin they showed that digitalis toxicity appeared earlier in hypokalaemic compared to normkalaemic dogs and was associated with a higher concentration of digoxin in the myocardium for the same administered dose.

Variation in individual susceptibility to digitalis can occasionally be very striking, some patients requiring and tolerating large doses of the drug, whereas others in the same age group may develop intoxication on very small doses. I have occasionally seen patients who develop toxic digitalis rhythms on doses as small as 0·25 mg digoxin twice a week. Age is a very important factor in digitalis intoxication; infants and children requiring relatively much larger doses of the drug than adults, while old age brings increasing susceptibility to intoxication. The presence of renal or hepatic dysfunction should always call for care in digitalis administration. Many of the examples of digitalis intoxication illustrated in the following pages were recorded from patients with raised blood urea levels.

Recognition of Potassium Depletion

Since potassium depletion is one of the most common predisposing causes to digitalis intoxication, it is clearly desirable to be able to recognize its presence. Unfortunately the serum level is often within the normal range in severely depleted patients. It is, however, worth estimating, for if it is low (for example, below 3·9 m equiv.) this is strong evidence for potassium loss. If the serum level is normal, potassium depletion may be suspected from a history of chronic purgation or prolonged therapeutic diuresis without adequate potassium supplements. Some idea of the potassium status of the patient may be obtained by measuring the output of potassium in the urine. This should be done over 24 hours without sodium restriction or potassium supplements or diuretics being given. An excretion of 20 m equiv. per litre or less is good evidence of serious depletion.

Causes of Intracellular Potassium Depletion

Severe intracellular potassium depletion can occur without being reflected in a low serum level. There are many causes of potassium depletion, including heart failure itself, but unquestionably the most common cause today in cardiac patients is the long continued use of modern diuretics with inadequate potassium supplements. A further important source of potassium loss is chronic purgation and it is always wise to exclude this before prescribing digitalis. It is perhaps not generally appreciated that the mucus in the loose stool following an aperient has an appreciable potassium content and daily purgation can lead to severe potassium depletion. A third cause of a negative potassium balance is steroid therapy. The correction of potassium depletion will be further discussed later.

CLINICAL FEATURES

Digitalis intoxication is generally associated with non-specific constitutional disturbances. These include weakness and apathy, nausea and vomiting, and commonly the onset or worsening of heart failure. It is important to remember that nausea and vomiting may be due to heart failure and may then disappear when the patient is digitalized. On the other hand, severe intoxication may be present without nausea and vomiting occurring. A common symptom, often not mentioned spontaneously by the patient, is disturbance of vision. This may take the form of blurred vision, flashes of light before the eyes or curious colour alterations, all objects appearing to be yellow or green (xanthopsia). Such symptoms are always associated with some disturbance of cardiac rhythm. The nature of the arrhythmia usually requires an electrocardiogram before it can be identified, but bigeminal rhythm due to a ventricular extrasystole following each beat of the dominant rhythm can usually be readily recognized at the bedside as 'coupled beats'.

Electrocardiography

Digitalis normally produces changes in the electrocardiogram in the majority of subjects. Such changes include shortening of the Q–T interval, sagging depression of the S–T segments and flattening or inversion of T waves. These changes do not indicate toxicity, nor are they a measure of therapeutic effect; they are simply evidence of digitalis administration. Digitalis intoxication is manifested in the electrocardiogram by a wide variety of disorders of rhythm. It has often been said that digitalis excess may result in almost any of the known dysrhythmias. The converse is also true; practically all arrhythmias which are known to be produced by digitalis intoxication have been recorded in undigitalized patients. The diagnosis of digitalis intoxication can usually be strongly suspected from the cardiogram alone, but a knowledge of the relevant clinical data is usually required for confirmation. Final proof of the aetiological role of digitalis is the disappearance of the arrhythmia when the drug is withdrawn.

CLASSIFICATION OF TOXIC DIGITALIS RHYTHMS

It is simplest to classify digitalis intoxication on an anatomical basis according to the main site of toxic action. Although this is convenient, in practice toxic action may be evident at more than one site. A classification of toxic digitalis rhythms on an anatomical basis is as follows.

Sino-atrial inhibition or block—This is usually associated with (1) junctional escape rhythms, and less often with (2) reciprocal beats.

Atrial arrhythmias—(1) Atrial tachycardia with block, (2) atrial fibrillation and (3) atrial flutter.

Atrioventricular junctional arrhythmias—(1) A.V. block, (2) junctional tachycardias and (3) A.V. dissociation, sometimes with accrochage.

Ventricular arrhythmias—(1) Bigeminy, (2) multiform ventricular extrasystoles, (3) bi-directional ventricular extrasystoles, (4) ventricular tachycardia, sometimes bi-directional, and (5) ventricular fibrillation.

Dual tachycardias—Simultaneous, independent, atrial and ventricular ectopic tachycardias.

The next few pages give examples of most of these toxic rhythms. In the interest of brevity, clinical details of the patients from whom these records were obtained is omitted except where relevant. In the majority of these examples, evidence for the aetiological role of digitalis was obtained by the disappearance of the arrhythmia when the drug was withdrawn and, in many instances, by its recurrence when digitalis was given again. In some cases the patient died before formal proof was obtained, but the inclusion of their records seems justified by strong circumstantial evidence that digitalis had been responsible.

Sino-atrial Block

A.V. Junctional Escape Rhythms—Reciprocal Beats

A common manifestation of digitalis intoxication is S.A. inhibition or block. An A.V. junctional escape rhythm then usually occurs and, if retrograde conduction is unimpaired, an A.V. junctional pacemaker may control both the atria and the ventricles. In the presence of a junctional rhythm, reciprocal beats may occur. *Figures 15.1* and *15.2* show two examples of S.A. block due to digitalis intoxication; reciprocal beats are present in *Figure 15.2.*

Atrial Arrhythmias

Atrial Tachycardia with Block

An important and dangerous manifestation of digitalis intoxication is atrial tachycardia with block. This arrhythmia is often referred to as paroxysmal atrial tachycardia with block, a term which is commonly shortened to P.A.T. with block. This terminology, however, is quite inappropriate. Digitalis induced atrial tachycardia with block commonly lasts for several days and, in this sense, is 'sustained' rather than paroxysmal. It is, moreover, important to appreciate that it is not just a static arrhythmia which appears suddenly, but it often has a gradual evolution over a period of several days.

Digitalis induced atrial tachycardia with block usually develops in patients who were in sinus rhythm; the resulting ventricular rhythm is fast and generally irregular, owing to varying degrees of A.V. block. Clinically it can readily be mistaken for atrial fibrillation and this may tempt the physician into increasing the dose of digitalis with disastrous results.

The same arrhythmia may also develop in patients with atrial fibrillation; when the arrhythmia is suppressed by appropriate measures, atrial fibrillation usually recurs, but some patients revert to sinus rhythm.

Electrocardiography in atrial tachycardia with block—The electrocardiogram in atrial tachycardia with block is usually distinctive. The atrial rate is generally between 150 and 250 per minute. Occasionally, particularly in the early stages, it is slower, between 100 and 150 per minute, but tends to accelerate if digitalis is continued. Atrial rates faster than 250 per minute sometimes occur and the record may closely simulate flutter. The P waves are often small in size and are generally best seen in right praecordial leads. They are always different in contour from P waves of the same patient in sinus rhythm. In the past, much emphasis has been laid on the presence or absence of isoelectrical intervals between the P waves in differentiating atrial tachycardia with block from atrial flutter. Such a differentiation implies that the two arrhythmias have a different mechanism. It was, however, pointed out in Chapter 7 that in the present state of our knowledge the main difference between the individual forms of atrial tachycardias is the atrial rate; the presence or absence of isoelectric intervals between the P waves is determined by two factors: the atrial rate and the width of the P

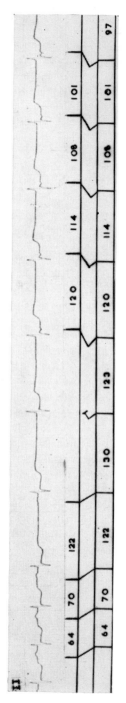

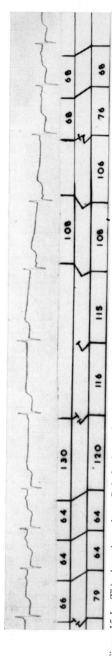

Figure 15.1.— This shows intermittent S.A slowing and arrest due to digitalis intoxication. The two rows are continuous. The first five beats of the upper row show progressive sinus slowing followed by sinus arrest. This is succeeded by a junctional escape rhythm, most of the junctional beats having a retrograde P wave in the ST segment. Sinus rhythm then transiently returns but there is again soon S.A. arrest. Normal sinus rhythm returned 24 hours after stopping digitalis

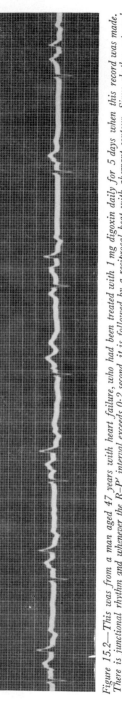

Figure 15.2.— This was from a man aged 47 years with heart failure, who had been treated with 1 mg digoxin daily for 5 days when this record was made. There is junctional rhythm and whenever the R–P' interval exceeds 0·2 second, it is followed by a reciprocal beat with aberrant contour. Sinus rhythm returned when digitalis was stopped. By courtesy of E. Fletcher

waves. When the P waves are wide, as they may be in mitral disease, they will merge together at slower rates than when they have a shorter duration. In *Figure 15.3* (from a patient with mitral stenosis) the atrial rate averages 150 per minute, but in lead II there are no isoelectric intervals between the P waves which are approximately 0·2 second in duration. It would seem a simple, if arbitrary, terminology to restrict the term 'flutter' to records with an atrial rate of 250–350 per minute, in which no isoelectric intervals are present between the P waves in at least one lead.

The atrial rhythm in atrial tachycardia with block is usually regular, but irregularity is not uncommon.

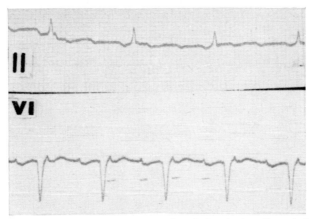

Figure 15.3—Atrial tachycardia with block due to digitalis intoxication. Sinus rhythm returned when digitalis was stopped and recurred again when digitalis was given a second time

A.V. block is a characteristic feature of digitalis induced atrial tachycardia. It is not necessarily present when the atrial rate is relatively slow but it usually appears with rates over 140 per minute. It may take the form of a Wenckebach type of conduction anomaly or there may be a simple fixed 2:1, 3:1 or 4:1 A.V. ratio.

Although atrial tachycardia with block is often due to digitalis intoxication, an identical arrhythmia may occur in undigitalized patients. In such patients, the ventricular rate can usually be easily controlled by digitalis therapy.

Figures 15.4–15.6 show four further examples of digitalis induced atrial tachycardia with block.

Atrial Fibrillation and Atrial Flutter

It is well documented that both atrial fibrillation and atrial flutter may be induced by digitalis intoxication and will then disappear when the drug is withdrawn. An example of digitalis induced atrial fibrillation is shown in *Figure 15.10* (page 276). It is probably associated with junctional tachycardia with block.

Atrioventricular Junctional Arrhythmias

Depression of conduction in the A.V. junction is a well known pharmacological effect of digitalis. In therapeutic doses, it slows the ventricular rate

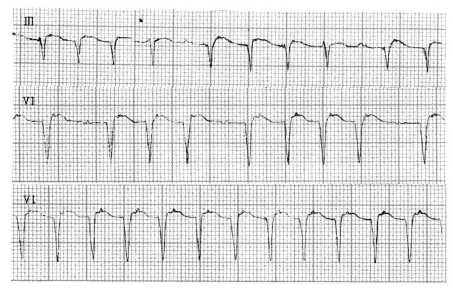

Figure 15.4—This record was obtained from a man with ischaemic heart disease who was admitted in left ventricular failure. It shows atrial tachycardia, at times with block, and at other times with 1:1 conduction. Normal sinus rhythm returned 24 hours after stopping digitalis

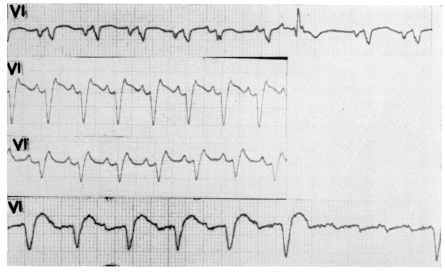

Figure 15.5—These four records were obtained from a man aged 67 years with anoxic cor pulmonale who had been treated with 0·75 mg digoxin daily. The upper record on admission shows basic sinus rhythm with occasional atrial extrasystoles. Following 2 ml mersalyl, the second electrocardiogram showed an atrial atachycardia with 2:1 block. Atrial rate 300 per minute. Digitalis was stopped and potassium was given by mouth. The third row, taken the following day, shows a slightly slower atrial rate (250 per minute); 48 hours later the bottom row was recorded. The atrial rate has slowed to 220 per minute with 2:1 A.V. block and occasional short periods of ventricular standstill. There is some QRS widening and the T waves have increased in size. The patient died suddenly, shortly after this record, presumably from potassium intoxication

in atrial fibrillation. In sinus rhythm, some lengthening of the P–R interval may occur without any other evidence of toxicity. In digitalis intoxication, more advanced degrees of A.V. block are fairly common. Complete A.V. block is unusual but has been reported following massive overdosage (McGuire and Richards, 1936). Partial A.V. block is more common and is usually associated with evidence of toxic action at some other site. *Figure 15.7*

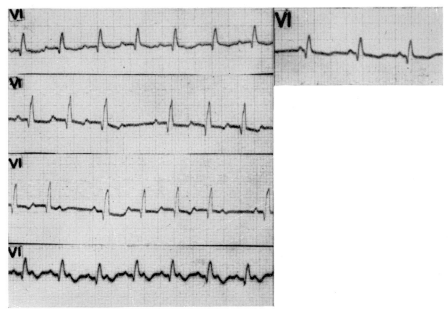

Figure 15.6—The four records on the left were taken at 2-day intervals and illustrate the evolution of digitalis induced atrial tachycardia with block. The upper record shows an atrial rate of 125 per minute, a prolonged P–R interval but no dropped beats. The P waves, however, are different in contour from those of the same patient in sinus rhythm illustrated on the right. The second row on the left shows an atrial rate of 143 per minute and a Wenckebach type of conduction anomaly. In the third row, the atrial rate has increased to 154 per minute and in the fourth row to 260 per minute with 2:1 A.V. block. Digitalis was then withdrawn and 2 days later sinus rhythm returned

shows an example of second-degree A.V. block with ventricular bigeminal rhythm due to multiform ventricular extrasystoles. After digitalis was withdrawn, the ventricular extrasystoles disappeared in three days, but partial A.V. block with Wenckebach periods persisted for several more days before normal conduction returned.

Pick, Langendorf and Katz (1961) have pointed out that in toxic doses digitalis may have a curious dual action on the A.V. junction. It both impairs conduction, particularly retrograde conduction, and at the same time often accelerates the rate of discharge of A.V. junctional pacemakers. The varied interplay of these two effects results in a wide spectrum of disorders of rhythm. When the patient is in sinus rhythm, a 'non-paroxysmal' form of junctional tachycardia with retrograde A.V. block results in A.V. dissociation, usually with capture beats. An example of this arrhythmia due to digitalis intoxication was shown in *Figure 10.2* (page 155).

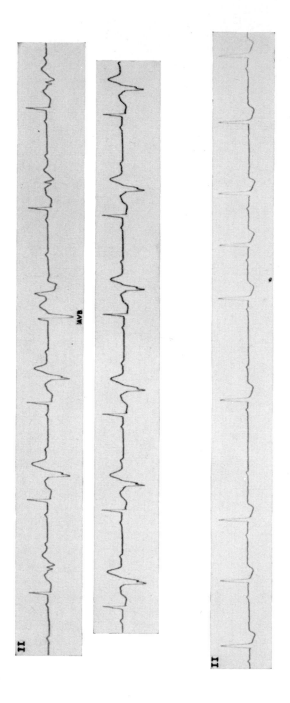

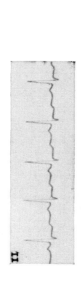

Figure 15.7—Digitalis-induced second-degree A.V. block with multiform ventricular extrasystoles (for fuller description see text)

Digitalis Intoxication in Atrial Fibrillation

In atrial fibrillation, the dual toxic action of digitalis on the A.V. junction may lead to A.V. dissociation with the ventricles controlled by an accelerated junctional pacemaker. The ventricular rhythm may then be quite regular and lead to the erroneous clinical impression that the patient has reverted to sinus rhythm. The upper record in *Figure 15.8* was from a patient with mitral valve disease who had been known to be fibrillating for years. She was admitted in heart failure with a regular ventricular rhythm of 95 per minute. Digitalis was stopped and three days later the lower record was made. The ventricular rate slowed to 82 per minute and the rhythm again became irregular. Whenever the ventricular rhythm of a digitalized patient in atrial fibrillation is found to be regular, digitalis intoxication should be suspected.

With more advanced intoxication the junctional rate may accelerate further and the ventricular rhythm may again become irregular owing to the development of block below the junctional pacemaker. An electrocardiographic diagnosis is only possible at this stage if the ventricular cycle lengths show the characteristic structure of Wenckebach periods (*see* page

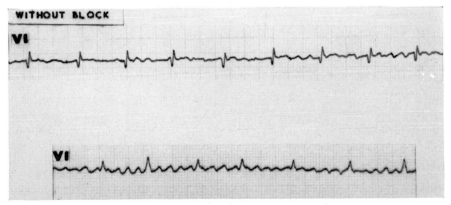

Figure 15.8—Digitalis-induced junctional tachycardia in a patient with atrial fibrillation (for further description see text)

27). *Figure 15.9* shows an example from a patient who developed a paradoxical acceleration of ventricular rate following an increase in digitalis dosage. The ventricular rate is 150 per minute. In the key below the record, a regular junctional tachycardia of 200 per minute is postulated with a Wenckebach type of conduction anomaly between the pacemaker and the ventricles. The conduction ratio varies from 3:2 to 5:4. This general pattern kept recurring consistently throughout a longish record. Digitalis was stopped and a few days later the ventricular rate had slowed to 90 per minute.

Unfortunately, in practice, it is uncommon to find this diagnostic pattern. More often, when a patient with atrial fibrillation develops a paradoxical acceleration in ventricular rate following an increase in digitalis dosage or diuretic therapy, the pattern of ventricular cycle lengths defies analysis. As Pick, Langendorf and Katz (1961) have pointed out, many complex factors, such as concealed conduction of atrial impulses or conduction during a

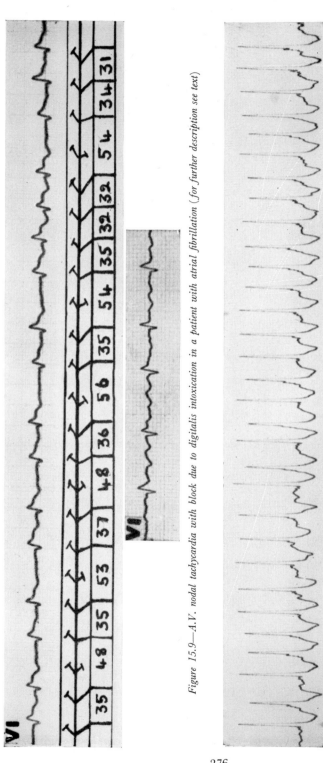

Figure 15.9—A.V. nodal tachycardia with block due to digitalis intoxication in a patient with atrial fibrillation (for further description see text)

Figure 15.10—Digitalis intoxication (for full description see text)

supernormal phase, may disturb the transmission of junctional impulses to the ventricles. The diagnosis of digitalis intoxication has then to be made on clinical grounds. *Figure 15.10* shows a characteristic example. The upper record was from a woman aged 76 years who, a year previously, had had an attack of atrial fibrillation which had spontaneously reverted to sinus rhythm. She had quite unnecessarily been maintained on digoxin 0·25 mg b.d. and an oral diuretic without potassium supplements ever since. This record was made 24 hours after she had again developed an irregular tachycardia with an apex rate of 150 per minute. Her dose of digoxin was immediately increased to 0·5 mg six hourly. After 3 doses had been given, the apex rate, instead of slowing, had risen to 200 per minute and her condition became critical. The record shows atrial fibrillation, but the ventricular cycle lengths have no recognizable pattern. A diagnosis of digitalis intoxication was made on clinical grounds; digoxin and diuretics were stopped and potassium was given by mouth. Within a few hours the heart rate began to slow progressively and 36 hours later the lower record was made showing reversion to sinus rhythm.

Whenever a digitalized patient with atrial fibrillation develops an unexpected increase in ventricular rate, the possibility of digitalis intoxication should always be considered.

Bi-directional Junctional Tachycardia

During the past 12 years, one of us has seen 10 examples of a substantially regular, bi-directional ectopic tachycardia without QRS widening. In each case, the rhythm had developed in patients who had been known to be in atrial fibrillation and there was good evidence that digitalis intoxication was responsible. All 10 records showed similar features. *Figures 15.11* and *15.12* show 2 examples. There is no evidence of atrial activity; all QRS complexes are normal in duration but alternate complexes are written in opposite directions in all leads except VR and V1. Six of these patients recovered, but 4 of them died.

Figure 15.13 shows the mean spatial direction of the vectors of the alternating QRS complexes. The outline surrounding them is a diagrammatic representation of the left ventricular muscle mass. It seems that the QRS forces are pointing alternately into the anatomical regions of distribution of the superior and inferior divisions of the left main bundle. It is therefore possible that this pattern is due to alternating block of the two divisions of the left main bundle.

Ventricular Arrhythmias

Three well recognized manifestations of digitalis intoxications are ventricular extrasystoles, ventricular tachycardia and ventricular fibrillation.

Since ventricular extrasystoles are common in heart disease (and may be suppressed by digitalis therapy), it is obviously important to be able to recognize when they are due to digitalis intoxication. There are no absolute criteria which enable this to be done but there are a number of highly suggestive indications.

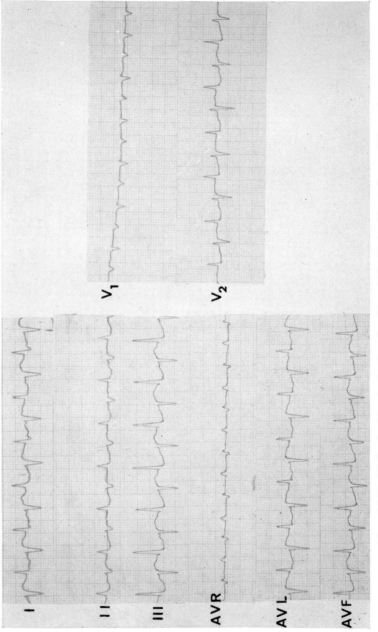

Figure 15.11—Bi-directional junctional tachycardia without QRS widening. Ventricular rate 190 per minute

Bigeminal Rhythm

Bigeminal rhythm due to an extrasystole occurring after every conducted beat is a common manifestation of digitalis intoxication. Although it may occasionally be due to heart disease and disappear when the patient is digitalized, its appearance for the first time in a digitalized patient strongly suggests intoxication. *Figure 15.14* shows a typical example in a patient with atrial fibrillation.

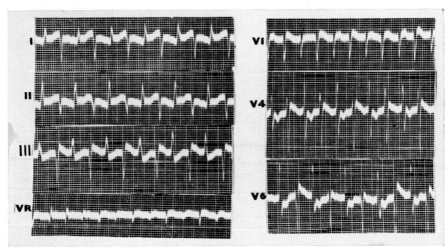

Figure 15.12—Bi-directional junctional tachycardia without QRS widening. Ventricular rate 168 per minute

Multiform Ventricular Extrasystoles

These are always strongly suggestive of digitalis intoxication. In *Figure 15.15,* the second, fourth, sixth and eighth QRS complexes are all ventricular extrasystoles. They all have different contours but each has precisely the

Figure 15.13—Spatial direction of the alternating QRS vectors (for further description see text)

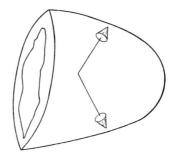

same coupling time to the preceding beat of 0·5 second. These should not be termed multifocal extrasystoles for the same coupling time strongly suggests that they all arise from the same focus, variations in contour reflecting variations in the pathway of conduction of the ectopic stimulus. A more appropriate term is multiform ventricular extrasystoles. Although

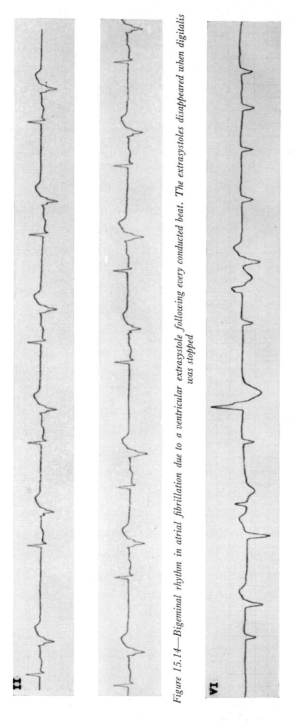

Figure 15.14—Bigeminal rhythm in atrial fibrillation due to a ventricular extrasystole following every conducted beat. The extrasystoles disappeared when digitalis was stopped

Figure 15.15—Multiform ventricular extrasystoles due to digitalis intoxication occurring in atrial fibrillation (for further discussion see text)

always very suggestive of digitalis intoxication, multiform ventricular extrasystoles occasionally occur in undigitalized patients.

Bi-directional Ventricular Extrasystoles

Bi-directional ventricular extrasystoles in which two or more successive ventricular ectopic beats are written in opposite directions, are always suggestive of digitalis toxicity. *Figure 15.16* shows atrial fibrillation with ventricular extrasystoles, often in pairs, following every conducted beat. When two consecutive extrasystoles occur, their main deflections are written in opposite directions. The extrasystoles disappeared a few days after digitalis was stopped.

Automatic ventricular beats terminating pauses, usually in atrial fibrillation, are common in digitalis intoxication. *Figure 15.17* shows an example of atrial fibrillation in which conducted beats are followed by multiform ventricular extrasystoles with a constant coupling time of 0·46 second. Two automatic ventricular beats (marked A.V.B.) occur in the strip; both are followed by ventricular extrasystoles with a slightly longer coupling time of 0·5 second. *Figure 15.17b* shows an electrocardiogram recorded one week after withdrawing digitalis. This shows atrial fibrillation with no ventricular ectopic beats.

Ventricular Tachycardia

This is a particularly dangerous complication of digitalis intoxication. There may be no specific features in the electrocardiogram to indicate the aetiological role of digitalis, but when this arrhythmia occurs in a digitalized patient, the drug should be withdrawn. Bi-directional ventricular tachycardia, in which alternate complexes are written in opposite directions, is usually due to digitalis intoxication, although it has been reported in undigitalized patients. This arrhythmia carries a high mortality. *Figure 15.18* shows a typical example from a patient who recovered when digitalis was withdrawn. No evidence of atrial activity is visible. The cycle lengths between the positive and negative deflections measure 0·44 second and between the negative and positive deflections 0·54 second. Neither QRS complex of the tachycardia resembles that of her 'normal' complexes after the tachycardia had ceased.

Ventricular Fibrillation

In the experimental animal, ventricular fibrillation can readily be produced by digitalis intoxication, and it is likely that death in clinical cases is commonly due to this cause. It has been recorded following intravenous administration of digitalis preparations, particularly in patients who had already received the drug by mouth.

Dual Tachycardias

Sometimes in digitalis intoxication, independent ectopic tachycardias may occur in both atria and ventricles simultaneously. There is usually A.V. dissociation, but capture beats or fusion beats may occur (*Figure 15.19* is reproduced by courtesy of A. Schott). The record shows both atrial and ventricular tachycardia. The atrial cycle length is about 0·64 second (rate

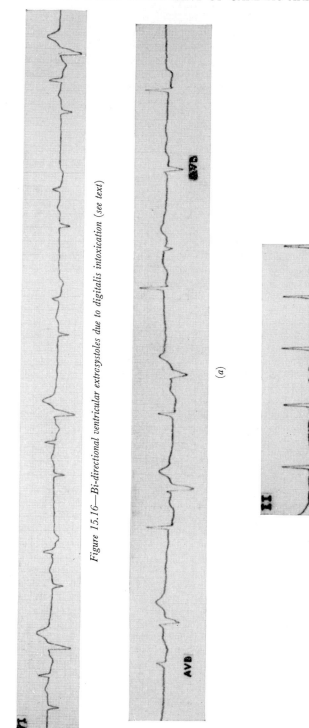

Figure 15.16—Bi-directional ventricular extrasystoles due to digitalis intoxication (see text)

(a)

(b)

Figure 15.17—Multiform ventricular extrasystoles with automatic ventricular beats due to digitalis intoxication (for further description see text)

of 94 per minute); the ventricular cycle length is 0·44 second (rate of 136 per minute). In lead V1 the ventricular complexes of every third beat have a slightly different contour and follow the preceding P wave after about 0·2 second. The appearances suggest these are fusion beats; their periodicity appears to be due to the fact that three times the ventricular cycle length closely approximates to twice the atrial cycle length.

TOXIC EFFECTS OF DIFFERENT DIGITALIS PREPARATIONS

It has already been pointed out that different digitalis preparations all have the same pharmacological effects and differ only in their rate of absorption and dissipation (*see* Chapter 13). Church and colleagues (1962) investigated the toxic effects of four different glycosides by producing deliberate intoxication. They concluded that there was no evidence that any of the oral preparations used tended to produce a pattern of intoxication different from that

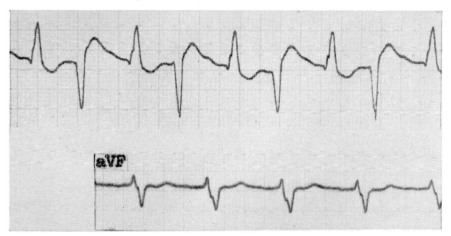

Figure 15.18—Digitalis-induced bi-directional ventricular tachycardia

of the others. When a patient was intoxicated for a second time, he was as likely to show different manifestations as he was to show the same, and this was independent of whether the same or different glycosides were used for the consecutive intoxications.

PREVENTION

Digitalis intoxication should rarely arise if adequate precautions are taken in the administration of the drug. Large doses should never be used to digitalize either elderly patients or subjects with renal disease associated with elevated blood urea levels. When it is necessary to give any diuretic more than twice a week, potassium supplements by mouth are mandatory. Several proprietary preparations of oral diuretics are available which contain incorporated potassium. This is claimed to act as a potassium supplement but in fact such preparations are valueless because the incorporated potassium is immediately lost in the diuresis. Whatever oral diuretic is used the whole dose should be given first thing on waking in the morning and

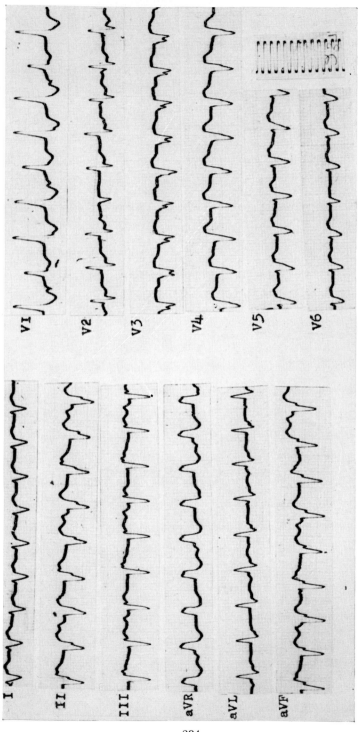

Figure 15.19—Simultaneous atrial and ventricular tachycardias due to digitalis intoxication (for further description see text). Reproduced by courtesy of Dr A. Schott

the supplementary potassium should then be taken later in the day when the diuresis is over. Potassium chloride is the most suitable preparation but in simple solution it is nauseating and poorly tolerated. Enteric coated tablets of potassium chloride are not absorbed, and uncoated tablets may produce bowel ulceration. A recent fashion for using 'effervescent' potassium tablets is undesirable because of their high bicarbonate content. The recently introduced compound 'Slow K' (Ciba) seems to provide potassium chloride in a suitable form for oral administration. Each tablet contains 600 mg of potassium chloride in a wax core designed for slow release. Two tablets, three times daily, is a suitable routine dose, but care is necessary in the presence of renal insufficiency to avoid hyperkalaemia. An occasional patient is encountered who proves intolerant of Slow K tablets, usually because of nausea. An alternative preparation of potassium chloride is Kloref made by Cox-Continental Ltd., Sussex.

TREATMENT

In the majority of cases of digitalis intoxication, the only treatment necessary is to stop the drug, withhold diuretics and, if necessary, to give potassium, usually by mouth. The necessity of withholding diuretics is perhaps not sufficiently well appreciated. In the days before oral diuretics were available, it was recognized that an injection of mersalyl could lead to digitalis intoxication. The phenomenon was termed 'Mercurial redigitalization'. At first, this was attributed to the diuresis mobilizing digitalis dissolved in oedema fluid. It was, however, shown later that potassium loss from the diuresis was the precipitating cause of digitalis toxicity (Lown and Levine, 1955). Exactly the same mechanism operates when oral diuretics are used and it is, therefore, essential to stop both digitalis and diuretics. Very frequently, as digitalis toxicity subsides, a spontaneous diuresis ensues. If the patient is not already receiving potassium, this should be given as 'Slow K', 1·2 g three or four times daily. After 2 or 3 days, if all evidence of toxicity has gone, digitalis may be re-started, but initially in half the dosage previously given. If necessary, diuretics may then be re-started. Sometimes, particularly in patients who have been on digitoxin (Nativelle's Digitaline), it may take 1–3 weeks before all evidence of intoxication has gone.

When the patient is more gravely ill with, for example, atrial tachycardia with or without A.V. block or ventricular tachycardia, termination of the toxic rhythm may be more urgent. If the blood urea is normal, the agent of choice is potassium chloride and it is quicker and safer to give this intravenously, provided there can be continuous electrocardiographic control. A solution containing 40 mEq of potassium chloride in 5 per cent dextrose is infused intravenously over a period of one hour. The drip should be stopped immediately if sinus rhythm returns or if there is any evidence of hyperkalaemia, such as 'peaking' or 'tenting' of the T waves. It may be necessary to give up to 120 mEq of potassium chloride in some cases of severe potassium depletion.

If, however, there is reason to suspect that renal function is poor and particularly if the blood urea is raised, intravenous potassium is too dangerous and diphenylhydantoin should be used instead, 250 mg being given slowly intravenously. In our opinion propranolol should not be used.

Occasionally, digitalis intoxication is due to frank overdosage in the absence of potassium depletion or other predisposing factors; this occasionally happens in attempted suicides or in children who have ingested large numbers of tablets mistaking them for sweets. Such patients usually present with nausea and vomiting and conduction disturbances in the A.V. junction. Ectopic arrhythmias are uncommon. If, however, they do occur, and we have encountered ventricular tachycardia in a child with a normal heart, the treatment of choice again is phenylhydantoin intravenously.

CHAPTER 16

ARRHYTHMIAS IN ACUTE MYOCARDIAL
INFARCTION

During the past 30 years, publications of series of acute myocardial infarction treated in hospitals have shown a virtually constant mortality rate of 30–40 per cent. The introduction and widespread employment of anticoagulant therapy does not appear to have achieved any significant reduction in this high death rate. Both in this country and in the United States of America, acute myocardial infarction is the commonest single cause of death today. The discovery that ventricular fibrillation, a common cause of sudden death in this condition, could, under favourable circumstances, be reverted to normal rhythm with resuscitation of the apparently 'dead' patient has led to a new approach in the management of these patients. The main emphasis now is on the prevention or immediate treatment of complications, particularly arrhythmias, by concentrating patients in special coronary care units where they can be continuously monitored during the dangerous phase of the illness. It is now established that the main mortality from myocardial infarction occurs in the first few days following an attack; 65 per cent of deaths occur in the first 3 days and 85 per cent in the first week.

INCIDENCE AND IMPORTANCE

The development of new techniques for continuously monitoring the electrocardiogram has revealed a far higher incidence of arrhythmias than had previously been realized. For example, Master, Dack and Jaffe (1937), who recorded daily electrocardiograms on their patients, reported an incidence of only 14 per cent, though they ignored isolated extrasystoles. Such records were necessarily short, and clearly many transient disturbances of rhythm were missed. With continuous monitoring Julian, Valentine and Miller (1964) reported that some disturbance of rhythm occurred in 95 of 100 consecutive patients. In 56 of these patients, the arrhythmias were potentially serious. Fluck and colleagues (1967) reported an incidence of 80 per cent of arrhythmias in 50 consecutive cases studied by continuous monitoring on magnetic tape. A similar high incidence has been reported by other workers.

Mower, Miller and Nachlas (1964) studied, retrospectively, the clinical features of 138 patients who had died following acute myocardial infarction. They divided the cases into three clinical groups, according to the main cause of death. One group died suddenly and often unexpectedly from an arrhythmia. A second group died from congestive heart failure and the third from hypotension or shock. If, when seen initially, the patient had both shock and an arrhythmia, he was included in the arrhythmia group, although it was not possible to know whether the arrhythmia had caused the hypotension or vice versa. On this basis they found that only 44 per cent of deaths were attributable to shock or congestive failure. On the other hand,

287

Lown and colleagues (1967) estimate that about 40 per cent of deaths are due to an arrhythmia. Two-thirds of these are due to ventricular fibrillation and one-third to bradycardia, heart block and asystole. They emphasize that it is well established that these 'electrical' deaths are not usually due to severe cardiac damage and that prompt treatment can usually restore normal heart action.

Classification

In several recent publications, sinus tachycardia has been cited as an arrhythmia occurring in acute myocardial infarction. It seems doubtful that this is justified, for sinus tachycardia is part of the complex compensatory mechanisms of the heart to offset impaired efficiency. On the other hand, sinus bradycardia is certainly not a compensatory mechanism and may perhaps justifiably be regarded as an abnormal rhythm. Otherwise it is again most convenient to classify the arrhythmias of myocardial infarction on an anatomical basis, as follows.

Sino-atrial disturbances—Sinus bradycardia or arrest, (*a*) with a junctional escape rhythm, or (*b*) with a wandering pacemaker.

Atrial arrhythmias—(1) Atrial extrasystoles, (2) atrial tachycardia, (3) atrial flutter, and (4) atrial fibrillation.

Atrioventricular junctional arrhythmias—(1) A.V. block, (2) junctional extrasystoles, and (3) junctional tachycardias, (*a*) with retrograde atrial activation, or (*b*) with A.V. dissociation.

Ventricular arrhythmias—(1) Ventricular extrasystoles, (2) ventricular tachycardia, (3) accelerated idioventricular rhythm, (4) ventricular parasystole and (5) ventricular flutter or fibrillation.

Pathogenesis of Arrhythmias in Acute Myocardial Infarction

A number of factors contribute to the high incidence of arrhythmias in acute myocardial infarction. Ischaemia-induced alterations in cardiac excitability may well contribute to ventricular ectopic activity. A further factor may be the increased sympatho-adrenal discharge which is known to occur in this condition, and which lowers the threshold to ventricular fibrillation. Cardiac reflexes may be responsible for the sinus bradycardia which occurs in about 20 per cent of patients. Necrosis and oedema, when involving pacemakers or conduction pathways, may compromise heart rhythm.

Relationship of Site of Infarction to Type of Arrhythmia

Note on Terminology

In writings on myocardial infarction, there is some variation in terminology. Infarcts characterized by Q waves and S–T, T changes in leads II, III and AVF are referred to by some authors as 'posterior', by some as 'diaphragmatic' and by others as 'inferior'. The term diaphragmatic will be used here.

There is a reasonably close correlation between the site of the infarct and the type of arrhythmia. Both atrial and ventricular extrasystoles and ventricular fibrillation may complicate acute myocardial infarction irrespective of its site. Sinus bradycardia, S.A. block and Wenckebach Type 1 A.V. block are usually associated with diaphragmatic infarction. Atrial arrhythmias and ventricular tachycardia are commonest in anterior myocardial infarction and when A.V. block complicates infarctions at this site it is usually of the Mobitz Type II variety due to involvement of both bundle branches. Left anterior hemi-block usually results from anterior infarcts. Many exceptions to these general rules occur.

Fluck and colleagues (1967) have suggested a classification of these arrhythmias based on the overall cardiac response to the dominant rhythm during the first 10 days following infarction. They introduce the term 'atrial

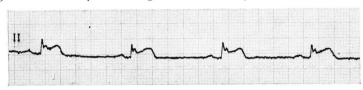

Figure 16.1—Sinus bradycardia in a patient with a recent diaphragmatic infarct. Rate approximately 50 per minute

transport dysfunction' for those A.V. junctional arrhythmias characterized by A.V. dissociation and junctional rhythm. They point out that when atrial and ventricular activation coincide in these arrhythmias, the loss of atrial contribution to ventricular filling leads to a fall in arterial blood pressure. It seems very doubtful that the description of an arrhythmia in terms of its haemodynamic effect is very helpful. For example, in atrial fibrillation, atrial contribution to ventricular filling is lost, so it too could be termed 'atrial transport dysfunction'. A logical extension of this type of terminology would be to call ventricular fibrillation 'ventricular transport dysfunction'.

Sino-Atrial Disturbances

Sinus Bradycardia or Arrest

Sinus bradycardia or arrest with a junctional escape rhythm or a wandering pacemaker between the sinus and A.V. junction may occur, particularly in diaphragmatic infarcts. It has been pointed out by Fluck and colleagues that these patients form a definite group, often with severe chest pain requiring frequent doses of morphia, and recurrent vaso-vagal attacks with a slow heart rate and hypotension. These episodes almost always develop during the first 48 hours following infarction. It is possible that in some the brady-cardia is due directly to morphine. During such attacks, the patients are pale, sweating, nauseated and often mentally confused. When the heart rate falls below 50 per minute the blood pressure may become unrecordable. *Figure 16.1* shows a sinus bradycardia of 50 per minute in a recent diaphragmatic infarct. *Figure 16.2* shows an example of junctional rhythm with a ventricular rate of 50 per minute from a patient with a recent diaphragmatic infarction. The primary disturbance is probably S.A. arrest or block.

Atrial Arrhythmias

Atrial extrasystoles when occurring infrequently, that is, 1 or 2 per minute, seem to have little significance. Bennett and Pentecost (1970) have shown that atrial extrasystoles with a short coupling time, that is when they fall in the vulnerable period of the atrium, may initiate atrial fibrillation. Atrial fibrillation, particularly when associated with a fast ventricular rate, may seriously reduce cardiac output. The same is also true of atrial tachycardia or atrial flutter. These atrial arrhythmias are generally transient but if the ventricular rate is fast they require treatment.

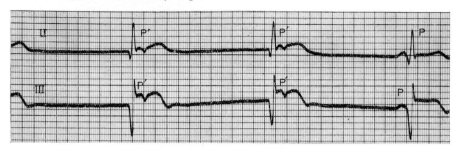

Figure 16.2—Recent diaphragmatic infarct, simultaneous recording of leads II and III. Time markings $\frac{1}{10}$ second. There is junctional rhythm. The first two complexes of the record have a retrograde P' wave in the ST segment. The last QRS complex is preceded by a sinus P wave but clearly it is not conducted, for the P–R interval is too short and it occurs at precisely the same time interval after the second QRS complex as does the second after the first

T. N. James (1961b) reported the autopsy findings on 11 patients with myocardial infarction and atrial arrhythmias. In each case, a coronary occlusion was found proximal to the origin of the sinus node artery and there was infarction of the sinus node. He concluded, however, that damage to the sinus node was only one of several factors responsible for the arrhythmias which included ischaemia of the A.V. node and atrial distension.

Atrioventricular Junctional Arrhythmias

Atrioventricular Block

A.V. block is a potentially serious complication of myocardial infarction. Continuous monitoring of the electrocardiogram has shown that it often occurs in progressive form, first-degree block increasing to second degree and then third degree. On the other hand, third-degree block may suddenly appear during normal conduction. Complete A.V. block may occur as an agonal event in patients dying of congestive heart failure. As a primary complication of infarction, its incidence has varied in different series between 2·5 and 8 per cent.

It is now well established that complete heart block when complicating acute myocardial infarction is more often associated with diaphragmatic infarction. Block results from inflammation and oedema in the region of the A.V. node. In the vast majority of these cases, the QRS complex in the electrocardiogram is normal in duration. On the other hand, when complete heart block is associated with anterior infarction, it is due to extensive necrosis of the ventricular septum involving both bundle branches and the electrocardiogram shows widened QRS complexes due to an idioventricular escape pacemaker. The mortality rate in these cases is very much higher, even when normal conduction returns. This is presumably due to the large size of the infarct.

Complete A.V. block usually develops between the first and fourth day following infarction. The mortality rate has been given as between 70 and 100 per cent in untreated cases. Its onset is usually associated with profound hypotension and a low cardiac output. Stokes–Adams attacks may occur, due either to asystole or ventricular fibrillation. It seems virtually certain that if the patient survives the illness, conduction almost always returns to normal. Two fatal cases studied histologically by Fluck and colleagues revealed no evidence of infarction of the A.V. node or bundle.

Junctional Tachycardia

Junctional tachycardia with a ventricular rate of 160–200 per minute is occasionally seen. *Figure 16.3* shows an example from a patient with a diaphragmatic infarct.

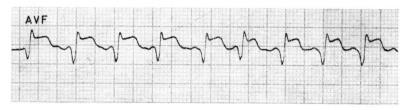

Figure 16.3—Junctional tachycardia from a patient with a recent diaphragmatic infarct. Ventricular rate 146 per minute

Atrioventricular Dissociation

A.V. dissociation with a ventricular rate faster than the sinus rate is a fairly common but transient arrhythmia occurring usually in diaphragmatic infarction. *Figure 16.4* shows an example with a ventricular capture by the sinus impulse. It is, of course, important not to mistake this arrhythmia for

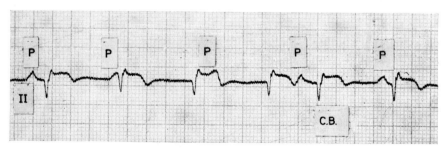

Figure 16.4—Recent diaphragmatic infarction. A.V. dissociation due to a non-paroxysmal nodal tachycardia. The fifth QRS complex (CB) is a capture beat by the sinus impulse

A.V. block. Fluck and colleagues have pointed out that when atrial and ventricular activation coincide, the blood pressure usually falls owing to the loss of atrial contribution to ventricular systole. The fall, however, is usually slight and A.V. dissociation is of little importance in prognosis.

Ventricular Arrhythmias

Ventricular arrhythmias are a particularly important and dangerous complication of myocardial infarction. They include ventricular extrasystoles, ventricular tachycardia, accelerated idioventricular rhythm, ventricular parasystole and ventricular flutter and fibrillation. The single, most frequent, disorder of rhythm in myocardial infarction is ventricular extrasystoles. At one time they were regarded as extremely benign, but it is now recognized that they commonly herald the onset of ventricular tachycardia or fibrillation. Lown and colleagues (1967) regard four characteristics of ventricular ectopic beats as particularly dangerous: (1) when they have a short coupling time, interrupting the T wave of the preceding beat, best expressed as the Q–R'/Q–T ratio which should measure more than 0·85 (*see* later); (2) when they occur in salvos of 2 or more in succession; (3) when they are multiform or multifocal and (4) when they occur at a greater frequency than 5 per minute.

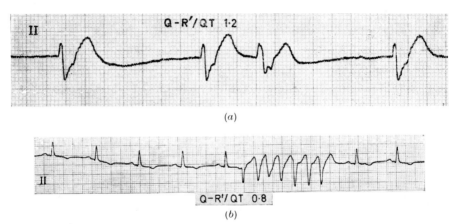

(a)

(b)

Figure 16.5—(a) The third QRS complex is a ventricular extrasystole with a relatively long coupling time giving a Q–R/Q–T ratio of 1·2. (b) Following the fifth beat, there is a short run of ventricular tachycardia. The Q–R/Q–T ratio of the first extrasystole of the tachycardia measures 0·8 second

Smirk (1949) first drew attention to the danger of ventricular extrasystoles with a coupling time so short that they interrupted the T wave of the preceding beat. Lown and colleagues (1967) suggest that this phenomenon is best expressed as the Q–R'/Q–T ratio. The Q–R' interval is measured from the commencement of the QRS complex of the preceding beat to the commencement of the R' of the extrasystole. The Q–T interval is measured in the usual way in a beat not followed by an extrasystole. When the Q–R'/Q–T ratio is less than one, the ectopic is clearly commencing on the previous T wave. According to Lown and colleagues Q–R'/Q–T ratios measuring between 0·60 and 0·85 entail the danger of ventricular fibrillation.

Figure 16.5a shows an isolated ventricular extrasystole with a Q–R'/Q–T ratio of 1·2. *Figure 16.5b* shows ventricular extrasystoles occurring in salvos with a short coupling time, giving a Q–R'/Q–T ratio of 0·8.

Although ventricular extrasystoles which interrupt the previous T wave are in general more dangerous than those with a long coupling time, this rule is by no means invariable. We have several times seen ventricular fibrillation develop following ventricular extrasystoles with a long coupling time.

Ventricular Tachycardia

This is the most frequent of the serious arrhythmias in myocardial infarction. Lown and colleagues (1967) observed an incidence of 29 per cent in 130 consecutive cases. They described two types; the most common variety consisted of brief, self-terminating paroxysms of 4–20 successive ectopic beats. These often commence with an ectopic interrupting a T wave. Although, at first, such episodes may be self-terminating, they may at any time progress to ventricular fibrillation. *Figure 16.8* shows the onset of ventricular fibrillation in a patient who had been having short runs of ventricular tachycardia.

The second type of ventricular tachycardia is sudden in onset, rapid in rate and is sustained. This is a malignant arrhythmia in myocardial infarction, leading to severe hypotension and congestive heart failure and demands immediate treatment.

Accelerated Idioventricular Rhythm

It is not uncommon during the acute stage of myocardial infarction to see a slow ventricular ectopic rhythm. Since the rate is slow, usually between 60 and 100 per minute, ventricular tachycardia is scarcely an appropriate term. Marriott (1968) has called it accelerated idioventricular rhythm. This name implies that an idioventricular centre has acquired a faster inherent rate than the A.V. junctional pacemaker and will thus escape if the sinus rate slows. A typical example is shown in *Figure 16.6*. The four rows are continuous and when in the top row the sinus cycle slows below 0·69 second (rate 85/minute) fusion beats with a ventricular ectopic focus appear and with further sinus slowing the ectopic cycle length is seen to be 0·72 second (rate 83/minute). In the fourth row, acceleration of the sinus rate enables sinus rhythm to become re-established after some further fusion beats. Rothfeld and colleagues (1968) reported that runs of accelerated idioventricular rhythm were usually short, varying from 4 to 30 beats. They terminated either as a result of acceleration of the sinus rate or slowing of the idioventricular rate.

In our experience accelerated idioventricular rhythm seems to be quite benign. However, Raftery and colleagues (1969) mention 11 patients, of whom 6 died. Pentecost and Bennett (1969) moreover have shown us a record with a similar rhythm terminating in ventricular fibrillation.

Ventricular Parasystole

In about 10 per cent of patients with ventricular ectopic beats, the rhythm shows all the characteristics of parasystole. An example of one recorded in the coronary care unit is shown in *Figure 16.7*. Such ectopic beats with a variable coupling time and a fixed inter-ectopic interval could well interrupt the T waves of the sinus beat and they always require immediate suppression.

Ventricular Fibrillation

Ventricular fibrillation is a common terminal rhythm in myocardial infarction. Meltzer and Kitchell (1966) have emphasized the importance of differentiating primary from secondary ventricular fibrillation. Primary

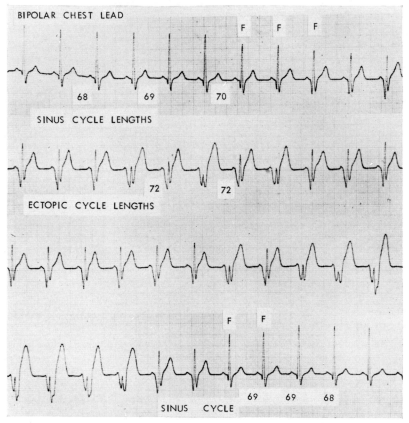

Figure 16.6—*Accelerated idioventricular rhythm. For fuller explanation, see text*

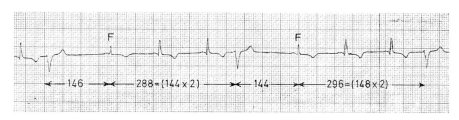

Figure 16.7—*Extract from bipolar chest lead. There is ventricular parasystole with two fusion beats*

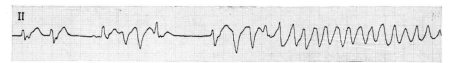

Figure 16.8—*This illustrates the onset of ventricular fibrillation in a patient who had been having short runs of ventricular tachycardia*

ventricular fibrillation is defined as an unexpected event occurring in the absence of shock or marked congestive failure. Secondary ventricular fibrillation is often the terminal rhythm in patients dying of circulatory failure. Primary ventricular fibrillation, if treated promptly, is potentially reversible. Secondary ventricular fibrillation is not.

MANAGEMENT

Coronary Care Unit

It is unfortunately true that the majority of deaths from myocardial infarction occur during the first hour following the onset of the attack. There is good reason to believe that many of these deaths are due to arrhythmias which are potentially reversible if skilled medical aid and equipment are available. 'Those who are admitted to hospital represent, in fact, the survivors of the storm which has already taken its main toll' (McNeilly and Pemberton, 1968). Unfortunately most of these deaths occur before the general practitioner has arrived or even been sent for.

Until a few years ago the mortality rate among patients admitted to hospital was still very high and had remained largely unchanged over the previous 30 years. Kurland and Pressman (1965) reported the mortality rate from 24 studies which had been published between 1937 and 1964 in patients with acute myocardial infarction treated in hospital. The total number of patients in these 24 studies was 11,153 and the mortality rate was 33·1 per cent. Although the death rates varied fairly widely between the individual series this seemed largely to reflect differences in diagnostic criteria adopted for the patient's entry into each study. There was certainly no evidence that the introduction and widespread use of anti-coagulant therapy in the early 1950s had had any appreciable effect. This rather dismal picture has been dramatically changed in the past few years by the introduction of the coronary care unit which has effected a substantial reduction in mortality rate from the arrhythmias occurring during the first few days.

Although such units still have little to offer to patients with severe cardiogenic shock, most units have reported a mortality rate of 20 per cent or less. Most such reports have come from teaching hospitals but it may be relevant here briefly to report the results obtained in a regional hospital. In September 1967, a coronary care unit was started in the North Staffordshire Hospital Group which serves a population of 500,000. All male patients admitted to hospital in the district with a diagnosis of myocardial infarction come into this unit.

Up till now only male patients have been accepted but with no upper age limit. In 1966, a retrospective study was carried out and this revealed that 300 male patients had been admitted to the medical wards in the district during the preceding year with a diagnosis of myocardial infarction. The mortality rate was over 30 per cent. During the first two years, 1,120 patients were admitted to the coronary care unit with a diagnosis of acute myocardial infarction. Investigations in the unit confirmed the diagnosis in 815 cases, or 72 per cent. This figure is substantially the same as that reported from other coronary care units.

The following criteria were adopted for the diagnosis of acute myocardial infarction. Acute transmural myocardial infarction was diagnosed from the presence of pathological Q waves in the electrocardiogram associated with transient ST segment elevation and subsequent T wave inversion. In the absence of pathological Q waves, cases were classed as acute restricted myocardial infarction, provided they fulfilled all the following three criteria: (1) A typical clinical presentation, (2) ST segment and T wave abnormalities showing serial changes in successive electrocardiograms, (3) a transient elevation of the SGOT to more than 50 units or of the SLD to more than 500 units. Other patients admitted with what appeared to be typical cardiac pain who did not fulfil these three criteria were classed as 'angina' and are not included in the results. The remaining patients were regarded as having non-cardiac pain. The mortality rate of the 815 patients who fulfilled the criteria for acute myocardial infarction was 18·8 per cent.

Equipment, Staffing and General Organization of the Coronary Care Unit

The general physicians generously allocated a 26-bedded ward for the unit. The patients are monitored for 72 hours and then, if all is well, are moved to an unmonitored bed in the same ward for the remainder of their hospital stay. Simple calculation suggested that if the admission rate was approximately constant, 300 patients a year could be monitored for 72 hours if four beds were equipped for this purpose.

It is convenient to consider the organization of the unit under four headings, namely: the equipment, the emergency call system, the nursing staff and the therapy employed.

Equipment

Initially the first two beds on each side of the ward were provided with monitors made by Cardiac Recorders. These continuously display the electrocardiogram and also show the heart rate on a simple dial. They can also be made to give an audible bleep with each heart beat and can sound an alarm if the heart rate rises above or falls below a predetermined level. In practice it was found that the continual bleeping of four monitors simultaneously served only to cause confusion and that the alarm system gave false alarms so frequently that neither of these facilities is now used. A simple bipolar chest lead is used for the purpose of monitoring. Three 3 mm Dracard electrodes* are employed, one being used for the earth lead. Two other essential pieces of equipment are a d.c. defibrillator and a direct-writing electrocardiographic machine. At the end of six months it became apparent that four monitored beds were insufficient for two reasons. Firstly, the daily administration rate fluctuated widely and secondly, the number of admissions rose steeply, presumably due to increasing awareness among local general practitioners of the existence of the unit. The number of monitored beds was then increased to six and this seemed adequate to cope with the increased admission rate. Since it proved virtually impossible for one observer to watch six monitors simultaneously, a six-channel 'slave' monitor was installed at the nurses' station where all six electrocardiograms are continuously displayed on a single cardioscope.

* Obtainable from Dracard Ltd., Boughton Monchelsea, Maidstone, Kent.

Emergency Call System

The emergency alarm utilizes the ordinary hospital bleep call system. There are a number of bleep receivers all on the same frequency which are known as the 'red bleeps'. Two members of the junior hospital staff are always on call for the unit and each carries one of these 'red bleeps' in addition to his ordinary one. It is his responsibility to hand it over to the next man on call when his period of duty is over. There is a simple bell-push in the coronary care unit which can be pressed in an emergency. When it is pressed a bell rings and a lamp lights on the hospital telephone switchboard. The operator then sends out a staccato call on the 'red bleep' frequency. An additional 'red bleep' is located in the ward so that the nursing staff knows that the call has gone out.

Nursing Staff

The present shortage of nurses in regional hospitals naturally poses a difficult problem in staffing a unit throughout the 24 hours. It is necessary always to have two people on the ward who have been trained in resuscitative techniques to deal with a cardiac arrest and who can recognize early changes in the electrocardiogram. There are three points worth emphasizing about nursing staff for a regional coronary care unit. First, the staff must as far as possible be permanent. It takes a little time to train staff for this kind of work and student nurses who only stay for a few weeks are of little help. However, this does not mean that it is necessary to have a large staff of state registered nurses, for it has proved surprisingly easy to teach most people of reasonable intelligence quickly to recognize significant changes in the electrocardiogram. As long as it can be arranged that one state registered nurse is always on duty, the remainder of the staff can be made up from state enrolled nurses or auxiliary nurses. A third point to be emphasized is that certain designated members of the nursing staff who have been adequately trained should be allowed to treat ventricular fibrillation immediately by direct current electric shock without waiting for medical help to arrive. Provided the consultant concerned is prepared to assume responsibility for this, there is no legal objection and the success rate of resuscitation is materially increased.

Drug Therapy

Since there is no evidence that anticoagulants are of any value in myocardial infarction they are not given routinely in this unit but only if there is some specific indication such as a deep vein thrombosis or a pulmonary embolus. Since it is often necessary during the first few days following myocardial infarction to give a variety of pharmacological agents intravenously, it is a good practice to have an intravenous route ready prepared. A useful device for this purpose is the Venflon needle illustrated in *Figure 16.9*. As soon as the patient is admitted, this needle is inserted into a suitable forearm vein. The inner needle is then withdrawn leaving the Teflon outer covering in situ in the vein. The end of this can then be closed with the bung. Five hundred units of heparin are then injected through the one-way valve in the hilt of the needle which will then remain patent for up to several days. Any necessary drugs can be injected as a bolus at any time through the valve or the bung can be removed and the male Luer fitting of an intravenous drip can be inserted for continuous intravenous infusion. A very useful additional device is the automatic drip counter made by Decca. This automatically

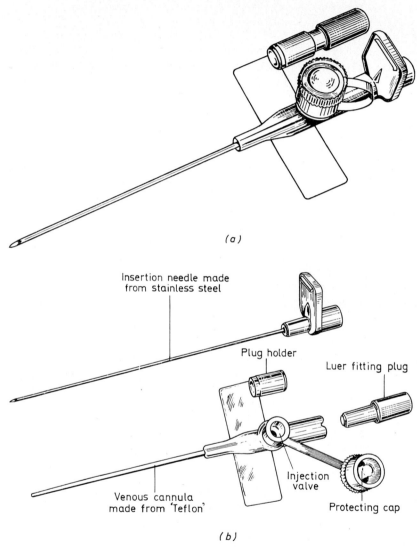

(a)

Insertion needle made
from stainless steel

Plug holder

Luer fitting plug

Venous cannula
made from 'Teflon'

Injection
valve

Protecting cap

(b)

Figure 16.9—The Venflon intravenous needle. (a) Shows the complete needle, (b) shows the needle dismantled

ensures that the drip rate will be constant at any chosen speed and saves a great deal of nursing time.

For the relief of pain, 6 mg heroin is given intravenously. Heroin has many advantages over morphia and the intravenous route ensures rapid action and avoids leaving unabsorbed depots of the drug in the subcutaneous tissues of patients with a low cardiac output.

Treatment of Individual Arrhythmias

Sinus Bradycardia

A slow heart rate of 60 or less should always be treated promptly. Atropine sulphate, 1 mg, given intravenously over about one minute will usually accelerate the heart rate to 80 or 90 beats a minute and the effect lasts two to four hours when, if necessary, the injection may be repeated. Hypotension associated with a bradycardia generally quickly improves as the heart rate increases. If there is no response to atropine, an intravenous drip of isoprenaline should be started using 4 mg dissolved in one litre of 5 per cent glucose.

Atrial arrhythmias

Occasional atrial extrasystoles can probably be disregarded; when however they are occurring at a rate of more than five per minute, they are probably best treated by practolol of which 5 mg should be given slowly intravenously over two to three minutes. This dose may be repeated until a response is obtained or a maximum of 25 mg has been given. Atrial tachycardia, flutter or fibrillation are usually transient disorders; when however they are associated with a rapid ventricular rate, practolol at present seems the best drug to use; again 5 mg is given intravenously over two to three minutes and this dose may be repeated until a response is obtained or a maximum of 25 mg has been given. (The average dose needed is in the region of 10 mg.) If no response to practolol occurs, the arrhythmia should be terminated by d.c. shock.

Atrioventricular Junctional Arrhythmias

First-degree heart block does not require treatment although its appearance should alert the physician to the possibility of more advanced block developing. With diaphragmatic infarcts, second-degree heart block often presents with Wenckebach periods, which may later progress to 2:1 block or complete block. Among the 815 patients with acute myocardial infarction who were admitted to the coronary care unit of the North Staffordshire Hospital Group during its first two years, 44 patients, or just over 6 per cent, developed complete heart block. At present it is generally recommended that such patients should be treated by electrical pacing after introducing a transvenous catheter into the right ventricle, using a portable image intensifier. When the coronary care unit in the North Staffordshire Hospital group was first started, a portable image intensifier was not available and all patients with complete heart block were treated by medical means alone. Sutton, Chatterjee and Leatham (1968) reported that in 55 patients with complete heart block following acute myocardial infarction, all of whom were electrically paced, 25 died giving a mortality rate of 45·5 per cent. In the North Staffordshire unit, 21 of the patients out of the total of 44 with complete heart block, all of whom were treated medically, died, giving a mortality rate of 47·5 per cent; thus it seems that the beneficial effects of electrically pacing these patients is at the most marginal only.

Medical treatment of acute heart block consists in giving 1 mg atropine intravenously straight away, and then an intravenous infusion of isoprenaline, using 4 mg in a litre of 5 per cent dextrose, is set up. The drip rate is adjusted to maintain a ventricular rate of 60 per minute. If more than 20 drops per minute is required, more isoprenaline is added to the Vaccolitre. When normal A.V. conduction returns, the drip should immediately be stopped to avoid sinus tachycardia.

Many centres continue to pace electrically with a demand pacemaker any patient with acute myocardial infarction and right bundle branch block and all patients with complete A.V. block, whether the infarct is anterior or diaphragmatic. However, Morris and his colleagues (1972) have recently stated, 'Neither prophylactic demand pacing for RBBB nor pacing for established A.V. block appeared to reduce the high hospital mortality rate, although pacing was considered to have been life saving in two patients. Pacing prolonged life for a few days in a large proportion of patients who died, however, and in several of these patients the conduction disturbances were reversible and death finally occurred from some other cause.'

We have heard Marriott state (1970) that electrical pacing appears only to bring comfort to the physician rather than benefit to the patient. It is our policy now only to pace patients with complete heart block who do not respond to medical measures with an adequate increase in heart rate or in whom isoprenaline induces ventricular arrhythmias or who continue to have Stokes–Adams attacks.

Reference was made in Chapter 14 (page 256) to the use of steroids in the treatment of A.V. block. In practice they had proved of no value in chronic forms of A.V. block but they are still employed by some authors in the treatment of A.V. block complicating acute myocardial infarction. The rationale of their use is that A.V. block is due to involvement of the conducting tracts by inflammation and oedema rather than necrosis. They should therefore be used in complete heart block complicating diaphragmatic infarction when the duration of the QRS complex is normal. A dose of 200 mg of hydrocortisone may be given intravenously, followed by 100 mg every 6 hours until normal conduction returns.

Atrioventricular Dissociation

A.V. dissociation due to a moderate junctional tachycardia with retrograde block is in my experience an innocuous arrhythmia and does not require treatment. Although intravenous atropine, by accelerating the sinus rate, may restore sinus rhythm, it necessarily produces a tachycardia and is best avoided.

Junctional Tachycardia

Junctional tachycardia with a rapid ventricular rate (*see Figure 16.3*) should be treated by intravenous practolol as described for supraventricular arrhythmias. If it fails to slow the ventricular rate the arrhythmia should be terminated by direct current shock followed by oral quinidine, 0·2 to 0·3 gm of quinidine sulphate every 4 hours.

Ventricular Arrhythmias

Perhaps the most valuable contribution of Lown and his colleagues (1967) has been to point out that although ventricular fibrillation is so common a cause of sudden and unexpected death, it often casts its shadows before it which may be picked up on the continuous monitor. To quote their words 'death, while sudden, is not unannounced'. The ventricular ectopic mechanisms which may herald the onset of ventricular fibrillation are ventricular extrasystoles showing one or more of the four characteristics described earlier, also ventricular tachycardia, accelerated idioventricular rhythm and ventricular parasystole.

Rare sporadic ventricular extrasystoles require no treatment. If one or more of the four dangerous characteristics is present, a single injection of 25 mg of 2 per cent lignocaine should be given intravenously. If the extrasystoles persist, a second injection is given, using a bolus of 50 mg. If this is successful, an intravenous drip is started, delivering 1 to 2 mg of lignocaine per minute, or enough to prevent recurrence of ectopic activity. If the larger injection of lignocaine should fail, procainamide should be tried next in a dose of 50 mg every two to three minutes until ectopic activity is abolished. It may then be possible to maintain the effect by a lignocaine drip. If both lignocaine and procainamide should fail to abolish ventricular extrasystoles, one of the other numerous anti-arrhythmic drugs should be used.

When, as is usual, lignocaine successfully suppresses extrasystoles, the intravenous infusion should be continued for two or three days but with a gradual reduction in dosage, after which anti-arrhythmic medication can be safely withdrawn.

Accelerated Idioventricular Rhythm

In our experience it is unwise to treat this arrhythmia with lignocaine. Since basically this arrhythmia is an escape rhythm, lignocaine or procainamide which tend to slow the sinus rate may only increase the frequency of the ectopic rhythm. We have found the most satisfactory treatment to be intravenous atropine which accelerates the sinus rate and the sinus impulse then keeps the idioventricular pacemaker suppressed.

Ventricular Parasystole

The management of this arrhythmia is exactly the same as that described for ventricular extrasystoles. It is usually promptly abolished by lignocaine.

Ventricular Tachycardia

Lown and his colleagues state that even if only a single short episode of ventricular tachycardia is observed, anti-arrhythmic measures should immediately be instituted and these are the same as described for ventricular extrasystoles. In the second, more persistent type of ventricular tachycardia, immediate termination should be aimed at. While preparations are being made for direct current reversion, drug therapy should be tried. A bolus of 100 mg lignocaine should be given intravenously; if this fails, practolol may be tried next but reversion with direct current shock under light general anaesthesia should not be delayed too long. Once sinus rhythm has been restored, an intravenous drip of lignocaine should be started.

Ventricular Fibrillation

According to Lown and his colleagues (1967) primary ventricular fibrillation should not occur if the foregoing measures are meticulously followed.

This however is not entirely true, because the abrupt onset of ventricular fibrillation has been observed in patients whose electrocardiogram was being continuously recorded on magnetic tape. There is no doubt however that the successful suppression of ventricular ectopic beats substantially reduces the incidence of ventricular fibrillation. When ventricular fibrillation occurs it should immediately be treated by direct current shock. An energy level of 100 watt-seconds is usually sufficient to terminate primary ventricular fibrillation and restore sinus rhythm. If no doctor is present on the unit at the time, a designated member of the nursing staff should be authorized to carry this out without delay. As soon as normal rhythm returns, 200 mEq sodium bicarbonate should be given intravenously to correct metabolic acidosis and should be followed by an intravenous lignocaine drip.

There can be little doubt that coronary care units can substantially reduce the mortality rate among patients with acute myocardial infarction admitted to hospital. Such units can be successfully run in regional hospitals without very elaborate or expensive equipment nor large numbers of highly qualified nursing staff.

There has been much talk recently of providing an ambulance service which would take the facilities of the coronary care unit to the patient's home. Such a service should be able to deal at once with dangerous arrhythmias before moving the patient to hospital. The staffing of such a service would almost certainly be beyond the resources of the average regional hospital.

REFERENCES

Abrams, L. D., Hudson, W. A. and Lightwood, R. (1960). 'A Surgical Approach to the Management of Heart Block, Using an Inductive Coupled Artificial Cardiac Pacemaker. *Lancet* **1,** 1372

Allen, J. D. and Shanks, R. G. (1969). 'The Effects of Bretylium, Lignocaine and Propranolol on Ventricular Fibrillation Threshold.' *Ir. J. med. Sci.* **2,** 252

— — and Saidi, S. A. (1969). 'A Comparison of the Effects of Bretylium, Lignocaine and Propranolol on Experimental Cardiac Arrhythmias.' *Br. J. Pharmac. Chemother.* **37,** 526

Alanis, J., Gonzalez, H. and Lopez, E. (1958). 'Electrical Activity of the Bundle of His.' *J. Physiol.* **142,** 127

Alexander, S., Kleiger, R. and Lown, B. (1961). 'Use of External Electric Counter-shock in Treatment of Ventricular Tachycardia.' *J. Am. med. Ass.* **177,** 916

Armbrust, C. A. and Levine, S. A. (1950). 'Paroxysmal Ventricular Tachycardia.' *Circulation* **1,** 28

Averill, K. H., Fosmoe, R. G., Lamb, J. and Lawrence, E. (1960). 'Symposium on Cardiology in Aviation.' *Am. J. Cardiol.* **6,** 108

Bacaner, M. B. (1966). 'Bretylium Tosylate for Suppression of Induced Ventricular Fibrillation.' *Am. J. Cardiol.* **17,** 528

— (1968). 'Treatment of Ventricular Fibrillation and other Acute Arrhythmias with Bretylium Tosylate.' *Am. J. Cardiol.* **21,** 530

Bachmann, G. (1916). 'The Interauricular Time Interval.' *Am. J. Physiol.* **41,** 309

Barker, P. S., Wilson, F. N. and Johnston, F. D. (1943). 'The Mechanism of Auricular Paroxysmal Tachycardia.' *J. Am. med. Ass.* **122,** 136

Beck, C. S. (1936). 'Resuscitation of Cardiac Standstill and Ventricular Fibrillation Occurring During Operations.' *Am. J. Surg.* **54,** 273

Beller, B. M., Frater, R. W. M. and Wulfsohn, N. (1968). 'Cardiac Pacemaking in the Management of Post-operative Arrhythmias.' *Ann. thorac. Surg.* **6,** 68

Bellet, S., Wasserman, F. and Brody, J. I. (1955). 'Treatment of Cardiac Arrest and Slow Ventricular Rates in Complete A.V. Heart Block.' *Circulation* **11,** 685

Bennet, D., Balcon, R., Hoy, J. and Sowton, E. (1970). 'Haemodynamic Effects of Dextro-propranolol in Acute Myocardial Infarction.' *Thorax,* **25,** 86

Bennett, M. A. and Pentecost, B. L. (1970). 'Pattern of Onset and Spontaneous Cessation of Atrial Fibrillation in Men.' *Circulation* **41,** 981

Bigger, J. T. Jr. and Goldreyer, B. N. (1970). 'The Mechanism of Supraventricular Tachycardia.' *Circulation* **42,** 673

Birchfield, R. I., Merefee, E. E. and Bryant, G. N. D. (1957). 'Disease of the Sino-atrial Node Associated with Bradycardia, Asystole, Syncope and Paroxysmal Atrial Fibrillation. *Circulation* **16,** 20

Black, J. W. and Stevenson, J. S. (1962). 'Pharmacology of a New Adrenergic Beta-receptor-blocking Compound (Nethelide). *Lancet* **2,** 311

Bouveret, L. (1889). 'De la Tachycardie Essentielle Parosystique.' *Revue Méd.* **9,** 755, 837

Bradley, S. M. and Marriott, H. J. L. (1958). 'Escape Capture Bigeminy.' *Am. J. Cardiol.* **1,** 640

Brashear, R. E. and Edmands, R. E. (1972). 'The Electrocardiographic Effects of Elevated Cerebrospinal Fluid Pressure: Wolff–Parkinson–White Type of Conduction Disturbance.' *Am. Heart J.* **84,** 653

Brown, A. K., Doukas, N., Riding, W. D. and Wyn Jones, E. (1967). 'Cardiomyopathy in Pregnancy.' *Br. Heart J.* **29,** 387

Burn, J. H. (1960). 'The Cause of Fibrillation.' *Br. med. J.* **1,** 1379

Burrell, Z. L. and Martinez, A. C. (1958). 'Chloroquine and Hydroxychloroquine in the Treatment of Cardiac Arrhythmias.' *New Engl. J. Med.* **258,** 798

Butler, S. and Levine, S. A. (1930). 'Diphtheria as a Cause of Late Heart Block.' *Am. Heart J.* **5,** 592

Butterworth, J. S. and Poindexter, C. A. (1942). 'Short P-R Interval Associated with Prolonged QRS Complex. A Clinical and Experimental Study.' *Archs intern. Med.* **69,** 437

Campbell, M. (1943). 'Congenital Complete Heart Block.' *Br. Heart J.* **5,** 13
— (1943). 'Latent Heart Block.' *Br. Heart J.* **5,** 163

Castellanos, A., Lunberg, L., Johnson, D. and Berkovits, V. B. (1966). 'The Wedensky Effect in the Human Heart.' *Br. Heart J.* **28,** 276

Chamberlain, D. A., Leinbach, R. C., Vassaux, C. E., Kastor, J. A., De Sanctis, R. W. and Sanders, C. A. (1970). 'Sequential Atrioventricular Pacing in Heart Block Complicating Acute Myocardial Infarction.' *New Eng. J. Med.* **282,** 577

Church, G., Schamroth, L., Schwartz, N. L. and Marriott, H. J. L. (1962). 'Deliberate Digitalis Intoxication. A Comparison of the Toxic Effects of Four Glycoside Preparations.' *Ann. intern. med.* **57,** 946

Cobb, F. R., Blunenschein, S. D., Sealey, W. C., Boineau, J. T., Wagner, G. S. and Wallace, A. G. (1968). 'Successful Surgical Interruption of the Bundle of Kent in a Patient with Wolff–Parkinson–White Syndrome.' *Circulation* **38,** 1018

Conn, H. L. (1966). In *Mechanisms of Quinidine Action. Mechanism and Therapy of Cardiac Arrhythmias* p. 594. Ed. by L. S. Dreifus, W. Likoff and J. H. Moyer. New York; Grune and Stratton

Conn, R. D. (1965). 'Diphenylhydantoin Sodium in Cardiac Arrhythmias.' *New Engl. J. Med.* **272,** 277

Cotton, R. P. (1867). 'Notes and Observations Upon a Case of Unusually Rapid Action of the Heart (232 per minute).' *Br. med. J.* **1,** 629

Damato, A. N., Lau, S. H., Helfant, R. H., Stein, E., Berkowitz, W. D. and Cohen, S. I. (1969). 'Study of Atrioventricular Conduction in Man using Electrode Catheter Recordings of His Bundle Activity.' *Circulation* **39,** 287

Davies, M. and Harris, A. (1969). 'Pathological Basis of Primary Heart Block.' *Br. Heart J.* **31,** 219

Davis, L. G. and Ross, I. P. (1963). 'Abnormal P waves and Paroxysmal Tachycardia.' *Br. Heart J.* **25,** 570

De Haan, R. L. (1961). 'Differentiation of the Atrioventricular Conducting System of the Heart.' *Circulation* **24,** 458

Deitz, G. W., Marriott, H. J. L., Fletcher, E. and Bellet, S. (1957). 'Atrial Dissociation and Uniatrial Fibrillation.' *Circulation* **15,** 883

Dewhurst, W. (1957). 'Malignant Auricular Arrhythmia.' *Br. Heart J.* **19,** 387

Diarz, F. V. (1950). 'Atebrin in Paroxysmal Tachycardia and Atrial Fibrillation.' *Br. Heart J.* **12,** 132

Dimond, E. G. and Hayes, W. L. (1958). 'An Electrocardiographic Demonstration of Atrial Dissociation.' *Am. Heart J.* **56,** 929

Dreifus, L. S., Bartolucci, G. and Likoff, W. (1960). 'Nodal Tachycardia, Aetiology and Therapy.' *Circulation* **22,** 741
— Nichols, H., Morse, D., Watanabe, Y. and Truex, R. (1968). 'Control of Recurrent Tachycardia of Wolff–Parkinson–White Syndrome by Surgical Ligature of the A.V. Bundle.' *Circulation* **38,** 1030

Durrer, D. and Roos, J. P. (1967). 'Epicardial Excitation of the Ventricles in a Patient with Wolff–Parkinson–White Syndrome (Type B).' *Circulation* **35,** 15
— Schoo, L., Schuilenburg, M. and Wellins, H. J. (1967). 'The Role of Premature Beats in the Initiation and Determination of Supraventricular Tachycardia in the Wolff–Parkinson–White Syndrome.' *Circulation* **36,** 644

Engelman, T. W. (1896). 'Über den Ursprung der Herzbewegung und die physiologischen Eigenschaften der Grossen Herznerven des Frosches.' *Archiv. ges. Physiol. (Bonn)* **65,** 109

Erlanger, J. (1910). 'Observations on Auricular Strips of the Cat's Heart.' *Am. J. Physiol.* **27,** 87

Evans, W. and Swann, E. (1954). 'Lone Atrial Fibrillation.' *Br. Heart J.* **16,** 189

Feldt, R. H., DuShane, J. W. and Titus, J. L. (1970). 'The Atrioventricular Conduction System in Persistent Common Atrioventricular Canal Defect.' *Circulation,* **42.** 437

Ferrer, I. N. (1967). 'New Concepts Relating to the Pre-excitation Syndrome.' *J. Am. med. Ass.* **201,** 162

REFERENCES

Fluck, D. C., Olsen, E., Pentecost, B. L., Thomas, M., Fillmore, S. J., Shillingford, J. P. and Mounsey, J. P. D. (1967). 'Natural History and Clinical Significance of Arrhythmias After Acute Cardiac Infarction.' *Br. Heart J.* **29,** 170

Fowler, P. B. S. (1962). 'A Syndrome Due to Changing or Transient Heart Block.' *Br. med. J.* **2,** 1638

Frey, W. (1918). 'Über Vorhofflimmern beim Menschen und seine Beseitigung durch Chinidin.' *Berl. klin. Wschr.* **55,** 417, 450

Friedberg, C. K., Jaffe, H. L., Pordy, L. and Chesky, K. (1962). 'The Two-step Exercise Electrocardiogram; A Double-blind Evaluation of Its Use in the Diagnosis of Angina Pectoris.' *Circulation* **26,** 1254

Froment, R., Gallavardin, L. and Cohen, P. (1953). 'Paroxysmal Ventricular Tachycardia.' *Br. Heart J.* **15,** 172

Gallagher, J. J., Damato, A. N., Varghese, P. J. and Lan, S. H. (1972). 'Localization of an Area of Maximum Refractoriness or "Gate" in the Ventricular Specialized Conduction System in Man.' *Am. Heart J.* **84,** 310

Gallavardin, L. (1920). 'Tachycardie parosystique ventriculaire.' *Archs Mal. Coeur* **13,** 121

— (1922). 'De la tachycardie parosystique à centre excitable.' *Archs Mal Coeur* **15,** 1

Gaskell, W. H. (1881). 'On the Innervation of the Heart with Special Reference to the Heart of Tortoise.' *J. Physiol. Lond.* **4,** 43

Ghose, R. R., Joekes, A. M. and Kyriacov, E. H. (1965). 'Renal Response to Paroxysmal Tachycardia.' *Br. Heart J.* **27,** 684

Gibson, D. G., Balcon, R. and Sowton, E. (1968). 'Clinical Use of I.C.I. 50, 172 as Antidysrhythmic Agent in Heart Failure.' *Br. med. J.* **3,** 161

Gilchrist, A. R. (1958). 'Clinical Aspects of High Grade Heart Block.' *Scott. med. J.* **3,** 53

Gillespie, W. J., Greene, D. G., Karatyas, N. D. and Lee, G. de (1967)., Effect of Atrial Systole on Right Ventricular Stroke Output in Complete Heart Block.' *Br. med. J.* **1,** 75

Goldsmith, C., Kapadia, G. G., Nimmo, L., Murphy, C., Moran, H. and Marcus, F. I. (1969). 'Correlation of Digitalis Intoxication with Myocardial Concentration of Tritiated Digoxin in Hypokalaemic and Normokalaemic Dogs.' *Circulation* Suppl. 3, **40,** 92

Grant, R. P. (1957). *Clinical Electrocardiography.* New York; McGraw-Hill

— Tomlinson, F. B. and van Buren, J. K. (1958). 'Ventricular Activation in the Pre-excitation Syndrome (Wolff–Parkinson–White)'. *Circulation* **18,** 355

Gross, H. and Jezzer, A. (1956). *Treatment of Heart Disease.* Philadelphia; Saunders

Halmos, P. B. (1966). 'Direct Current Conversion of Atrial Fibrillation.' *Br. Heart J.* **28,** 302

— Davies, M., Redwood, D., Leatham, A. and Siddons, H. (1969). 'Aetiology of Chronic Heart Block.' *Br. Heart J.* **31,** 206

Hamilton, S. D., Hartley, T. D., Miller, R. H., Scheibler, G. L. and Marriott, H. J. L. (1968). 'Disturbances in Atrial Rhythm and Conduction following the Surgical Creation of an Atrial Septal Defect by the Blalock–Hanlon Technique.' *Circulation* **38,** 73

Harris, A., Bluestone, R., Busby, E., Davies, G., Leatham, A., Siddins, H. and Sowton, E. (1966). 'The Management of Heart Block.' *Br. Heart J.* **27,** 469

— Davies, M., Redwood, D., Leatham, A. and Siddons, H. (1969). 'Aetiology of Chronic Heart Block: A Clinicopathological Correlation in 65 Cases.' *Br. Heart J.* **31,** 206

Harris, A. S. and Kokenot, F. H. (1950). 'Effects of Biphenylhydantoin Sodium (Dilantin Sodium) and Phenobarbital Sodium upon Ectopic Ventricular Tachycardia in Acute Myocardial Infarction.' *Am. J. Physiol.* **163,** 505

Harrison, D. C., Sprouse, J. H. and Morrow, A. G. (1963). 'The Anti-arrhythmic Properties of Lidocaine and Procaine Amide. *Circulation* **28,** 486

Harvey, W. P. (1959). 'What's New in Arrhythmias?' *Circulation* **20,** 286

Hay, J. (1906). 'Bradycardia and Cardiac Arrhythmia Produced by Depression of Certain Functions of the Heart.' *Lancet* **1,** 139

Helfant, R. H., Scherlag, B. J. and Damato, A. N. (1967). 'Protection from Digitalis

Toxicity with the Prophylactic use of Diphenylhydantoin Sodium. An Arrhythmic–Inotropic dissociation.' *Circulation* **36**, 119

Herman, G. R., Park, H. M. and Hejtmanciak, M. R. (1959). 'Paroxysmal Ventricular Tachycardia.' *Am. Heart J.* **57**, 166

Hill, I. G. W. (1963). 'Some Less Familiar Forms of Heart Disease.' *Scott. med. J.* **8**, 331

His, W. (1893). 'Die Thätigkeit des embryonalen Herzens und deren Bedeutung für die Lehre von der Herzbewegung beim Erwachsenen.' *Arb. med. Klin. Lpz.* **14**

Hoffman, B. F. and Cranefield, P. F. (1960). *Electrophysiology of the Heart.* New York; McGraw-Hill

Hoffman, P. (1964). 'Behandlung Koronarer Durchblutingsstörungen mit Isoptin in der Praxis.' *Medsche Klin.* **59**, 1387

Hoffman, S. A., Wallace, H. W., Baue, A. E., Blakemore, W. S. and Zinsser, H. F. (1969). 'Postoperative Ventricular Arrhythmias Caused by Isoproterenol: Conversion with Insulin.' *J. thorac cardiovasc. Surg.* **58**, 664

Holzmann, M. and Scherf, D. (1932). 'Uber Elektrokardiogramme mit verkurtzer Vorhof-Kammer-Distanz und positiven P-Zacken.' *Ztschr. J. klin. Med.* **121**, 404

Howitt, G., Husaini, N., Rowlands, D. J., Logan, W. F. W. E., Shanks, R. G. and Evans, N. G. (1968). 'The Effect of the Dextro-isomer of Propranolol on Sinus Rate and Cardiac Arrhythmias.' *Am. Heart J.* **76**, 736

Hudson, R. E. B. (1960). 'The Human Pacemaker and Its Pathology.' *Br. Heart J.* **22**, 115

Hunt, D., Sloman, G. and Westlake, G. (1969). 'Ventricular Aneurysmectomy for Recurrent Tachycardia.' *Br. Heart J.* **31**, 264

Hunt, N. C., Cobb, F. R., Waxnan, M. B., Zeft, H. J., Peter, R. H. and Morris, J. J. (1968). 'Conversion of Supraventricular Tachycardias with Atrial Stimulation. Evidence for Re-entry Mechanisms.' *Circulation* **38**, 1060

Hutchinson, E. C. and Stock, J. P. P. (1960). 'The Carotid Sinus Syndrome.' *Lancet* **2**, 445

Iliescu, C. C. and Sebastiani, A. (1923). 'Notes on the Effects of Quinidine upon Paroxysms of Tachycardia.' *Heart* **10**, 223

Imperial, E. S., Carballo, R. and Zimmerman, H. A. (1960). 'Disturbances of Rate, Rhythm and Conduction in Acute Myocardial Infarction: A Statistical Study of of 153 Cases.' *Am J. Cardiol.* **5**, 24

James, T. N. (1961a). 'Morphology of Human Atrioventricular Node, With Remarks Pertinent to its Electrophysiology.' *Am. Heart J.* **62**, 756

— (1961b). 'Myocardial Infarction and Atrial Arrhythmias.' *Circulation* **24**, 761

— (1963). 'The Connecting Pathways between the Sinus Node and A.V. Node and between the Right and Left Atrium in the Human Heart.' *Am. Heart J.* **66**, 498

Jerrell, A. and Lange-Nielsen, F. (1957). 'Congenital Deaf-mutism, Functional Heart Disease with Prolongation of the Q T Interval and Sudden Death.' *Am. Heart J.* **54**, 59

Jewitt, D. E., Mercer, C. J. and Shillingford, J. P. (1969). 'Practolol in the Treatment of Cardiac Dysrhythmias due to Acute Myocardial Infarction.' *Lancet* **2**, 227

Johnson, R. L., Averill, K. H. and Lamb, L. E. (1960). 'Electrocardiographic Findings in 67,375 Asymptomatic Subjects.' *Am. J. Cardiol.* **6**, 153

Jose, A. D. (1966). 'Effect of Combined Sympathetic and Parasympathetic Blockade on Heart Rate and Cardiac Function in Man.' *Am. J. Cardiol.* **18**, 476

Julian, D. G., Valentine, P. A. and Miller, G. G. (1964). 'Disturbance of Rate, Rhythm and Conduction in Acute Myocardial Infarction.' *Am J. Med.* **37**, 915

Katz, L. N. and Pick, A. (1956). *Clinical Electrocardiography.* London; Kimpton

Keith, A. and Flack, M. W. (1907). 'The Form and Nature of the Muscular Connections Between the Primary Divisions of the Vertebrate Heart.' *J. Anat. Physiol., Lond.* **41**, 172

Kelly, D. T., Brodsky, S. J., Mirowski, M., Krovetz, J. and Rowe, R. D. (1972). 'Bundle of His Recordings in Congenital Complete Heart Block.' *Circulation* **45**, 277

Kent, A. F. S. (1893). 'Researches on the Structure and Function of the Mammalian Heart.' *J. Physiol., Lond.* **14**, 233

Kistin, A. D. (1963). 'Multiple Pathways of Conduction and Reciprocal Rhythm with Interpolated Ventricular Extrasystoles.' *Am. Heart J.* **65**, 162

REFERENCES

— (1965). 'Atrial Reciprocal Rhythm.' *Circulation* **32,** 687

— and Landowne, M. (1951). 'Retrograde Conduction from Premature Ventricular Contractions; A Common Occurrence in the Human Heart.' *Circulation* **3,** 738

Kleiger, R. and Lown, B. (1966). 'Cardioversion and Digitalis.' *Circulation* **33,** 878

Kline, S. R., Dreifus, L. S., Watanabe, Y., McGarry, T. F. and Likoff, W. (1962). 'A Valuation of the Antiarrhythmic Properties of Antazoline.' *Am. J. Cardiol.* **9,** 564

Kreus, K. E., Salokannel, S. J. and Woris, E. K. (1966). 'Non-synchronised and Synchronised Direct-current Countershock in Cardiac Arrhythmias.' *Lancet* **2,** 405

Kulbertus, H. and Collignon, P. (1969). 'Association of Right Bundle Branch Block with Left Superior or Inferior Intraventricular Block.' *Br. Heart J.* **31,** 435

Kurland, G. S. and Pressman, D. (1965). 'The Incidence of Arrhythmias in Acute Myocardial Infarction Studied with a Constant Monitoring System.' *Circulation* **18,** 834

Langendorf, R., Pick, A. and Katz, L. N. (1965). 'Ventricular Response in Atrial Fibrillation. Role of Concealed Conduction in the A.V. Junction.' *Circulation* **32,** 69

— — and Winternitz, M. (1955). 'Mechanisms of Intermittent Ventricular Bigeminy. 1. Appearance of Ectopic Beats Dependent on Length of the Ventricular Cycle, the "Rule of Bigeminy".' *Circulation* **11,** 422

Lepeschkin, E. (1964). 'The Electrocardiographic Diagnosis of Bilateral Bundle Branch Block in Relation to Heart Block.' *Prog. cardiovasc. Dis.* **6,** 445

Lev, M. (1964). 'Anatomic Basis for Atrioventricular Block.' *Am. J. Med.* **37,** 742

— and Lerner, R. (1955). 'The Theory of Kent. A Histological Study of the Normal Atrioventricular Communication of the Human Heart.' *Circulation* **12,** 176

— Widron, J. and Erickson, E. E. (1951). 'A Method for the Histopathological Study of the Atrio-ventricular Node, Bundle and Branches.' *Archs Path.* **52,** 73

— Leffler, W. B., Langendorf, R. and Pick, A. (1966). 'Anatomic Findings in a Case of Ventricular Pre-excitation (W.P.W.) Terminating in Complete Atrioventricular Block.' *Circulation* **34,** 718

Levine, S. A. and Harvey, W. P. (1949). *Clinical Auscultation of the Heart.* Philadelphia; Saunders

Levy, A. G. (1915). 'The Genesis of Ventricular Extrasystoles under Chloroform; With Special Reference to Consecutive Ventricular Fibrillation.' *Heart* **5,** 299

Lewis, T. (1911). 'Premature Contractions Arising in the Junctional Tissues.' *Q. Jl. Med.* **5,** 1

— (1920). 'Observations upon Flutter and Fibrillation.' *Heart* **7,** 293

— (1925). *The Mechanism and Graphic Registration of the Heart Beat.* London; Shaw

— (1933). *Diseases of the Heart.* London; Macmillan

Lian, C., Cassimatis and Hebert (1952). 'The Value of the Auricular Praecordial Lead S5 in the Diagnosis of Disorders of Auricular Rhythm.' *Archs Mal. Coeur* **45,** 481

Linenthal, A. J. and Zoll, P. J. (1963). 'Prevention of Ventricular Tachycardia and Fibrillation by Intravenous Isoproterenol and Epinephrine.' *Circulation* **27,** 5

Ling, G. and Gerard, R. W. (1949). 'The Normal Membrane Potential of Frog Sartorius Fibres.' *J. cell. Comp. Physiol.* **34,** 383

Lloyd-Mostyn, R. H., Kidner, R. H. and Oram, S. (1973). 'Sino-atrial Disorder including the Brady-tachycardia Syndrome. A Review with Addition of 11 Cases.' *Q. Jl Med.* **42,** 41

Lopez, J. F. (1969). 'Electrocardiographic Findings in Patients with Complete Atrioventricular Block.' *Br. Heart J.* **30,** 20

— Edelist, A. and Katz, L. N. (1963). 'Slowing of the Heart Rate by Artificial Electrical Stimulation with Pulses of Long Duration in the Dog.' *Circulation* **28,** 759

Lown, B. (1967). 'Electrical Reversion of Cardiac Arrhythmias.' *Br. Heart J.* **29,** 469

— and Levine, S. A. (1955). *Current Concepts in Digitalis Therapy.* London; Churchill

— and Newman, J. (1962). 'New Method for Terminating Cardiac Arrhythmias.' *J. Am. med. Ass.* **182,** 548.

— Ganong, W. F. and Levine, S. A. (1952). 'Syndrome of Short P–R Interval, Normal QRS Complex and Paroxysmal Rapid Heart Action.' *Circulation* **5,** 693

— Ehrlich, L., Lipschultz, B. and Blake, J. (1961). 'Effect of Digitalis in Patients Receiving Reserpine.' *Circulation* **24,** 1185

— Falsho, A. M., Hood Jnr., W. B. and Thorn, G. W. (1967). 'The Coronary Care Unit.' *J. Am. Med. Ass.* **199,** 156
— Arons, W. L., Ganong, W. F., Vazifdar, J. P. and Levine, S. A. (1955). 'Adrenal Steroids and Atrio-Ventricular Conduction.' *Am. Heart J.* **50,** 760
Lucchesi, B. R. (1965). 'Effects of Pronethalol and its Dextroisomer upon Experimental Cardiac Arrhythmias.' *J. Pharmac. exp. Ther.* **148,** 94
McGuire, J. and Richards, C. E. (1936). 'Fatal Digitalis Poisoning Occurring in a Normal Individual.' *Am. Heart J.* **12,** 109
Mackenzie, J. (1908). *Diseases of the Heart.* Oxford; Oxford University Press
McKussick, V. (1966). '*Mendelian Inheritance in Man*, pp. 136, 137. London; Heinemann
McMichael, J. and Sharpey-Schafer, E. P. (1944). 'Action of Intravenous Digoxin in Man.' *Q. Jl. Med.* **13,** 123
McNeill, R. S. (1964). 'Effect of a beta-Adrenergic Blocking Agent, Propanolol, on Asthmatics.' *Lancet* **2,** 1101
McNeilly, R. H. and Pemberton, J. (1968). 'Duration of Last Attack in 998 Fatal Cases of Coronary Artery Disease and its relation to possible Cardiac Resuscitation.' *Br. med. J.* **3,** 139
Magidson, O. (1969). 'Resection of Postmyocardial Infarction Ventricular Aneurysm for Cardiac Arrhythmias.' *Dis. Chest* **56,** 211
Mahaim, I. (1947). 'Kent's Fibres and the A.V. Paraspecific Conduction Through the Upper Connections of the Bundle of His.' *Am. Heart J.* **33,** 651
Marriott, H. J. L. (1957). 'Interactions between Atria and Ventricles During Interference Dissociation and Complete A.V. Block.' *Am. Heart J.* **53,** 884
— (1968). Personal Communication
— (1969). 'Ways and Means of Communication.' *Dis. Chest* **55,** 93
— (1970). Personal communication
— (1972). *Workshop in Electrocardiography.* Oldsmar, Florida; Tampa Tracings
— and Bradley, S. M. (1957). 'Main-stem Extrasystoles.' *Circulation* **16,** 544
Master, A. M., Dack, S. and Jaffe, H. L. (1937). 'Disturbances of Rate and Rhythm in Acute Coronary Artery Thrombosis.' *Am. intern. Med.* **11,** 735
Meltzer, L. E. and Kitchell, J. B. (1966). 'The Incidence of Arrhythmias Associated with Acute Myocardial Infarction.' *Prog. cardiovasc. Dis.* **9,** 50
Mendel, D. (1966). Personal Communication
Mendez, C., Aceves, J. and Mendez, R. (1961). 'The Anti-adrenergic Action of Digitalis on the Refractory Period of the A.V. Transmission System.' *J. Pharmac. exp. Ther.* **131,** 199
Miller, R. and Sharrett, R. H. (1957). 'Interference Dissociation.' *Circulation* **16,** 803
Mines, G. R. (1913). 'On Dynamic Equilibrium in the Heart.' *J. Physiol., Lond.* **46,** 349
Mobitz, W. (1924). 'Über die unvollstandige Störung der Er egungsüberleitung zwischhen Vorkof und Kammer des menschüchen Herzens.' *Z. gest exp. Med.* **41,** 180
Moe, G. K., Childers, R. W. and Merideth, J. (1968). 'An Appraisal of "Supernormal" A.V. Conduction.' *Circulation* **38,** 5
— Preston, J. B. and Burlington, H. (1956). 'Physiological Evidence for a Dual A.V. Transmission System.' *Circulation Res.* **4,** 357
Morris, J. J., Peter, R. H. and McIntosh, H. D. (1966). 'Electrical Conversion of Atrial Fibrillation.' *Ann. int. Med.* **65,** 216
— Estes, E. H., Whalen, R. E., Thompson, H. K. and McIntosh, M. D. (1964). 'P Wave Analysis in Valvular Heart Disease.' *Circulation* **29,** 242
Morris, R. M., Mercer, E. J. and Croxton, M. S. (1972). 'Conduction Disturbances due to Anteroseptal Myocardial Infarction and their Treatment by Endocardial Pacing.' *Am. Heart J.* **84,** 4, 560
Mower, M. M., Miller, D. I. and Nachlas, M. M. (1964). 'Clinical Features Relevant to Possible Resuscitation in Death after Acute Myocardial Infarction. *Am. J. Cardiol.* **67,** 437
Nadas, A. S., Daechner, S. W., Roth, A. and Blumenthal, S. L. (1952). 'Paroxysmal Tachycardia in Infants and Children.' *Paediatrics, Cairo* **9,** 167
Narula, O. S., Samet, P. and Javier, R. P. (1972). 'Significance of the Sinus Node Recovery Time.' *Circulation* **45,** 1972
— Cohen, L. S., Samet, P., Lister, J. W., Scherlag, B. and Hildner, F. J. (1970).

REFERENCES

'Localization of A.V. Conduction in Defects in Man by Recording of His Bundle Electrogram.' *Am. J. Cardiol.* **25,** 228

Newman, B. J., Donosco, E. and Friedburg, C. K. (1966). 'Arrhythmias in the W. P. W Syndrome.' *Prog. cardiovasc. Dis.* **9,** 147

Öehnell, R. F. (1940). 'Postmortem Examination and Clinical Report of a Case of the Short P–R Interval and Wide QRS Wave Syndrome (W.P.W.).' *Cardiologia* **4,** 249

— (1944). 'Pre-excitation. A Cardiac Abnormality.' *Acta med. scand.* Suppl. 152

Otto, H. L. and Gold, H. (1926). 'Persistent Premature Contractions.' *Archs intern. Med.* **38,** 186

Papp, C. (1969). 'A New Look at Arrhythmias.' *Br. Heart J.* **31,** 267

Papp, J. Gy. and Vaughan Williams, E. M. (1969). 'The Effect of Intracellular Atrial Potentials of Bretylium in Relation to its Local Anaesthetic Potency.' *Br. J. Pharmac. chemother.* **35,** 352

Parkinson, J. and Papp, C. (1947). 'Repetitive Paroxysmal Tachycardia.' *Br. Heart J.* **9,** 241

Parkinson, J., Papp, C. and Evans, W. (1941). 'The Electrocardiogram of Stokes-Adams' Attack.' *Br. Heart J.* **3,** 171

Pentecost, B. L. and Bennett, M. A. (1969). Personal Communication

Penton, G. B., Miller, H. and Levine, S. A. (1955). 'Some Clinical Features of Complete Heart Block.' *Circulation* **13,** 801

Peter, R. H., Morris, J. J. and McIntosh, H. D. (1966). 'Relationship of Fibrillatory Waves and P Waves in the Electrocardiogram.' *Circulation* **38,** 599

Phibbs, B. (1963). 'Paroxysmal Atrial Tachycardia with Block Around the Ectopic Pacemaker.' *Circulation* **38,** 949

Pick, A. (1956). 'Aberrant Ventricular Conduction of Escape Beats. Preferential and Accessory Pathways in the A.V. Junction.' *Circulation* **13,** 702

— and Dominguez, P. (1957). 'Non-paroxysmal A.V. Nodal Tachycardia.' *Circulation* **16,** 1022

— and Katz, L. M. (1955). 'Disturbance of Impulse Formation and Conduction in the Pre-excitation (W.P.W.) Syndrome. Their Bearing on its Mechanism.' *Am. J. Med.* **19,** 759

— Langendorf, R. and Katz, L. N. (1961). 'A.V. Nodal Tachycardia with Block.' *Circulation* **24,** 12

— — — (1962). 'The Supernormal Phase of Atrio-ventricular Conduction.' *Circulation* **26,** 388

Prinzmetal, M., Corday, E., Brill, I. C., Oblath, R. W. and Kruger, H. E. (1952). *The Auricular Arrhythmia.* Springfield; Thomas

Purkinje, J. E. (1845). 'Mikroskopische neurologische Beobachtungen.' *Archs Anat. Physiol. wissensch. Med.* **281,** 1845

Raftery, E. V., Rehman, M. F., Banks, D. C. and Oran, S. (1969). 'Incidence and Management of Ventricular Arrhythmias after Acute Myocardial Infarction.' *Br. Heart J.* **31,** 273

Richman, J. L. and Wolff, L. (1954). 'Left Bundle Branch Block Masquerading as Right Bundle Branch Block.' *Am. Heart J.* **47,** 383

Rodensky, P. L. and Wasserman, F. (1961). 'Observations on Digitalis Intoxication.' *Archs intern. Med.* **108,** 171

Roelandt, J., Schamroth, L., Draulans, J. and Hugenholtg, J. G. (1973). 'Functional Characteristics of the Wolff–Parkinson–White Bypass.' *Am. Heart J.* **85,** 260

Rokseth, R., Hatle, L., Gedde-Dahl, D. and Foss, P. O. (1970). 'Pacemaker Therapy in Sino-atrial Block Complicated by Paroxysmal Tachycardia. *Br. Heart J.* **32,** 93

Rosen, K. M., Ehsani, A. and Rahimtoola, S. H. (1972). 'H.V. Intervals in Left Bundle Branch Block. Clinical and Electrocardiographic Correlations.' *Circulation* **46,** 717

— Loeb, H. S., Gunnar, R. M. and Rahimtoola, S. H. (1971a). 'Mobitz Type II Block Without Bundle Branch Block.' *Circulation* **44,** 1111

— Mehta, A., Rahimtoola, S. H. and Miller, R. A. (1971b). 'Sites of Congenital and Surgical Heart Block as Defined by His Bundle Electrography.' *Circulation* **44,** 833

Rosenbaum, F. F., Hecht, H. H., Wilfsun, F. N. and Johnston, F. D. (1945). 'The

Potential Variations of the Thorax and Oesophagus in Anomalous Atrioventricular Excitation (Wolff–Parkinson–White Syndrome).' *Am. Heart J.* **29,** 281

Rosenbaum, M. B., Elizari, M. V. and Lazzari, J. O. (1968). *Los Hemibloqueos.* Buenos Aires; Paidós

— Halpern, M. S., Nan, G. J., Elizari, M. V. and Lazzari, J. O. (1970). 'The Mechanism of Narrow Ventricular Ectopic Beats.' In *Symposium on Cardiac Arrhythmias, Elsinore, Denmark.* Ed. E. Sandoe, E. Flensted-Jensen and K. H. Olesen. Sodertalje, AB Astra

— Gerardo, J. N., Levi, R. J., Halpern, M. S., Elizari, M. V. and Lazzari, J. O. (1969). 'Wenckebach Periods in the Bundle Branches.' *Circulation* **40,** 79

Rothfeld, E. L., Zucker, I. R., Parsonnet, V. and Alinsonorin, C. A. (1968). 'Idioventricular Rhythm in Acute Myocardial Infarction.' *Circulation* **37,** 203

Sandler, A. and Marriott, H. J. L. (1965). 'The Differential Morphology of Anomalous Ventricular Complexes of Right Bundle Branch Block Type in Lead VI. Ventricular Ectopy Versus Aberration.' *Circulation* **31,** 551

Sandler, G., Clayton, G. A. and Thornicroft, S. G. (1968). 'Clinical Evaluation of Verapamil in Angina Pectoris.' *Br. med. J.* **3,** 224

Sarnoff, S. J., Brockman, S. K., Gilmore, J. P., Linden, R. J. and Mitchell, J. H. (1960). 'Regulation of Ventricular Contraction. Influence of Cardiac Sympathetic and Vagal Nerve Stimulation on Atrial and Ventricular Dynamics? *Circulation Res.* **8,** 1108

Schamroth, L. (1962). 'Ventricular Parasystole with Slow Manifest Discharge.' *Br. Heart J.* **24,** 731

— (1966). 'Genesis and Evolution of Ectopic Ventricular Rhythm.' *Br. Heart J.* **28,** 244

— (1971). *The Disorders of Cardiac Rhythm.* Oxford; Blackwell Scientific Publications

— and Chesler, E. (1963). 'Phasic Aberrant Ventricular Conduction.' *Br. Heart J.* **25,** 219

— and Dove, E. (1966). 'The Wenckebach Phenomenon in Sino-atria Block. *Br. Heart J.* **28,** 350

— and Friedberg, H. D. (1966). 'Significance of Retrograde Conduction in A.V. Dissociation.' *Br. Heart J.* **27,** 896

— and Marriott, H. J. L. (1961). 'Intermittent Ventricular Parasystole with Observations on its Relationship to Extrasystolic Bigeminy.' *Am. J. Cardiol.* **7,** 799

— — (1964). 'Concealed Ventricular Extrasystoles.' *Circulation* **27,** 1043

— and Yoshonis, K. (1969). 'Mechanisms of Reciprocal Rhythm.' *Am. J. Cardiol.* **24,** 224

— Krikler, D. M. and Garrett, C. (1972). 'Immediate Effects of Intravenous Verapamil in Cardiac Arrhythmias.' *Br. med. J.* **1,** 660

Schellong, F. (1924). 'Die Allorhythmien des Herzens infolge Störung der Reizbildung und der Reizübertragung.' *Ergebn. inn. Med. Kinderheilk.* **25,** 477

Scherf, D. (1944). 'Alteration in the Form of the T Waves with Changes in Heart Rate.' *Am. Heart J.* **28,** 332

— and Bornemann, C. (1961). 'Parasystole with a Rapid Ventricular Centre.' *Am. Heart J.* **62,** 320

— and Dix, J. H. (1952). 'The Effects of Posture on A.V. Conduction.' *Am. Heart J.* **43,** 494

— and Schott, A. (1953). *Extrasystoles and Allied Arrhythmias.* London; Heinemann

— — (1959). 'Mechanism of Origin of Ectopic Beats.' *Am. J. Cardiol.* **3,** 351

— Romano, F. J. and Terranova, R. (1948). 'Experimental Studies on Auricular Flutter and Auricular Fibrillation.' *Am. Heart J.* **36,** 241

Scherlag, B. J., Samet, P. and Helfant, R. H. (1972). 'His Bundle Electrogram. A Critical Appraisal of its Uses and Limitations.' *Circulation* **46,** 601

— Lan, S. H., Helfant, R. H., Berkowitz, W. D., Stein, E. and Damato, A. N. (1969). 'Catheter Technique for the Recording of His Bundle Activity in Man.' *Circulation* **39,** 13

Schiebler, G. L., Adams, P., Anderson, R. C., Amplatz, K. and Lester, R. G. (1959). 'Clinical Study of 23 Cases of Ebstein's Anomaly of the Tricuspid Valve.' *Circulation* **19,** 165

Schneider, R. G. (1969). 'Familial Accounts of Wolff–Parkinson–White Syndrome.' *Am. Heart J.* **78,** 34

REFERENCES

Schott, A. (1955). 'Disorders of Auricular Rhythm Associated with Bundle Branch Block Simulating Ectopic Ventricular Tachycardia.' *Cardiol. prat.* **26,** 353

— (1964). 'Observations on Digitalis Intoxication—A Plea.' *Post-grad. med. J.* **40,** 628

Seaton, A. (1966). 'Quinidine Induced Paroxysmal Ventricular Fibrillation Treated with Propranolol.' *Br. med. J.* **1,** 1522

Segers, M. (1946). 'Les phenomènes de synchronisation au niveau du coeur.' *Archs int. Physiol.* **54,** 87

— Lequime, J. and Denolin, H. (1947). 'Synchronisation of Auricular and Ventricular Beats During Complete Heart Block.' *Am. Heart J.* **33,** 685

Sherf, L. and James, T. N. A. (1969). 'New Electrocardiographic Concept. Synchronized Sinoventrical Conduction.' *Dis. Chest.* **55,** 127

Singer, R. and Winterberg, H. (1920). 'Extrasystolen als Interferenzersheinung.' *Wien Arch. inn. Med.* **1,** 391

Smirk, F. H. (1949). 'R Waves Interrupting T Waves.' *Br. Heart J.* **11,** 23

Sowton, E. (1965). 'Artificial Pacemaking and Sinus Rhythms.' *Br. Heart J.* **27,** 311

— Leatham, A. and Carson, P. (1964). 'The Suppression of Arrhythmias by Artificial Pacemaking.' *Lancet* **2,** 1098

— Balcom, R., Preston, T., Leaver, D. and Yacoub, M. (1969). 'Long-term Control of Intractable Supraventricular Tachycardia by Ventricular Spacing.' *Br. Heart J.* **31,** 700

Spach, M. S., Huang, S., Armstrong, S. I. and Canent, R. V. (1963). 'Demonstration of Peripheral Conduction System in Human Hearts. *Circulation* **28,** 333

Stern, S. (1966). 'Synergistic Action of Propranolol and Quinidine.' *Am. Heart J.* **72,** 569

— (1967). 'Conversion of Chronic Atrial Fibrillation to Sinus Rhythm with combined Propranolol and Quinidine Treatment.' *Am. Heart J.* **74,** 170

— (1971). 'Treatment and Prevention of Cardiac Arrhythmias with Propranolol and Quinidine.' *Br. Heart J.* **33,** 522

Stock, J. P. P. (1966). 'Beta-adrenergic Blocking Drugs in the Clinical Management of Cardiac Arrhythmias.' *Am. J. Cardiol.* **18,** 444

— and Dale, N. (1963). 'Beta-adrenergic Receptor Blockade in Cardiac Arrhythmias.' *Br. med. J.* **2,** 1230

Sutton, R. and Davies, M. (1968). 'The Conduction System in Acute Myocardial Infarction Complicated by Heart Block.' *Circulation,* **38,** 987

— Chatterjee, K. and Leatham, A. (1968). 'Heart Block Following Acute Myocardial Infarction.' *Lancet* **2,** 645

Swanick, E. J., La Camera, F. and Marriott, H. J. L. (1972). 'Morphologic Features of Right Ventricular Ectopic Beats.' *Am. J. Cardiol.* **30,** 8, 888

Swiderski, J., Lees, M. H. and Nadas, A. S. (1962). 'The Wolff–Parkinson–White Syndrome in Infancy and Childhood.' *Br. Heart J.* **24,** 561

Tawara, S. (1906). *Das Reizleitungsystem des Saugertierherzens.* Jena; Fischer

Thomas, M. and Woodgate, D. (1966). 'Effect of Atropine on Bradycardia and Hypotension in Acute Myocardial Infarction.' *Br. Heart J.* **28,** 409

Thompson, G. W. (1956). 'Quinidine as a Cause of Sudden Death.' *Circulation* **14,** 757

Thorel, C. (1910). 'Uber den Aufbau des Sinus Knotens und seine Verbindung mit der Cava superior und den wenckebachschen Bundeln.' *Münch. med. Wschr.* **57,** 183

Trendelenberg, W. (1903). 'Untersuchungen über das Verhalten des Herzmuskels bei rhythmischer elektrischer Reizung.' *Arch. Anat. Physiol.* p. 271

Uhley, H. N. and Rivkin, L. M. (1959). 'Visualisation of the Left Branch of the Human Atrioventricular Bundle.' *Circulation* **20,** 419

Unger, P. N., Lesser, M. E., Kugel, V. H. and Lev, M. (1958). 'The Concept of "Masquerading" Bundle Branch Block. An Electrocardiographic-pathologic Correlation.' *Circulation* **17,** 397

Vassaux, C. and Lown, B. (1969). 'Cardioversion of Supraventricular Tachycardias.' *Circulation* **39,** 791

Vaughan Williams, E. M. (1958). 'The Action of Quinidine Interpreted from Intracellular Potentials of Single Cardiac Fibres.' *Lancet* **1,** 943

— (1966). 'Mode of Action of Beta-receptor Antagonists on Cardiac Muscle.' *Am. J. Cardiol.* **18,** 399

— and Sekiya, A. (1963). 'Prevention of Arrhythmias due to Cardiac Glycosides by Block of Beta-sympathetic Receptors.' *Lancet* **1**, 420

Ward, O. C. (1964). 'A New Familial Cardiac Syndrome in Children.' *J. Ir. med. Ass.* **54**, 103

Warner, A. O. and McKussick, V. A. (1958). 'Wolff–Parkinson–White Syndrome. A Genetic Study.' *Circulation Res.* **6**, 18

Watanabe, Y. and Dreifus, L. S. (1967). 'Second Degree Atrioventricular Block.' *Cardiovasc. Res.* **1**, 150

— Josipovic, V. and Dreifus, L. S. (1968). 'Electrophysiological Mechanisms of Bretylium Tosylate.' *Circulation* **38**, Suppl. VI, 202

Wedensky, N. E. (1887). 'Über die Beziehung zwischen Reizung und Erregung im Tetanus.' *Ber. Akad. Wiss. St. Petersburg* **54**, 96 Appendix No. 3

Wellens, H. J. J. (1971). *Electrical Stimulation of the Heart in the Study and Treatment of Tachycardias.* Leiden; H. E. Stenfert Kroese N.V.

— and Durrer, D. (1968). 'Supraventricular Tachycardia with Left Aberrant Conduction due to Retrograde Invasion into the Left Bundle Branch.' *Circulation* **38**, 474

— Peinier, M., Schuilenburg, M. D. and Durrer, D. (1972). 'Electrical Stimulation of the Heart in Patients with Ventricular Tachycardia.' *Circulation* **46**, 216

Wenckebach, K. F. (1899). 'Zur Analyse des unregelmässigen Pulses. II Über den regelmässig intermittirenden Puls.' *Z. klin. Med.* **39**, 475

Wenckebach, K. F. (1907). 'Beitrage zur Kenntriss des menschlichen Herztäligkeit.' *Arch. Anat. Physiol.* **1-2**, 1.

— (1914). *Die unregelmässige Herztätigkeit und ihre klinische Bedeutung,* Leipzig; Engelmann p. 125

— (1923). 'Cinchona Derivatives in Treatment of Heart Disorders.' *J. Am. Med. Ass.* **81**, 472

— and Winterberg, H. (1927). *Die Unregelmässige Herztätigkeit.* Leipzig; Engelmann

Williams, D. O. (1973). 'Supernormal Phase of A.V. Conduction. A Study during —Heart Block and Endocardial Pacing.' *Br. Heart J.* **35**, 365

  Jones, E. L., Nagel, R. E. and Smith, B. S. (1972). 'Familial Atrial Cardiomyo-Wpathy with Heart Block.' *Q. Jl Med.* **41**, 491

Wilson, F. H. (1915). A Case in which the Vagus Influenced the Form of the Ventricular Complex of the Electrocardiogram.' *Archs intern. Med.* **16**, 1008

Winton, S. S. (1948). 'Sino-auricular Block. An Analysis of Eleven Cases.' *Acta cardiol.* **3**, 108

Wolff, L., Parkinson, J. and White, P. D. (1930). 'Bundle Branch Block with Short P–R Interval in Healthy Young People Prone to Paroxysmal Tachycardia. *Am. Heart J.* **5**, 685

Wood, P. (1963). 'Polyuria in Paroxysmal Tachycardia, Paroxysmal Atrial Flutter and Fibrillation.' *Br. Heart J.* **25**, 273

Zoll, P. M. and Linenthal, A. J. (1963). 'A Program for Stokes-Adams' Disease and Cardiac Arrest.' *Circulation* **27**, 1

— — Gibson, W., Paul, M. H. and Norman, L. R. (1956). 'Termination of Ventricular Fibrillation in Man by Externally Applied Electric Countershock.' *New Engl. J. Med.* **254**, 727

— — — — — (1958). 'Intravenous Drug Therapy of Stokes-Adams' Disease.' *Circulation* **17**, 325

INDEX